Picturing the Lame in Italian Art from Antiquity to the Modern Era

The presence of the orthopedically impaired body in art is so pervasive that, paradoxically, it has failed to attract the attention of most art historians. In *Picturing the Lame in Italian Art from Antiquity to the Modern Era*, Livio Pestilli investigates the changing meaning that images of individuals with limited mobility acquired through the centuries. This study evinces that, in distinct opposition to the practice of Classical artists, who manifested a lack of interest in the subject of lameness since it was considered "a defect or a deformity" and deformity a "want of measure, which is always unsightly," their Early Christian counterparts depicted them profusely, because images of the miraculous healing of the lame became the reassuring sign of universal acceptance and the promise of a more equitable existence in this life or the next. Subsequently, in the Middle Ages, when voluntary poverty came to be associated with the necessary condition of faithfulness to Christ, the indigent lame, along with others who were forced to beg for a living, became the image of the *alter Christus*. This view was to change in the Renaissance and Baroque periods, when, with the resurgence of Classical and Pauline ideals that condemned the idle, representations of the orthopedically impaired became associated with swindlers, freeloaders and parasites. This fascinating story came basically to an end in the eighteenth century, when, with the revival of the Greek ideal of the Beautiful, the lame gradually left center stage to be relegated again to the margins of the visual arts. A coda provides an overview of the "state of the art" in contemporary Italy.

Livio Pestilli is Director and Professor of Art History at Trinity College Rome Campus, Italy. He is the author of *Paolo de Matteis: Neapolitan Painting and Cultural History in Baroque Europe* (Ashgate, 2013) and co-editor of *"Napoli è tutto il mondo": Neapolitan Art and Culture from Humanism to the Enlightenment*, Pisa and Rome (2008).

Picturing the Lame in Italian Art from Antiquity to the Modern Era

Livio Pestilli

Routledge
Taylor & Francis Group
LONDON AND NEW YORK

First published 2017
by Routledge

2 Park Square, Milton Park, Abingdon, Oxfordshire OX14 4RN
52 Vanderbilt Avenue, New York, NY 10017

Routledge is an imprint of the Taylor & Francis Group, an informa business

First issued in paperback 2018

British Library Cataloguing in Publication Data
A catalogue record for this book is available from the British Library

Library of Congress Cataloging in Publication Data
A catalog record for this book has been requested

ISBN: 978-1-4724-6978-6 (hbk)
ISBN: 978-0-367-20026-8 (pbk)

Typeset in Perpetua
by Swales & Willis Ltd, Exeter, Devon, UK

For Wendy
Che fortuna averti incontrata!

Contents

Plates

The colour plates can be found between pp. 114 and 115

Figures

Acknowledgments

I would like to express my gratitude to all of those individuals who through the years helped, directly or indirectly, with the gestation and completion of this project. Particular thanks to Fr. Achille Bonazzi, Jean Cadogan, Francesca Campana, Fr. Alberto Coratti, Henry DePhillips, Gabriele Fabbrici, Cristiana Filippini, Julia Hairston, Philine Helas, Andrew Hopkins, Pamela Jones, Helen and Anthony Langdon, Mons. Vittorio Lanzani, Giovanna Mori, Ana González Mozo, Tom Nichols, Kirstin Noreen, Steven Ostrow, Valentino Pace, Borden Painter, Annie Ravenhill-Johnson, Silvia Rizzo, Ingrid Rowland, Walter Stephens, William Wallace, Inge Weustink, Thomas Willette, Gerhard Wolf, Maria Wyke and Mark Zucker (d. 2013).

I would also like to express my gratitude to Erika Gaffney, formerly at Ashgate, for her editorial vision, and to Trinity College (Hartford, Connecticut) and the Cesare Barbieri Endowment for Italian Culture for their generous subsidy of this project.

Finally, I would like to thank my muses: Wendy, Federico and Daniele. *Haec ornamenta sunt mea*.

Introduction

About twenty-five years ago, when visiting the Norman cathedral of Monreale just outside of Palermo, besides being impressed by the sheer beauty and magnitude of the overall mosaic decoration, I was particularly struck by the moving scene of *Christ Healing the Infirm* (Plate 4). In the Sicilian mosaic, the reassuring blessing hand of Christ, dramatically designed to act as a contrapuntal detail to the supplicating gestures of ailing humans, was a reminder that the people they represented had reverted to a metaphysical solution to their physical problems. This touching encounter between the majestic figure of the Savior and the diminutive, frail, suffering humanity represented by lame, blind and hunchbacked individuals gave me pause to ponder how different city streets must have looked before modern medicine helped to prevent, limit or cure such physical impairments and how frequently a number of persons affected by such ailments must have turned to begging as a means of survival. It was at this time that I began paying more attention to the representation of the orthopedically impaired body in Italian art and I quickly became aware that its presence was much more pervasive than I had realized.[1]

When years later I participated in a conference on the subject of *Roman Bodies: Metamorphoses, Mutilation, and Martyrdom*, I decided to further investigate how motor impairment had been represented in Western art.[2] To my surprise, I learned that while physical conditions such as gibbosity and dwarfism had been represented with some regularity, human lameness had seldom been represented in the Classical period. The under-representation of the lame in Greek and Roman art was a clear indication that Classical artists reflected the distinct concerns of pagan societies that perceptibly differed from those that characterized Christian communities in later centuries. Even though I was unable to tackle the project for some time, I decided that a more thorough study of the subject was in order. When in more recent times I returned to the task, I became aware that the field of physical disability, especially since the promulgation of the 1964 Civil Rights Act and the Americans with Disabilities Act (ADA) of 1990, had flourished extensively and had engendered a wide-ranging body of literature.[3]

My goal with the present volume is to contribute both to this important field of research and to a specific socio-anthropological theme in Italian art by limiting my investigation to images that focus strictly on bodies whose mobility has been curtailed partially or totally. Thus, the substantive "lame" that appears in the title of the book is meant to symbolize synecdochically bodies with impaired locomotion, including the mutilated, the genetically altered body and the paralytic. The reasons for focusing on this type of disability and restricting the research to only one geographical area are easily told. First and foremost, the topic would quickly mushroom to unwieldy dimensions if other ailments were included – such as blindness, muteness, epilepsy and leprosy – or if the historical investigation were extended to the art of more than one country. Second, since images of the orthopedically impaired in Western art occur prevalently in depictions of miracles, and given that the majority of wondrous healings recorded in processes of canonization in the Middle Ages or in the *Lives* of saints pertain indeed to people affected by motor problems, focusing on the representation of such individuals promised to be a more effective field of research.[4] Third, given that able-bodied members of society, in past as in contemporary societies, are frequently skeptical of individuals who, to make ends meet, publically exhibit their physical ailments in the hope of receiving alms, and assuming that lameness is one of the impairments more easily simulated by pseudo-disabled persons, studying such images ensured a better understanding of how "normal" society viewed these persons and how their opinions shifted in the course of history.[5] That is, by studying images of the orthopedically impaired one learns "more about the viewer than about the person using a cane or a wheelchair."[6] And although surely not for everyone, but certainly for a number of individuals of the lower classes, since the loss of full mobility often resulted in the inability to maintain a productive role in society, the subject of human lameness will constructively lead to an inquiry of the corollary topic of poverty and mendicancy.[7] However, it should be clear at the outset that the picture that results from an investigation of images of the lame is a biased view of the phenomenon since the majority of the population, typically from the lower rungs of the social ladder, hardly left any documentation that may inform us of their views on this matter. Our impressions, in other words, remain partial as we can only view them through the lenses of the upper classes.[8] And even though orthopedic impairment affected all members of the social pyramid, the disabled elite not only found ways of compensating for their disability but, more importantly for this study, did not attract the artists' attention.

To this "outsider" approaching disability studies from an art historical perspective, a few observations seem necessary. First of all, it is by now clear that disability is a protean concept that changes depending on time and place, and that it is "a socially driven relation to the body that became relatively organized in the eighteenth and nineteenth centuries."[9] Indeed, if in preindustrial societies the disabled person, although perhaps treated unkindly, was integrated in the community, the "kinder" treatment of impaired individuals in postindustrial societies ultimately marginalized these same persons "through the discursivity of disability."[10] It is also evident that the able-bodied, perhaps better defined as TABs ("temporarily able-bodied"),[11] in all periods of history have frequently neglected to tackle the concerns of the impaired.[12] Moreover, it is apparent that the very terminology they have used to describe situations and events, as well as bodily and psychological conditions concerning the physically disadvantaged, has revealed some deep-seated prejudices and misunderstandings. Consequently, the adoption of better-suited terms to define people with physical, psychological or neurological conditions that are perceived by mainstream society as straying from the "norm" is a welcome change. In this study, therefore, I will generally adopt the sensible linguistic differentiation between "impairment" and "disability" that has recently been suggested – the former being a somewhat neutral term describing a physical, medical condition and the latter being a psychologically charged word that may imply the inability on the part of the impaired to perform the way able-bodied people do and suggest their possible dependence on society.[13] However, since there is now a well-established discipline of Disability Studies and a reputable Society for Disability Studies that without reserve address issues pertaining to impairments by referring to them as "disabilities,"[14] one should be reminded that neologisms and euphemisms at times create their own linguistic barriers and convolutions.[15] In truth, one is particularly aware that acceptable terms used in discussing the representation of disability today may be criticized, if not at present, certainly in the future and that even well-meaning words and interpretations may be sanctioned by others.[16] Nonetheless, especially since many of the sources consulted or quoted in this book employ terms that are historically apposite – even if nowadays considered politically incorrect or offensive – words such as *cripple* or *lame* to describe someone who has impaired locomotion will be retained.[17]

As a premise to the study of how orthopedic impairment was depicted in Italian art, the book will begin by analyzing the reasons why Classical pagan artists shunned the representation of the lame body while their Early Christian counterparts exploited it to its utmost potential to promote the new religion. I will then move chronologically from the Middle Ages, when the disabled was considered more positively, at least by some sectors of society, as an *alter Christus* (another Christ) – that is, as an individual who truly embodied the suffering Christ – to the Renaissance, when some deep-seated prejudices already present in ancient societies resurfaced with greater intensity. Next I will investigate how in the transitional period between the Renaissance and the Baroque the orthopedically impaired were more frequently stigmatized by being depicted as rogues, swindlers and cheats. Finally the narrative will lead to the following century, when, with the advent of Neoclassicism, the lame in Italian art tend to disappear, as the depiction of the human body reverted to those ideals championed by Classical Greek artists. A coda will look at a few significant examples that give an indication of how images of the orthopedically impaired were employed in the twentieth century and conclude with an overview of "the state of the art" in contemporary Italy.

Through the years, many studies have appeared that deal with disabilities and poverty. Very few art historians, however, have been attracted by these topics and those scholars who have investigated them have done so by considering diverse types of physical impairments or representations of the poor within a limited historical period. The present volume is the first to make a systematic art historical investigation of a specific physical condition, the way it has been depicted through the ages in one country and the changing significance it acquired with the passage of time. The hope is that this study will serve as a catalyst to others who feel compelled to cross their professional boundaries into the crucial and growing field of Disability Studies.

Notes

1 The same phenomenon occurs in literature. "Disabled peoples' social invisibility has occurred in the wake of their perpetual circulation throughout print history." See David T. Mitchell and Sharon L. Snyder, *Narrative Prosthesis: Disability and the Dependencies of Discourse*, Ann Arbor, 2000, p. 52.

2 The conference, organized at the British School at Rome in association with the American Academy, the Istituto Olandese di Roma, Palazzo delle Esposizioni and the British Council, took place on March 29–31, 2001. The proceedings of the conference were ultimately published in the volume

Roman Bodies: Antiquity to the Eighteenth Century, Andrew Hopkins and Maria Wyke (eds.), London, 2005. See Livio Pestilli, "Disabled Bodies: The (Mis)Representation of the Lame in Antiquity and their Reappearance in Early Christian and Medieval Art," in ibid., pp. 85–97.

3 For a useful résumé of the primary literature on the historiography of disability and the "state of the art," see Irina Metzler, *Disability in Medieval Europe: Thinking about Physical Impairment during the High Middle Ages, c. 1100–1400*, London and New York, 2006, pp. 1–37.

4 See André Vauchez, *Sainthood in the Later Middle Ages*, Cambridge, 1997, pp. 468–469, and Metzler, *Disability in Medieval Europe*, pp. 132–133.

5 For a comparable assessment with regard to the disabled at large see Peggy Phelan, *Unmarked: The Politics of Performance*, London, 1993, quoted by Ann Millett-Gallant, *The Disabled Body in Contemporary Art*, New York, 2000, p. 147.

6 Lennard J. Davis, "Dr. Johnson, Amelia, and the Discourse of Disability in the Eighteenth Century," in *"Defects": Engendering the Modern Body*, Helen Deutsch and Felicity Nussbaum (eds.), Ann Arbor, 2000, p. 56.

7 Indeed, as pointed out in Rosemary Garland-Thomson, *Extraordinary Bodies: Figuring Physical Disability in American Culture and Literature*, New York, 1997, p. 35, "Perhaps the most enduring form of segregation has been economic: the history of begging is virtually synonymous with the history of disability."

8 With specific reference to the ancient world, though the same idea applies to many societies in subsequent centuries, Harriet I. Flower, "Elite Self-Representation in Rome," in *Social Relations in the Roman World*, Michael Peachin (ed.), Oxford, 2011, p. 271, rightly points out, "It was the elites who defined Rome, its character and place in the world, and within the European cultural imagination."

9 Lennard J. Davis, *Enforcing Normalcy: Disability, Deafness and the Body*, London and New York, 1995, p. 3. Among others underscoring this fact see Garland-Thomson, p. 41.

10 Davis, *Enforcing Normalcy*, p. 3.

11 As it has been rightly stated: "The fact that we will all become disabled if we live long enough is a reality many people who consider themselves able-bodied are reluctant to admit." Garland-Thomson, p. 14. For TABs, ibid., p. 141, n. 14.

12 David T. Mitchell and Sharon L. Snyder, *The Body and Physical Difference: Discourses of Disability*, Ann Arbor, 2004, p. 4, point out that according to a study by the World Health Organization disabled people comprise 6 to 7 percent of any given society and that there are about 240 million disabled people in the world. According to other statistics, the figure of severely impaired people in the world is 500 million. See Davis, *Enforcing Normalcy*, p. 7, quoting O. Shirley's *A Cry for Health: Poverty and Disability in the Third World*, Rome, 1983.

13 This differentiation was first introduced in the field of British Disability Studies. As pointed out by Mitchell and Snyder, *Narrative Prosthesis*, p. 179: "British disability studies has offered up the important distinction between 'impairment' and 'disability' in order to differentiate between material and ideological experiences." Millett-Gallant, p. 7: "The culturally ubiquitous medical model views disability as a set of medical and corporeal 'problems' and works to cure, fix, or eliminate the 'problems' and consequently, disabled people, from the population. In contrast, disability studies strives to establish a social model for disabled people as an oppressed group and forges alliances with theories and positions of other socially marginalized groups .... Whereas the medical model locates disability on and in the body as 'abnormality' and privileges normalization or standardization of all bodies, a social model asserts that disability is constructed through environmental, social, and political apparatuses that work to exclude disabled people." See also Metzler's recap of the theoretical issues at stake in *Disability in Medieval Europe*, pp. 20–22 and idem, *A Social History of Disability in the Middle Ages: Cultural Considerations of Physical Impairment*, New York and London, 2013, p. 5.

14 See, for example, the Society for Disability Studies' (SDS) mission statement on the website at http://www.disstudies.org/about (accessed March 4, 2016).

15 Comparable linguistic calisthenics, to use an example totally unrelated to Disability Studies, is the current trend in English-language publications to employ the acronyms CE (Common Era) and BCE (Before the Common Era) instead of the traditional BC (Before Christ) and AD (Anno Domini)

when dating events. Since events labeled BCE and CE are computed starting from the reputed date of Christ's birth, the whole linguistic undertaking is simply a futile exercise in political correctness.

16 See Mitchell and Snyder, *Narrative Prosthesis*, p. 41.

17 In fact, there are people who favor the appellation "cripple" so as to seek recognition for the otherness of one's body and personal identity in the face of "normalcy." See Nancy Mairs, "On Being a Cripple," in *Plaintext: Essays*, Tucson, 1986, p. 9, as quoted by Garland-Thomson, p. 25 and p. 145, n. 15.

1 Classical and Early Christian precedents

> Are bodily defects, if very conspicuous, to offend us, but not a deformity of character?
>
> (Cicero, *Laws*, I, xix, 51)

It must not have been particularly edifying for the young Claudius to hear his mother Antonia call him "a monster of a man, not finished but merely begun by Dame Nature" or to be used as the negative term of comparison when she accused someone of being "a bigger fool than her son Claudius."[1] Although of a sickly nature, with shaky head and hands and a faltering voice, his intellect was sharp and sufficiently cultivated to write historical treatises.[2] Thus, despite his physical impairments and psychological problems, at the age of fifty-one this man became Rome's fourth emperor (ruled AD 41–54). Understandably, at a time when court portraiture was characterized by idealized beauty, physical perfection and perennial youth, no image of Claudius exists where he appears as anything less than a perfect specimen of the human race or a divinity (Plate 1).[3] Nevertheless, despite his (accidental) rise to fame, the social reality surrounding physical impairment caused a sense of unease in members of the able-bodied society who often forced disabled individuals onto the psychological, if not the physical, margins of society.[4] The disabled elite, of course, were socially and financially better protected from the consequences of infirmity.[5] Nonetheless, proof of this general disquiet is a letter reputedly written by the first of the Roman emperors, Augustus (ruled 27 BC to AD 14), to his wife Livia about the appropriateness of a public role for her grandson in which it is clear that for the Romans lameness, along with other physical impairments, was a matter of ridicule and derision. Indeed, public opinion could be unkind with a man whose gait was gravely affected by weak knees that "gave way under him."[6] Augustus asks:

> Now we [Augustus and Tiberius] are both agreed that we must decide once and for all what plan we are to adopt in his [Claudius's] case. For if he be sound and so to say complete, what reason have we for doubting that he ought to be advanced through the same grades and steps through which his brother has been advanced? But if we realize that he is wanting and defective in soundness of body and mind, we must not furnish the means of ridiculing both him and us to a public which is wont to scoff at and deride such things.[7]

It is irrelevant whether Augustus actually wrote the letter and truly believed the whole imperial family would be ridiculed by Claudius's physical appearance or it was all invented by

Suetonius, the first-century biographer of *The Lives of the Caesars*.[8] The fact that this mind-set was expressed at all in an official historical account implies that there must have been sufficient members of the able-bodied society for whom physical impairments were worthy of derision.[9] Seneca the Younger, for example, in his essay *On Benefits* seems to reflect exactly this attitude when he says, "this one [Claudius] is deformed in body, hideous in aspect, and will bring ridicule upon the insignia of his office."[10] Even so, since this seems to have been a common sentiment in literary sources, one wonders if ancient artists reflected such an attitude and whether the Classical Roman world differed in this respect from its Greek counterpart. Additionally, it is important to inquire whether the visual and social values upheld in antiquity with regard to lameness were transmitted to succeeding centuries.

If, as some maintain, "those members of society castigated for their 'otherness' ... are relegated to the margins of the community in an effort to ignore their existence," and if it is true that art mirrors "with varying iconography and creative emphasis" the changes that distinguish the societies in which they are produced,[11] then the attentive viewer will discover that, while in antiquity the malformed, dwarfs, hunchbacks and those with abnormal bodies were abundantly depicted on various artifacts, the lame, or those affected by motor impairment, were not just relegated to the margin of the ancients' visual field but to an artistic limbo from which they were only to be rescued with the rise of Christianity.[12]

* * *

There is no doubt that in antiquity there were individuals who considered orthopedic impairment a pitiable misfortune, as one gathers from Lysias's oration *For the Disabled Man*.[13] Indeed, for Plato lameness is metaphorically connected to an imperfect soul. In his view, if the external sensations and affections that enter the human soul after its encasement in man's mortal body "combine in him with any true nurture or education, he attains the fullness and health of the perfect man, and escapes the worst disease of all, but if he neglects education he walks lame to the end of his life and returns imperfect and good for nothing to the world below."[14] Still, there were many individuals with impaired mobility who, despite their physical ailment, were prominent citizens and achieved great success, such as Artemon "Periphoretus" (the "immobile" or, more accurately, the "Carried-Around"), Pericles's lame engineer who was brought about on a stretcher;[15] Philip of Macedonia, father of Alexander the Great, who suffered numerous mutilations, including that of his leg;[16] Tyrtaeus, the seventh-century Spartan poet who "with his verses fired manly hearts for battles of Mars,"[17] yet whose every member was disfigured;[18] and Agrippa, Augustus's admiral and son-in-law, whose youth was made "unhappy by lameness."[19] However, when congenital defects were detected immediately after birth, serious problems arose. Indeed, a topos of Classical Greek society is that a malformed child was exposed at birth and left to die.

It is not known whether in cases of infant deformity the practice of death by exposure (*apothesis*) was indeed a reality in Athens, but in the *locus classicus* for this assumption, Plutarch's life of *Lycurgus* (16.1–2), one learns that the Spartan state actually demanded it:[20]

> Offspring was not reared at the will of the father, but was taken and carried by him to a place called Lesche, where the elders of the tribes officially examined the infant, and if

> it was well-built and sturdy, they ordered the father to rear it, and assigned it one of the nine thousand lots of land; but if it was ill-born and deformed, they sent it to the so-called Apothetae, a chasm-like place at the foot of Mount Taygetus, in the conviction that the life of that which nature had not well equipped at the very beginning for health and strength, was of no advantage either to itself or the state.[21]

Although there are numerous Greek and Roman references to the elimination of unwanted children that range from drowning and strangulation to infant exposure, care should be taken not to make anachronistic assumptions.[22] Nevertheless, one would suspect that if different writers in various parts of the Mediterranean included references to this practice, it must not have been a total mental construct. Plato, for instance, mentions in his *Republic* that in the ideal state there is no room for "the offspring of the inferior, and [that] any of those of the other sort who are born defective" must thus be eliminated secretly.[23] In the *Theaetetus* he further declares that intellectual progeny, like real human beings, should be looked at carefully from every angle to ascertain whether or not it is "a lifeless phantom not worth the rearing," who ought to be exposed.[24] Comparably, while in discussing his version of the ideal state, Aristotle also argues in favor of the promulgation of a law to suppress the deformed child,[25] the second-century Greek doctor Soranus of Ephesus, after having described the various steps that must be taken to ascertain the good health of the child, claimed that the unhealthy infant was not worth rearing.[26]

As to the Romans, Dionysius of Halicarnassus asserted that Romulus forbade his countrymen to suppress any child under the age of three unless they were maimed or monstrous from their very birth. In such cases, parents were allowed to expose their progeny, so long as their five nearest neighbors also approved.[27] Also supporting the view that the Romans were prone to eliminate defective children is Livy's story about a newly born who was the size of a four-year-old. The child, who was considered an ominous portent not so much for his dimensions but because of his "uncertain" gender, was removed from Roman territory and drowned at sea.[28] Cicero, for his part, refers to the Twelve Tables and their dictate that "terribly deformed infants shall be killed" (*Laws*, 3.8, 19). Finally, Seneca the Elder, who devoted a whole declamation to a hypothetical legal case on crippled beggars (*mendici debilitati*), in which arguments are made for and against a man who crippled children who had been exposed and deprived them of the alms they collected, has Clodius Turrinus perorate in favor of the man, who is charged for having harmed the state.[29]

While all of the foregoing literary evidence, it has been argued, is insufficient "to conclude that their [the deformed children's] destruction was standard practice" in Greece,[30] others have claimed, "it should be clear that in Roman culture the killing of defective newborns was common."[31] Scholarly opinions on this subject vary[32] and although it is difficult to learn much about disabilities, in general, and lameness, in particular, from ancient medical texts,[33] it is significant that infant exposure is actually one of the discriminating features by which an anonymous second-century author differentiates Christians from pagans.[34] In fact, it is the argument in favor of the "sanctity of life" that distinguishes the writings of all Christian apologists, from Justin Martyr (*The First Apology*, 27), to Clement of Alexandria (*Christ the Educator*) and Tertullian (*Ad nationes*, I.15; *Apology*, 9).[35] Lactantius summed up their view most explicitly: "For they are not of our number … who either strangle their sons born from themselves, or if they are too pious, expose them."[36]

The sort of humane and economic justification for infanticide that Plutarch and other sources provide – that is, exposure is in the interest of both the deformed child and society – may be questioned.[37] Yet, it is a fact that in Greek culture lameness was associated with deviancy and viewed as a threat to the established order, as demonstrated by the Labdacids' line in Thebes: Labdacus (the lame) engendered Laius (the left-handed), whose lineage is cursed to extinction because of his homosexual and violent behavior; Oedipus (swollen foot), the son of Laius, commits patricide and incest; and Eteocles and Polyneices, the sons of Oedipus, kill each other.[38] Even if such evidence is only based on literary sources, it is indisputable that "social constructions are as important as effective practices in representing a society."[39]

If one considers the emphasis the Greeks placed on the Beautiful (*To Kalon*) in the arts, and given that for some influential thinkers such as Plato lameness was "a defect or a deformity,"[40] and deformity defined as a "want of measure, which is always unsightly,"[41] it comes as no surprise that Classical artists had very little interest in portraying the lame body. Even in the rare depictions of Homer's Thersites, "the ugliest man who came beneath Ilion," who was "bandy-legged and went lame of one foot,"[42] the physical impairment is nowhere explicitly portrayed.[43] Indeed, although there are some Greek and Hellenistic examples of deformed or infirm humans, the representation of lame mortals in the visual tradition is virtually absent.[44] In fact, images of the orthopedically impaired body that have survived from the Classical world are basically limited to those of the smith-god Hephaistos, "the very renowned Lame One,"[45] whose characteristic trait was the deformation of his feet.

Although congenital, Hephaistos's malformation was not hereditary, since his parents, Zeus and Hera, were perfectly formed.[46] According to the Homeric tradition, the defect caused great embarrassment to his mother, who lamented that the son whom she bore "was weakly among all the blessed gods and shriveled of foot, a shame and a disgrace to me in heaven, whom I myself took in my hands and cast out so that he fell in the great sea."[47] Thus, at least in this tradition, it should be clear that Hephaistos's lameness was the cause of his having been cast down from Mount Olympus and not the outcome of his fall. Furthermore, the Greeks' and Romans' discomfiture with what they considered the aberrant body may be detected not only in the fact that Classical culture generated only one disabled god, but even more by the extent to which artists felt compelled to camouflage his lameness.[48]

In his *Guide to Greece*, Pausanias informs his readers that in Athens there was a temple dedicated to Hephaistos in which the statue of the smith-god was flanked by one of Athena.[49] Arguing against the ancients' anthropomorphic view of the gods, the Roman orator Cicero expands our knowledge of the statue of Vulcan (the Roman counterpart for Hephaistos) by noting that at Athens there was a standing statue of Vulcan made by Alcamenes that, though draped, displayed a slight lameness, "though not enough to be unsightly."[50]

A student of Phidias, the great sculptor and architect of the Parthenon, Alcamenes was thus extolled by the informed viewer for his sense of measure and decorum in the representation of this god's disability. In truth, this sculptor's sensibility is better understood when looking at depictions of Vulcan dating to the sixth century BC in which this god's disfigurement was overly explicit. These images, closely following Homer's epithets for the god ("the crook-foot" or "lame"), do in fact represent one or both of Vulcan's feet withered or deformed.[51]

Perhaps the earliest of these images, from about 570 BC, is on the François Vase in the Florence Archaeological Museum (Figure 1.1). Here the artist, Kleitias, painted on the body

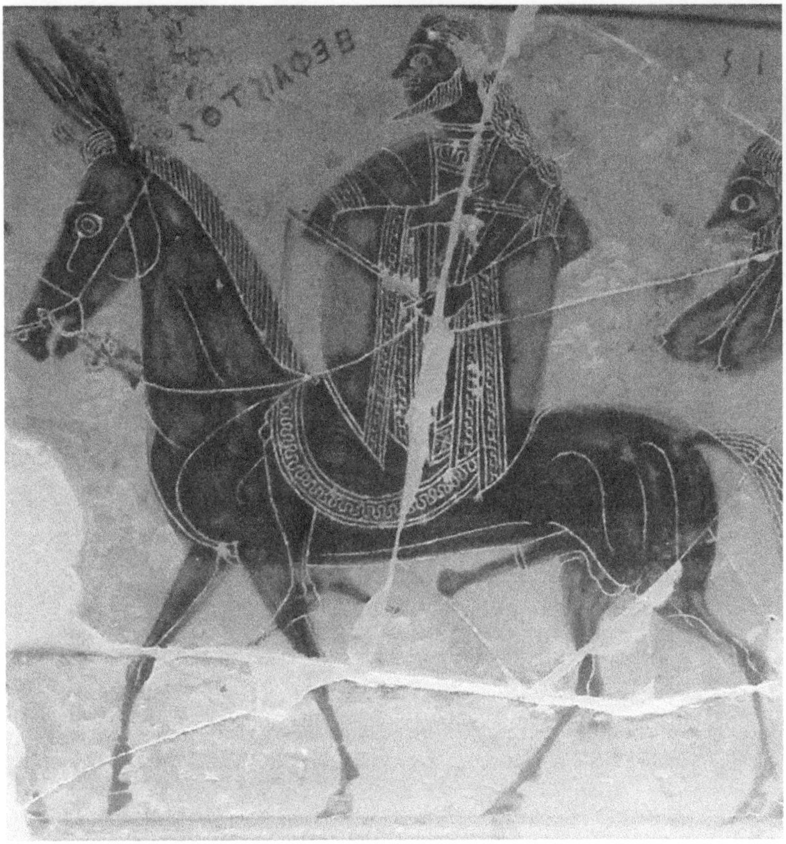

Figure 1.1 *Hephaistos*, François Vase, sixth century BC, Florence Archaeological Museum. Photo: author

of the volute crater the return of Hephaistos to Olympus in the midst of a Dionysiac procession, or thiasos. Although not immediately apparent, the god's impairment is signaled by a twisted, backward right foot on the far side of his mount.[52] A similar approach was adopted by the painter of an Attic vase from the end of the sixth century where Hephaistos is present at the birth of Athena in his role as "midwife" (Figure 1.2). On the right of the seated Zeus, the lame god is shown standing with a twisted foot.[53] However, the most indicative examples of this stark realism are found on a vase in the Kunsthistorisches Museum, Vienna, depicting *The Return of Hephaistos to Olympus* (Plate 2), and in a very small scarab representing Hephaistos's counterpart, the Etruscan Sethlans (Figure 1.3), both dated to about 520 BC. In the former, Dionysos greets the donkey-riding Hephaistos, whose feet are severely distorted and turned backwards;[54] in the latter, comparably explicit in representing his physical anomaly, Sethlans is pictured holding a shield and standing between Thetis and her son Achilles with upturned feet, as though performing a precarious balancing act.[55]

In Roman art Vulcan is mostly depicted in his smith's clothes, with a cap and short tunic (*pilos* and *exomis*). Given that his legs are typically in sight, one would expect artists to make

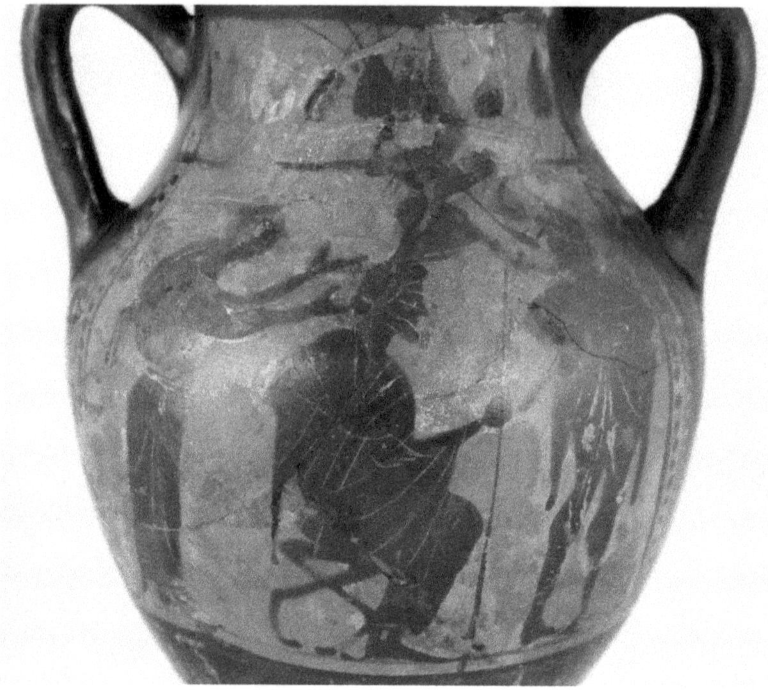

Figure 1.2 Greek amphora, *Hephaistos as Midwife*, Lyman Allyn Art Museum, New London, Connecticut. Photo: Lyman Allyn Art Museum, New London, Connecticut

some reference to his disability. Instead, his lameness, if represented, follows Alcamenes's understatement and not the deformed, backward twist of the feet present in the Greek archaic tradition, as witnessed by a statuette of the god found in Ostia (Figure 1.4). Indeed, the difficulty in discerning any reference to Vulcan's disability is such that at times one is left in doubt as to whether the seeming disparity in the rendition of the right and left leg is an artistic aberration or is meant to hint at the god's impairment. This is the case with the Albani Puteal (second century AD) in the Capitoline Museum (Figure 1.5), where Vulcan's disability might be indicated by a slight inward twist of the left or "sinister" foot and an underdeveloped calf muscle.[56]

Although there are some Roman works that portray Vulcan's lameness as well as some Greek and Hellenistic examples of deformed or infirm humans, there are no Roman artifacts that attest to a presence of lame *mortals* in the visual tradition.[57] This paucity of artistic evidence is certainly at odds with the historical reality of communities where, if nothing else, wars must have altered human bodies permanently. One interesting exception is attested by a *denarius* of about 85–83 BC, coined for Publius Furius Crassipes or Crassupes (Splay Foot), which commemorates his curule aedileship by showing on the obverse a small deformed foot, with three toes turned upwards, next to the head of a turreted female head of Cybele, the Phrygian Mother Earth (Figure 1.6).[58] This, however, is merely a synecdochical representation of the disabled body in which a part (the splayed foot) stood for the whole (the lame body) and does not portray an actually orthopedically impaired anatomy. In an age when

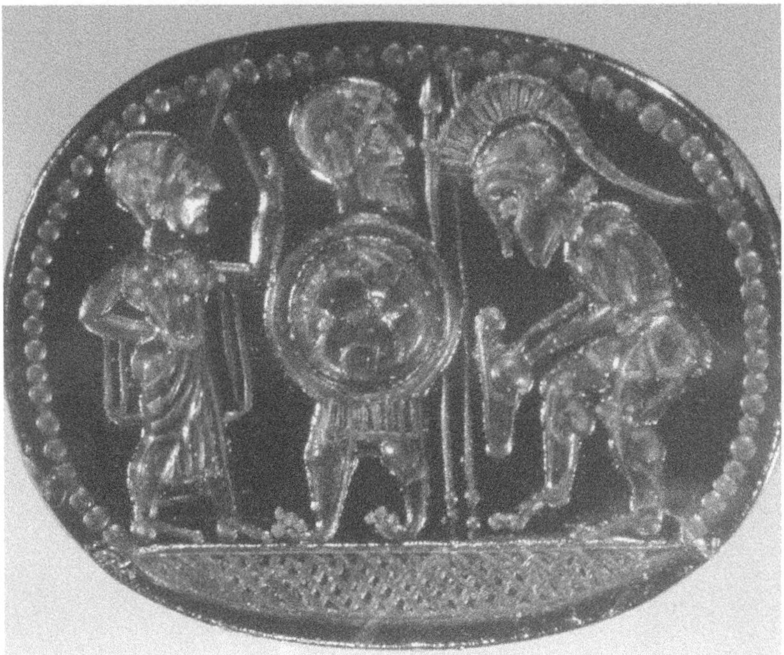

Figure 1.3 Master of the Boston Dionysos, Sethlans scarab, ca. 520–510 BC, J. Paul Getty Museum, Malibu. Photo: J. Paul Getty Museum

humans were even less protected than nowadays by modern medicine against congenital deformities, disfigurations, diseases, illnesses and mutilations, the very scarcity of such images is an indication of a society that generally did not feel compelled to represent the less-than-perfect body. In this regard, Cicero's view may be taken as indicative of the Roman *forma mentis*. In an attempt to prove that just as the body suffers disease, sickness and defect, so too does the soul, the orator expressed his distaste for lameness by stating that "defect [is the term used] when the parts of the body are not symmetrical with one another and there ensue crookedness of the limbs, distortion, ugliness."[59]

Given the obdurate, even contemptuous, response of ancient artists and societies to the orthopedically impaired body, the appearance of the lame and the paralytic in the third century is all the more striking.[60] The drastic change raises a question about the circumstances that encouraged the retrieval of images of people whose mobility was partially or totally impaired from the margins of art and prompts one to ask what these depictions reveal about the social order that produced them. In fact, the issue is of great significance because the increasing occurrence of representations of the disabled in general in the visual arts corresponds to a change from the pagan to the Christian worldview.[61] Indeed, the appearance of individuals whose ambulatory facility was curtailed by congenital impairments, disease or amputation flourished in art only when their presence was appropriated by artists for the ideological needs of the Christian Church. Even though Christians, as much as their pagan predecessors, equated the beautiful with the good (*kalos kagathos*), the frequent depiction of

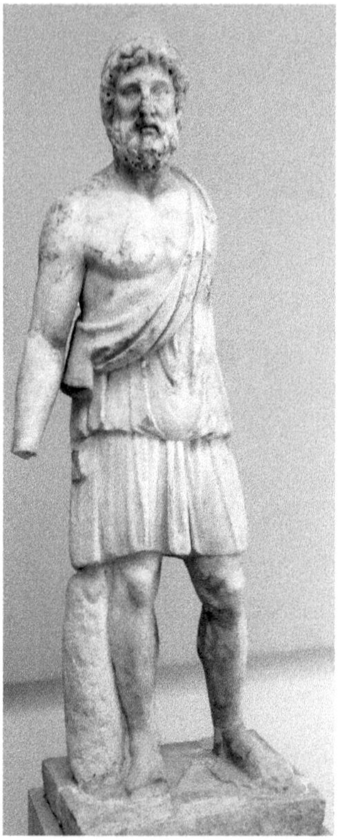

Figure 1.4 Vulcan, Ostia Antica Museum. Photo: author

immobile individuals or those with limited mobility became for the faithful a reassuring sign of universal acceptance and the promise of a more equitable existence in the next life if not in the earthly one.[62] Certainly, since human experience more often than not witnesses the disabled body's "resistance to cure or successful rehabilitation,"[63] the miraculous events depicted by the Christian artists were a true innovation. In other words, although in New Testament scenes the cure of cripples still presupposed their inclusion in the new religious group only after the elimination of their physical differences,[64] the orthopedically impaired body that pagan artists had mostly chosen to ignore became, at the hands of craftsmen with an innate talent for narrative painting, a poignant reinforcement of Christian beliefs for the faithful and a persuasive tool of proselytization for the clergy.

* * *

The baptistery frescoes from the Dura Europos "Christian House" at the Yale University Art Gallery, originally from the Syrian Desert near the River Euphrates, represent one of the earliest testimonies of Christian art. Among these frescoes is a fascinating panel that represents the *Miracle of the Paralytic*, in which a beardless Christ gestures towards a figure who is lying in

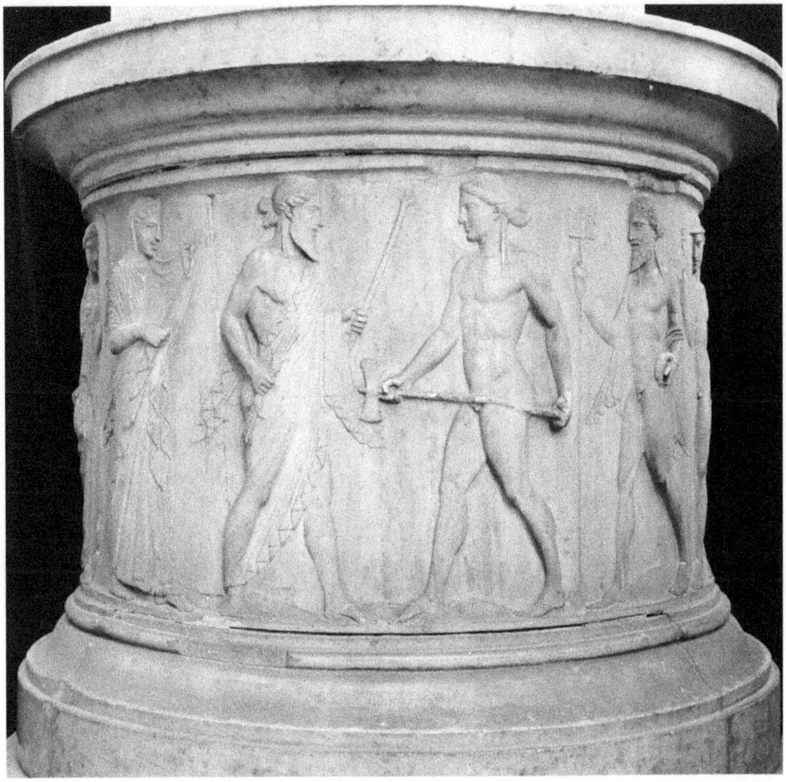

Figure 1.5 Vulcan, Albani Puteal, Capitoline Museum, Rome

bed while, within the same scene, the figure is also shown walking away with the bedstead on his shoulders, cured of his infirmity (Figure 1.7).[65] Like other frescoes in the baptistery, this depiction of the miracle attests to Christ's healing powers. Furthermore, for a religion that promised eternal life and equality after death, the miracle probably spoke more directly than others to the neophyte because miracles involving the physically impaired became a promise of reparation in the next life.[66]

Miracles, of course, also occurred in the pagan world. One often learns of wondrous cures in relationship to the cults of the gods Asklepios and Isis. In healings ascribed to the divine intervention of Asklepios at Epidauros, for example, the array of ailments spans from baldness to pregnancies, tumors, infertility and tuberculosis.[67] Still, most common of all in the Hellenistic period are references to injured or disfigured limbs, wounds caused by weapons and blindness.[68] The cure for these conditions seems to have come in the form of an epiphany or a dream while the infirm pilgrim spent the night in a sacred precinct, but there is no indication that the supplicants experienced "a spiritual transformation or a promise of anything transcendent."[69] According to Suetonius, such was the case with a seemingly successful cure of a blind man and a lame man who went to Vespasian asking that they be delivered of their disorders. As promised them by Serapis in a dream, Vespasian restored the eyes by spitting upon them and the leg by touching it with his heel.[70] Indeed, the significance

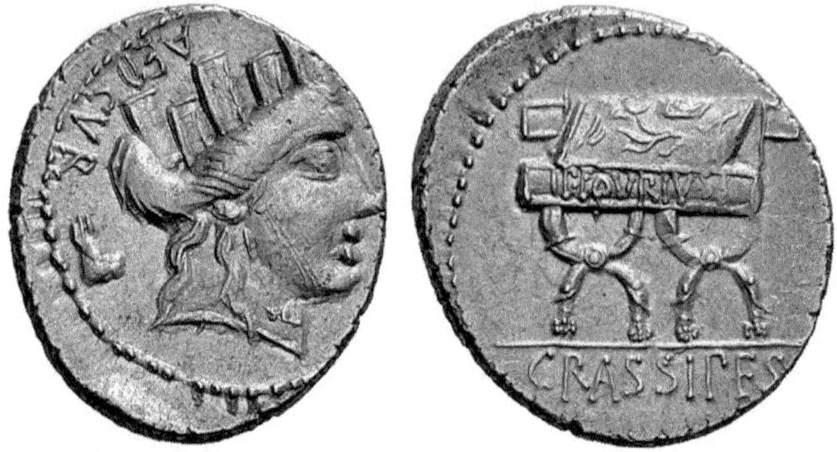

Figure 1.6 *Denarius* of Crassipes, 84 BC. Photo: from Edward Allen Sydenham, *The Coinage of the Roman Republic,* London, 1952, pl. XVIII

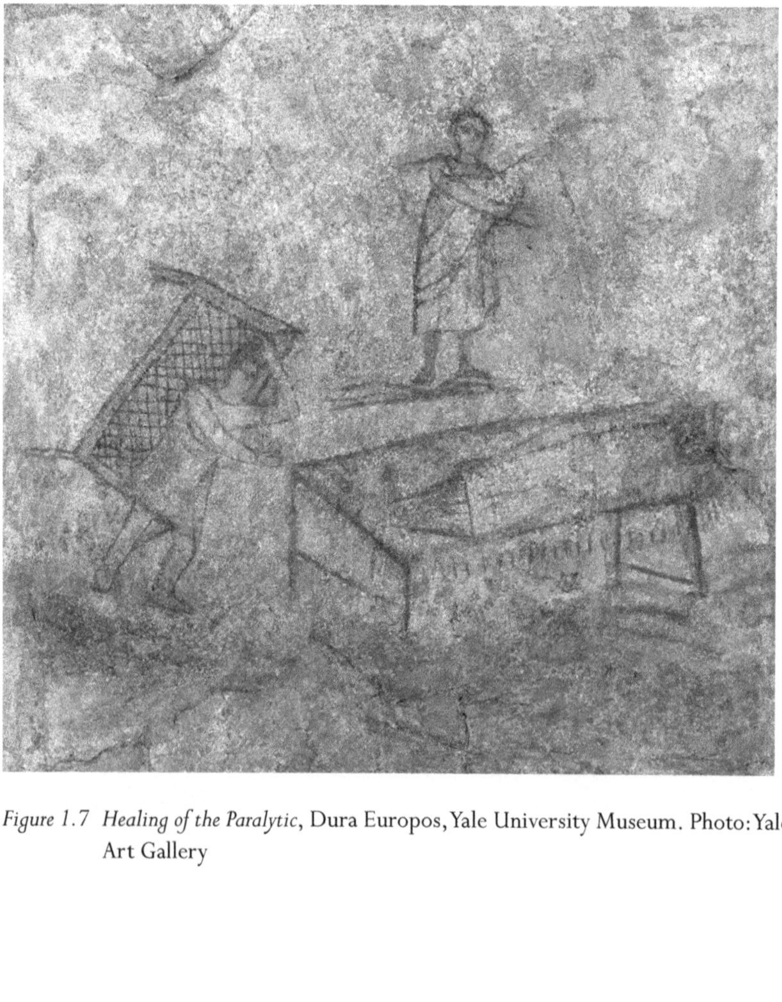

Figure 1.7 *Healing of the Paralytic*, Dura Europos, Yale University Museum. Photo: Yale University Art Gallery

of these events was limited to the earthly realm, even if a perceptible change did take place in the late first and early second centuries with the cult of Isis. Apparently, the upper classes saw in this deity more "the medicine of immortality" than a physical healer.[71] Nonetheless, pagan "healing iconography" is practically non-existent.[72]

Miracles are also described in the Old Testament. Healing miracles through the intercession of a human being or his earthly remains, however, are limited to only one incident involving the prophet Elijah's disciple, Elisha.[73] Although Elijah had raised the dead son of the widow of Zarephath (1 Ki 17:17–24), and Elisha himself similarly resuscitated the dead son of the Shunammite woman (2 Ki 4:32–37) and the corpse of a dead man who was flung into the prophet's tomb ("the man had no sooner touched the bones of Elisha than he came to life and stood up on his feet," 2 Ki 13:21), these three miracles involved resurrections more than the actual healing of a living individual. The only Old Testament miracle that truly involves the healing of an infirm person through the intervention of another human being has to do with the leper Naaman, who is told by Elisha to immerse himself seven times in the Jordan "and his flesh became clean once more like the flesh of a little child" (2 Ki 5:14).

In the New Testament, however, references to the infirm become much more frequent and the sheer number of instances in which the disabled or miracles are mentioned is an indication of the greater attention they received from Christian observers. In truth, by consulting a concordance of the Bible one becomes aware of the dimensions of such a phenomenon. The noun "halt" appears twice in the Old Testament while four in the New; the verb "healed" thirty-two in the Old and forty-six in the New Testament; the substantive "infirmities" twelve in the New and none in the Old, whereas the singular form "infirmity" appears three times in the Old Testament and seven in the New Testament; "maimed" only once in the Old and six in the New; while, focusing on the orthopedically impaired, the word "lame" appears eighteen times in the Old Testament and ten in the New, and "palsy," that is paralysis, thirteen times in the New and none in the Old Testament.[74] Most indicative of all, however, is the fact that the word "miracle" is utilized only once in the Old Testament and nine times in the New, while the plural "miracles" appears a mere four times in the Old and twenty-three in the New Testament.[75]

In fact, for the Early Christians miracles involving the healing of incurable ailments, such as blindness and lameness, gave hope not only in this world but also, more importantly, in the next. In many ways, miracles had a universal and eternal resonance for the Christians. Therefore, while referring to Christ's healing power over body and soul, the miracle of the paralytic was also interpreted as a wondrous event that most tangibly gave hope for a more equitable world.[76] Moreover, although even in the New Testament there are traces of a mindset that sees disease as a punishment for those who disobey divine law, it is obvious that Christ "neither directly or indirectly considers illness as a consequence of a moral transgression or a sin."[77] Thus Jesus set a new course for his community whereby, in Diego Gracia's words: "the ill person is not looked upon as an impure being that must be excluded from the cultural and social community, but a privileged place or object for the manifestation of the salvific work of God. This work is Jesus, the Saviour whose practice overrules and surpasses the Old Testament practices. And this new practice is essentially practice with outsiders, the poor, and the ill."[78] Consequently, when seen against the Judaic tradition that connected defect to sin,

Christ's miracles involving the disabled were a revolutionary way of breaking the link between disability and individual fault.[79]

Despite Christianity's more accepting view of the disabled, most Early Christian art does not depict the body with limited mobility. In images that represent the *Miracle of the Paralytic* in a wide range of media and geographical sites, such as the fourth-century bowls now in the Corning Museum of Glass and the Römisch-Germanisches Zentralmuseum in Mainz (Figure 1.8),[80] a Roman ivory plaque dated to 410–420 with miracles of Christ at the Louvre in Paris (Figure 1.9),[81] or the later sixth-century mosaic with the "Healing of the Paralytic at Capernaum" in the church of Sant'Apollinare Nuovo in Ravenna and the early eighth-century fresco of the same subject from the oratory beneath the Roman basilica of San Saba (Plate 3), the disability of the orthopedically impaired may only be inferred from the bedridden figure or the healed paralytic as he walks away carrying his bed.[82] These depictions indicate that representations of the paralytic from late antiquity to the end of the second phase of Early Christian art – which extends from the beginning of the fourth- to about the end of the fifth century – and beyond involve a visual prolepsis;[83] they are abridged representations that project the formerly ill or disabled as already admitted into "normal," healthy society.[84]

Thus, when the unaccustomed Early Christian viewers came upon the kind of images of the lame and disabled that began permeating their visual world at the beginning of the sixth century, they must have been as surprised by the novelty of this graphic approach as reassured

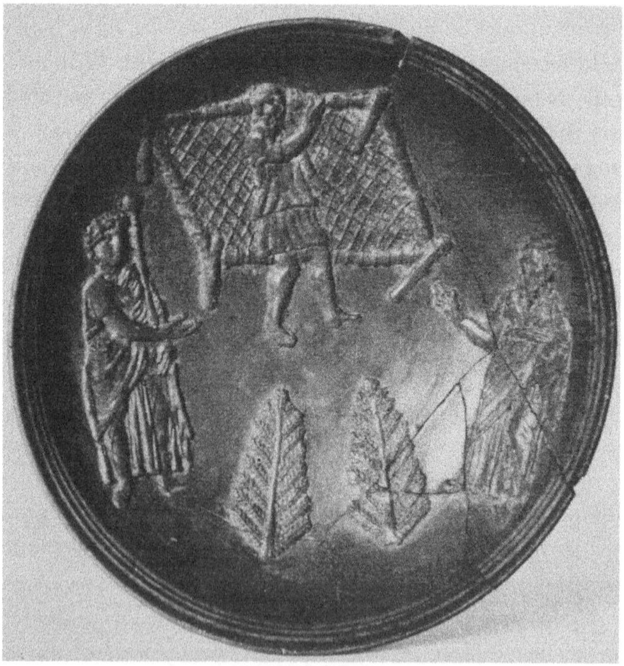

Figure 1.8 Bowl with the *Healing of the Paralytic*, Römisch-Germanisches Zentralmuseum, Mainz/Lübke & Wiedemann, Studios für Fotografie, Stuttgart

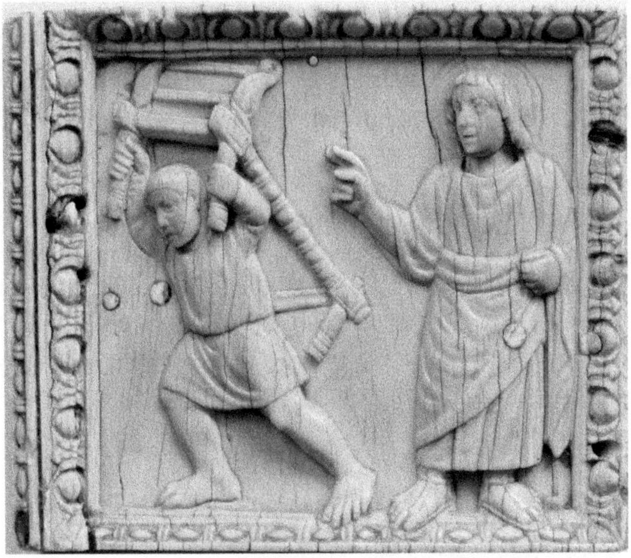

Figure 1.9 *Miracle of the Paralytic*, ivory plaque, Musée du Louvre, Paris. Photo: ©RMN-Grand Palais (musée du Louvre)/Daniel Arnaudet

by the ostensible clarity of the religious message. If on the one hand the realistically rendered infirmity shown prior to any miraculous cure reminded viewers of the vulnerability of the human condition, on the other hand it also gave tangible form to the wondrous, redressing the powers of Christ the healer.[85]

The more realistic portrayal of disabled bodies probably first occurred in depictions of the *Healing of the Infirm*, in which the lame, the crippled, the blind and other suffering humans appeared in New Testament cycles illustrating the life of Christ.[86] While in the first phase of Christian art (ca. AD 200–313) the primary approach to the pictorial subject was one that favored "image-signs" that abbreviated as much as possible the content of the story depicted, by the fifth and into the sixth century there had been a move towards a more descriptive type of art through which the artists included more details that would intensify the lifelike quality of the evangelical scenes.[87] One good example of this verism is the sixth-century throne of Maximian in the Museo Arcivescovile in Ravenna (AD 546–556). In the panel representing *Christ Healing the Blind Man* (Figure 1.10), the depiction of the cripple is comparable to the realistic rendition of Hephaistos's infirmity as executed in the archaic Greek tradition previously discussed (Figures 1.1 and 1.2 and Plate 2). In this ivory carving the artist represented a youthful, clean-shaven Christ touching the eyes of the blind man while a cripple raises his left leg with a conspicuously deformed foot. With his lifted, supplicating right hand the cripple waits his turn to be delivered from his affliction as the bearded figure of a bystander (probably the prophet Isaiah), with a book in his left hand and raised right hand, stands behind him and bears witness to the miracle. In this instance, there is no allusion or cosmetic camouflage to gloss over the true nature of the lame man's impairment as there had been with the depictions of the *Miracle of the Paralytic*. The viewer is confronted directly with a manifestation of typically irreversible orthopedic conditions and the expectation of the miraculous, imminent cure.

On a symbolical level, of course, the stark reality of the physical ailments illustrated on the throne of Maximian only intensified the efficacy of the message. In fact, the pairing of the blind and the lame in Western art had a long tradition that, as exemplified by the first-century *Apocryphon of Ezekiel*, represented the doctrine of the resurrection of *both* body and soul, with the blind "standing" for the body and the lame representing the soul.[88] Just as significantly, the presence of the bearded bystander in this same panel was a clear reference to Matthew 8:16–17, where Christ's cure of the infirm was seen as a fulfillment of Isaiah's prophecy ("He took our sicknesses away and carried our diseases for us") and Matthew 11:5–6: "the blind see again, and the lame walk, lepers are cleansed, and the deaf hear, and the dead are raised to life and the Good News is proclaimed to the poor; and happy is the man who does not lose faith in me."[89]

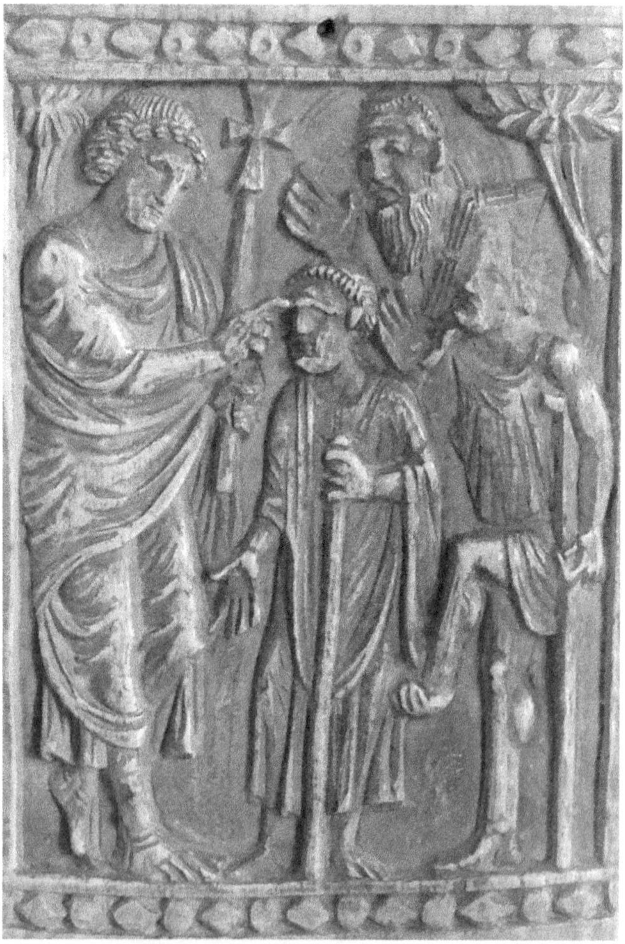

Figure 1.10 Healing of the Infirm, Throne of Maximian, Ravenna. Photo: author

This greater interest in a more realistic representation of infirm individuals in a narrative context may be seen in illuminated manuscripts that were executed in the Byzantine East and "imported" in the West, such as the sixth-century Rabbula Gospels in the Laurentian Library in Florence (Figure 1.11), the ninth-century *Parisinus Graecus* 923 (Figure 1.12) in the Bibliothèque Nationale in Paris, the eleventh-century *Parisinus Graecus* 74 (Figure 1.13), or the eleventh/twelfth-century Tetra-Gospel from the Laurentian Library (Figure 1.14). In all of these manuscripts the illuminators not only rendered quite graphically the twisted limbs of the lame, but also included the cripples with their contorted feet and legs who, crawling on the ground, make their way towards Christ aided by their wooden trestles, or mini-crutches; a striking way of representing an ailing humanity.[90]

It was through such exportable Middle Eastern artifacts that the depiction of the disfigured body most likely made its way to the West and affected the local tradition.[91] The reason why the artists' descriptive creativity was elicited in these manuscripts is probably due to the fewer spatial restrictions implicit in the medium of painting itself, which allowed for a fuller account of Christ's miracles.[92] Therefore, alongside the "before and after" narration of

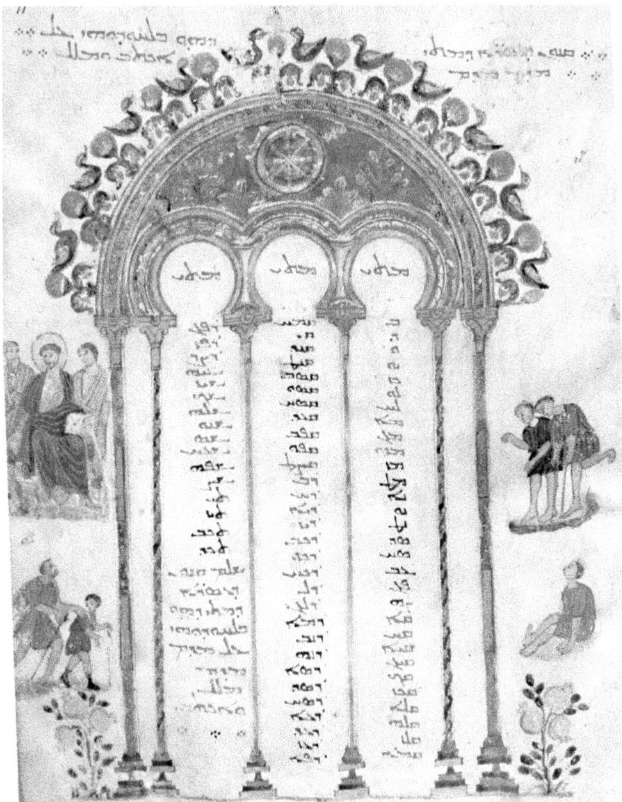

Figure 1.11 *Healing of the Infirm, Rabbula Tetragospels*, Laurenziana Library, Florence. Photo: Firenza, Biblioteca Medicea Laurenziana, Ms. Plut. 1.56, c. 11r, su concessione del MiBACT

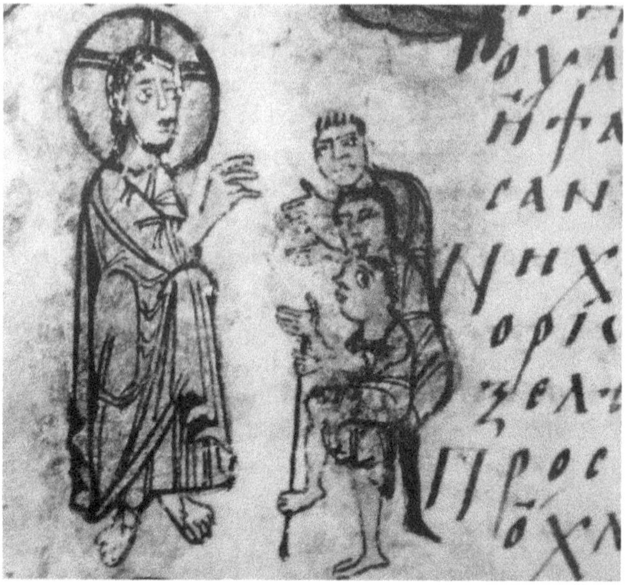

Figure 1.12 *Healing of the Infirm*, *Parisinus Graecus* 923. Photo: from Kurt Weitzmann, *The Miniatures of the Sacra Parallela Parisinus Graecus 923*, Princeton, 1979, fig. 425

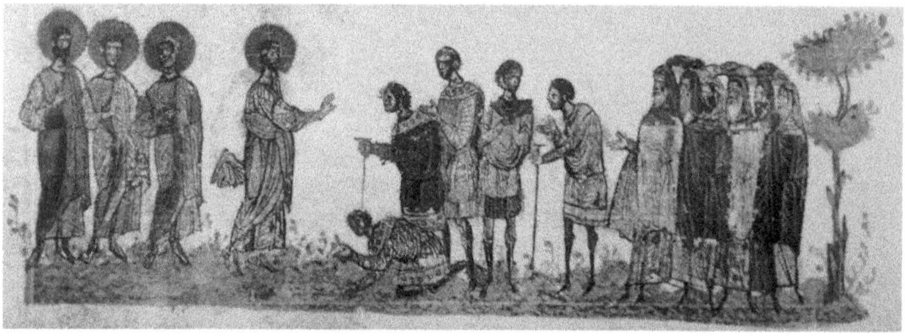

Figure 1.13 *Healing of the Infirm*, *Parisinus Graecus* 74. Photo: from Henry A. Omont (ed.), *Évangiles avec peintures byzantines du XIe siècle*, 2 vols., Paris, 1908, II, pl. 35

the *Miracle of the Paralytic*, artists could now give vent to a more narrative emphasis in representing all of those infirm members of humankind who sought a miraculous cure. Truly, this might have been the case on the walls of the Roman church of San Saba, since the patrons of the fresco cycle were an immigrant monastic community that had left the Holy Land and established itself in Rome. Even though there is no evidence among the fragments that have come to light from this church that *The Healing of the Infirm* was represented, the fact that these frescoes so closely reflect Palestinian art of the mid-seventh century makes the likelihood of the inclusion of this particular scene in this fresco cycle feasible.[93] In these Middle Eastern works the realistic representation of the lame is consistently differentiated from the proleptic depictions of the paralytic. Ultimately, it was this starker realism of the illuminated

Figure 1.14 *Healing of the Infirm*, *Tetra-Gospel*, Laurentian Library. Photo: from Tania Velmans, *Le Tétraévangile de la Laurentienne*, Paris, 1971, fig. 65

manuscript tradition that was transmitted to the art of the late Middle Ages, as indicated by the cripple who drags his body with the aid of trestles in the mosaics in the cathedral of Monreale of 1182 (Plate 4) or in an Italian fourteenth-century manuscript of the *Meditations on the Life of Christ*.[94]

* * *

To better understand the appearance of the lame in Western art and the socio-historical context that sustained such depictions, one must pause and reflect on the collateral problems of poverty – since some of those individuals who, because of their social and physical condition, were unable to sustain themselves financially were destined to a life of mendicancy - and the perception society had of able-bodied idlers, especially when believed to be simulating physical disabilities.

A penetrating analysis of the rapport between the rich and poor in pagan and Christian societies has indicated that, contrary to what Christian homiletics would lead one to believe, pagan societies were not frigid towards the marginalized and that "there was no lack of outreach to the distressed."[95] Just like the later Christian beggars, the pagan mendicants who lingered around temples in the hope of receiving coins or some food from the sacrificial offerings "were not totally ignored."[96] It is just that almsgiving for the pagans, especially in the Roman world, was focused on "civic euergetism," the practice of doing good deeds for one's city.[97] What was lacking to the non-Christian practice of *humanitas* – "the humane treatment which one person shows to another because of the common bond of a shared human nature"[98] – was a clear focus. As Peter Brown points out: "A general ideal of humanity was widespread, but the actions that sprang from that ideal were scattered erratically throughout society. They never congealed into a single social action that summed up everyone's ideal of a signal act that combined generosity and humanity in the way that almsgiving to the poor was consistently exalted in Jewish and Christian circles as the pious act par excellence."[99] What instead clearly defined and differentiated Christian from even Jewish almsgiving – for whom the poor faced the rich not so much asking for alms as in search of justice – was that even the smallest of gifts opened up a path to heaven.[100] As Brown aptly points out, "gifts to the poor could be seen as loans to God.

God would repay them with unimaginable interest."[101] What distinguished the Christians approach to almsgiving, in other words, was "the supernatural efficacy of the Christian gift."[102] Complications, of course, arose when the person asking for alms was perceived to be a freeloader.

It has been noted that the able-bodied in Classical Greece and Rome, as well as Christians in late antiquity, were typically suspicious of idlers.[103] Plato, for instance, was most categorical in his planning of the ideal state: "There should be no begging in the state. If anyone attempt it and seek to scrape up a living by his incessant entreaties, he shall be expelled from the marketplace by the commissioners of the market and from the city by the urban commission, and escorted over the borders by the rural police, that our land may be entirely cleaned of such creatures."[104] However, matters changed in time in the gradual transition from a more distanced pagan attitude to the Christian greater forbearance towards the marginalized. Thus, by the fourth century, while the pagans had referred to the poor as "base" or "ignoble," Christians instead spoke of them as "the meek" and "the afflicted," focusing more on their material needs than on their social status.[105] This transformation may be exemplified by comparing the antithetical responses to destitute beggars by the pagan judicial system that was inherited by the first Christian emperors and the Early Christian Fathers. Indeed, just two years after Christianity had been made the official state religion, in an imperial decree issued in 382 under the emperors Gratian, Valentinian and Theodosius, which would eventually be included in *The Code of Justinian*, one finds the following ruling:

> All those who adopt the uncertain calling of public beggars shall be examined and their physical condition and age be ascertained, and if they have been reduced to this state through idleness, and not by disease, those of them who are slaves shall become the property of the person who detected them. Where, however, they are free by birth, they shall be subjected as vassals to whoever has exposed them and proved their imposture. If they are fugitives, or others have advised them to adopt the profession of beggars, the rights of action of their masters shall remain unimpaired.[106]

However, even allowing for the rhetorical nature of the homiletics of the Early Church Fathers,[107] it is enlightening and symptomatic of the Christian worldview to read what authors such as John Chrysostom had to say about the beggars who must have abundantly populated the late-antique urban fabric. In delivering one of his homilies in the winter of 387 in Antioch, Chrysostom declared:

> We must open our hearts, then, to all the poor, to those suffering evil for any reason at all, according to the Scripture that commands us to "rejoice with those who rejoice and weep with those who weep." Because we are human beings, we must offer the favor of our kindness first of all to other human beings, whether they need it because they are widows or orphans or because they are exiles from their own country, or because of the cruelty of their masters or the harshness of their rulers or the inhumanity of their tax-collectors, or because of the bloody violence of robbers or the insatiable greed of thieves, or because of the legal confiscation of their property, or shipwreck – all are wretched alike, and so all look towards our hands, as we look towards God's, for the things we need.[108]

It is irrelevant, in other words, whether the mendicants who beg are disabled or able-bodied; the mere fact that these individuals humble themselves by asking for alms is sufficient reason for the Christian to donate liberally, without preconditions, as opposed to what the *Code of Justinian* decreed. But all the more, continues Chrysostom, should one's heart open up to those who beg because of physical ailments or diseases. He therefore denounces the apparent turning of a deaf ear to the plight of the least fortunate members of society, even by members of the Christian community. Having gone through the marketplace at a time when even Nature herself seemed to have withdrawn her "hand" because of the inclement weather, he states:

> Today, I stand before you to make a just, useful, and suitable intercession. I come from no one else; only the beggars who live in our city elected me for this purpose, not with words, votes, and the resolve of a common council, but rather with their pitiful and most bitter spectacles. In other words, just as I was passing through the marketplace and the narrow lanes, hastening to your assembly, I saw in the middle of the streets many outcasts, some with severed hands, others with gouged-out eyes, others filled with festering ulcers and incurable wounds, especially exposing those body parts that, because of their stored-up rottenness, they should be concealing. I thought it the worst inhumanity not to appeal to your love on their behalf, especially now that the season forces us to return to this topic.[109]

Similarly, Gregory of Nazianzus moves his hearers to a comparable compassion in Oration 14 ("On the Love of the Poor") when, with a masterful *ekphrasis*, he verbally depicts the disfigured bodies of the mendicants as vividly as a painter (Plate 5). In describing the tribulations that ensue when illness is added to poverty, he affirms:

> For most people, only one thing causes misery: something is lacking. Perhaps time, or hard work, or a friend, or a relative, or the passing of time has taken it away. But for the people I am speaking of, misery is present even more abundantly, in that the resources to work and to help themselves in need have been taken away along with their flesh, and the fear of growing weaker is always greater to them than the hope of recovery .... There stands before our eyes a terrible, pitiable sight, unbelievable to anyone who did not know it was true: human beings both dead and alive, mutilated in most parts of their body, scarcely recognizable either for who they are or where they come from; they are, rather, wretched remnants of once-human beings .... They are truncated human beings, deprived of possessions, family, friends and their very bodies, distinctive in being able both to pity themselves and hate themselves at once. They are uncertain whether to lament for the parts of their bodies that no longer exist, or for those that remain – those which the disease has consumed, or those left for the disease to work on.[110]

John Chrysostom also parries accusations of idleness and simulation of physical impairments addressed to the beggars by respectable citizens by clarifying his Christian stance on such issues: "I do not say these things haphazardly now, but rather because many are often overly investigative toward the needy; they examine their lineage, life, habits, pursuit, and the vigor of their body. They make complaints and demand immense public scrutiny of their health. For this precise reason, many of the poor simulate physical disabilities, so that by dramatizing their misfortunes they may deflect our cruelty and inhumanity."[111] Given the mendicants' destitute state, even simulation is a fair tactic if it helps to soften the hearts of the able-bodied citizens. Nothing justifies the worst of all possible crimes in their regard: insensitivity. Taking Lazarus as his "brother and teacher," Chrysostom clarifies: "In adversity, the absence of those who might help us does not dismay us as much as the indifference of those who, though present, refuse to reach out to us."[112]

The change from the pagan to a Christian worldview was brought about by something that undermined the establishment to its very foundations. Even more than Christianity's belief in and a promise of an afterlife, it was in the here and now that the new religion challenged the Classical world, since for the Christians "only one thing is sacred, and that is human fellowship."[113] Actually, if previously the care of the disabled had been primarily a family concern, for the Christians it became a "communal responsibility."[114] In his treatise "On Works and Alms," St. Cyprian put it most concisely: "How more could He (the Lord) stimulate the works of our righteousness and mercy, than by saying that whatever is given to the needy and poor is given to Himself, and by saying that He is aggrieved unless the needy and poor be supplied? So that he who in the Church is not moved by consideration for his brother, may yet be moved by contemplation of Christ; and he who does not think of his fellow servant in suffering and in poverty, may yet think of his Lord, who abideth in that very man whom he is despising."[115]

In a world founded on a slave-based economy in which social disparity was deeply rooted, to declare "the last shall be first,"[116] extol the "bond among human beings"[117] and emphasize the importance of fraternal love represented a significant reversal from the religious, social and political views of the pagan world. The appearance of the lame body in Early Christian art testifies to this transformation.

Notes

1 For Antonia's reputed repulsion for her son, see Suetonius, *The Lives of the Caesars*, 2 vols., John Carew Rolfe (tr.), Cambridge and London, 1979, V, iii, 2. J.P. Balsdon, in *The Oxford Classical Dictionary*, Oxford, 1984, p. 245, describes the impairment as being "some sort of paralysis." Susanna Morton Braund and Paula James, "*Quasi Homo*: Distortion and Contortion in Seneca's *Apocolocyntosis*," *Arethusa*, 31 (1998): 287, claim Claudius's infirmities to have been "variously diagnosed as poliomyelitis and as cerebral palsy." Of course, the choice of the emperor's name could not have been more apposite, for the verb *claudĕre* in Latin means *to limp*. See also Robert Graves's literary characterization in *Claudius the God*, London, 1966, p. 1: "I, Tiberius Claudius Drusus Nero Germanicus, the cripple, the stammerer, the fool of the family, whom none of his ambitious and bloody-minded relatives considered worth the trouble of executing, poisoning, forcing to suicide, banishing to a desert island or starving to death."

2 Dio Cassius, *Roman History*, 9 vols., Earnest Cary (tr.), London and New York, 1924, VII, lx, p. 369. Claudius's ailments have also been variously diagnosed as meningitis, pre-natal encephalitis, multiple sclerosis. See Michael Grant, *The Twelve Caesars*, London, 1975, p. 129.

3 On imperial imagery at the time of Augustus, see Paul Zanker, *The Power of Images in the Age of Augustus*, Alan Shapiro (tr.), Ann Arbor, 1988.

4 The information one may rely on, of course, reflects the views of the upper classes since that is the only information available to us. For a succinct recap of the Romans' response to disability, see

Johannes Stahl, "Physically Deformed and Disabled People," in *Social Relations in the Roman World*, Peachin (ed.), Oxford, 2011, pp. 715–33.

5 Ibid., p. 731: "In short, disabled persons in the Roman world were in almost all situations pushed to the margins of society, or were integrated only by virtue of being made the butts of mockery and abuse. The only thing that might come to the rescue of such a person, again, generally speaking, was high social status."

6 Suetonius, V, iii, 9.

7 Ibid., V, iv, 9–11.

8 No doubt these reports were anecdotal and invented by the historian, who employs physical deformities to reflect the moral and political defects of a ruler. See Braund and James, n. 1.

9 For the use of deformed individuals at the Roman imperial court for amusement, entertainment and derision, and the employment of the deformed to characterize "bad" emperors in Suetonius and the *Scriptores Historiae Augustae*, see Lisa Trentin, "Deformity in the Roman Imperial Court," *Greece and Rome*, 58 (2011): 195–208. Cicero, *De Oratore*, 2 vols., E.W. Sutton and H. Rackham (trs.), Cambridge, MA, and London, II, p. 239: "In ugliness too and in physical blemishes there is good enough matter for jesting, but here as elsewhere the limits of license are the main question." On a similar note, Quintilian reminds his readers, "For, as Cicero says, 'Laughter has its basis in some kind or other of deformity or ugliness.'" See Robert Garland, *The Eye of the Beholder: Deformity and Disability in the Graeco-Roman World*, Ithaca, NY, 1995, pp. 73–86.

10 Seneca, *De Beneficiis*, IV, xxxii, 3, in *Moral Essays*, John W. Basore (tr.), Cambridge and London, 1989: "Hic corpore deformis est, adspectu foedus et ornamenta sua traducturus." It is assumed that Seneca is alluding to Claudius. Ibid., p. 270, note *a*.

11 Priscilla Baumann, "Margins/Outsiders," in *Encyclopedia of Comparative Iconography: Themes Depicted in Works of Art*, 2 vols., Helene E. Roberts (ed.), Chicago, 1998, II, pp. 545–551, esp. pp. 547 and 550.

12 For depictions of dwarfism and other human features worthy of derision, see Alexandre G. Mitchell, *Greek Vase-Painting and the Origins of Visual Humour*, Cambridge, 2009. For an exceptional sculpture of a hunchback at Villa Albani and its possible function within the Baths of Caracalla, where it was found, see Lisa Trentin, "What's in a Hump? Re-examining the Hunchback in the Villa Albani-Torlonia," *Cambridge Classical Journal*, Proceedings of the Cambridge Philological Society, 55 (2009): 130–156.

13 Lysias, "For the Disabled Man," Stephen Charles Todd (tr.), Austin, 2000, pp. 252–259. Stahl, p. 717: "Yet in Roman times, a right-sided paralysis was much more negatively judged than was one on the left side of the body, and an encounter with someone crippled on the right side was held to be an evil omen." Ibid., p. 722: "But in particular epileptics and people lame in the right foot were regularly shunned .... Should it so happen that contact with such a person could not be avoided, one might protect oneself by spitting in front of, or on, the person in question (cf. Plin. *Nat.* 28.35; Apul. *Apol.* 44)."

14 Plato, *Timaeus*, in *The Collected Dialogues of Plato*, Edith Hamilton and Huntington Cairns (eds.), Princeton, 1985, p. 1172, 44c.

15 *Plutarch's Lives*, Bernadotte Perrin (tr.), III, London, 1996, p. 79. Since physical disability in ancient Greece was considered in relationship to the person's role in society, that is, "the criteria of physical disability rested not on one's ability to function as an individual but on one's functional ability within the community," and given that there were many who continued working and being self-sufficient despite their physical ailments, being impaired did not qualify one as the "unable" (*adunatous*). To qualify as such, one had to be a poor, physically impaired person who was unable to work. To these individuals the Athenian state granted a small pension after an annual inspection by the council of citizens, the Boule, as indicated by Aristotle (*Constitution of Athens*, in *The Complete Works of Aristotle*, Jonathan Barnes (ed.), 2 vols., Princeton, 1985, II, p. 2372) and as argued by Lysias in favor of a client in the late fifth century BC, "On the Refusal of a Pension", W.R.M. Lamb (tr.), Cambridge, MA, and London, 1943, 22–23, pp. 539–531 (Lysias 24). See Martha L. Edwards, "Constructions of Physical Disability in the Ancient Greek

World: The Community Concept," in *The Body and Physical Difference*, Mitchell and Snyder (eds.), pp. 35–50, esp. pp. 35–38.

16 Demosthenes, *De Corona*, Charles Anthony Vince and James Herbert Vince (trs.), London and New York, 1926, p. 61.

17 Horace, *Ars Poetica*, in *Satires, Epistles and Ars Poetica*, Henry Rushton Fairclough (tr.), London and Cambridge, MA, 1978, p. 483, lines 401–403.

18 Pomponius Porphyro, *Commentum in Horatium Flaccum: de arte poetica*, Alfred Holder (ed.), Innsbruck, 1894, lemma 402, line 2: "omni parte membrorum deformis." Tyrtaeus was originally an Athenian who "is excluded from Athens because he is lame, stupid, of low birth and mad; he is in fact given to Sparta as a joke." See Todd Merlin Compton, *Victim of the Muse*, Cambridge and London, 2006, pp. 119–129.

19 Pliny, *Natural History*, 10 vols., Horace Rackham (tr.), London and Cambridge, MA, 1947, VII, xlv, p. 537. For literary reference to orthopedically impaired individuals who were still able to function in some military capacity in the Greek world, see Edwards, "Constructions of Physical Disability," pp. 39–41.

20 Henri-Jacques Stiker, *A History of Disability*, Ann Arbor, 1999, p. 50: "*Apothesis* was the term reserved for the exposure of infants born deformed, as distinct from *ekthesis*, which referred to fatal exclusion for other reasons as determined by the male head of the family."

21 *Plutarch's Lives, Lycurgus*, Bernadotte Perrin (tr.), London and New York, 1914, I, 1–2, p. 255; Robert Garland, *The Greek Way of Death*, London, 1985, pp. 80–81.

22 Emiel Eyben, "Family Planning in Graeco-Roman Antiquity," *Ancient Society*, 11–12 (1980–1981): 12–13. For the references, see especially p. 15, nn. 36 and 37. Martha L. Rose, *The Staff of Oedipus: Transforming Disability in Ancient Greece*, Ann Arbor, 2003, pp. 31–33, admonishes caution in interpreting the ancients' elimination of defective babies since the major sources adduced to support the Greeks' recourse to this practice are four other literary references besides Plutarch. For a comparable recap, see also Christian Laes, "Learning from Silence: Disabled Children in Roman Antiquity," *Arctos*, 42 (2008): 92–99.

23 Plato, *The Republic*, in *The Collected Dialogues of Plato*, Hamilton and Cairns (eds.), 460c, p. 699.

24 Plato, *Theaetetus*, in *The Collected Dialogues of Plato*, Hamilton and Cairns (eds.), 161a, p. 866.

25 Aristotle, *Politics*, in *The Complete Works of Aristotle*, Barnes (ed.), VII, 1335b, lines 20–26, p. 2119.

26 *Soranus' Gynecology*, Owsei Temkin (tr.), Baltimore and London, 1991, II, 10, p. 80. To these commonly cited Greek sources Darrel W. Amundsen adds Epictetus (*Discourses*, I, 23) – who, in answer to Epicurus's "Let us not bring up children", retorts that not even the sheep or wolves abandon their offspring – and a number of Classical authors who reported practices in other cultures where this child exposure was condemned. Among these authors he enlists Heliodorus (*An Ethiopian Romance*), Tacitus (*Germania*, 19), Philo Judaeus, Josephus (*Against Apion*, 2.24), Diodorus Siculus (*Library of History*, 40.3). See Darrel W. Amundsen, *Medicine, Society, and Faith in the Ancient and Medieval Worlds*, Baltimore and London, 1996, pp. 55–56.

27 Dionysius of Halicarnassus, *Roman Antiquities*, Earnest Cary (tr.), London and Cambridge, 1937, II.15.

28 Livy, *Histories*, 13 vols., Frank Gardner Moore (tr.), Cambridge, MA, and London, 1950, VII, xxvii, 37.

29 Seneca the Elder, *Controversiae*, Michael Winterbottom (tr.), Cambridge and London, 1974, 10.4.16, p. 439.

30 Rose, p. 48: "In summary, the source material that discusses deformed offspring in the ancient Greek world is too thin to conclude that their destruction was a standard practice. The cultural atmosphere into which such babies were born was one in which deformed people were not categorically deemed evil, worthless, or ill." See note 22.

31 Amundsen, p. 60.

32 For a useful recap of the "state of the scholarship" on this issue, see the useful essay by Ville Vuolanto, "Infant Abandonment and the Christianization of Medieval Europe," in *The Dark Side*

of Childhood in Late Antiquity and the Middle Ages, Katariina Mustakallio and Christian Laes (eds.), Oxford, 2011, pp. 3–19.

33 See Christian Laes's short but valuable contribution to this subject, "Raising a Disabled Child," in *The Oxford Handbook of Childhood and Education in the Classical World*, J.E. Grubbs and T. Parkin (eds.), Oxford, 2013, pp. 125–144. Hippocrates (460–370 BC), in his chapter on leg fractures, relates how supposedly the Amazons dislocated the male offsprings' knees or hips, making them lame and incapable of plotting against the females. He writes that he is not sure about the truth of such reports but that he knew "that such would be the result of dislocating the joints of young infants." *Hippocrates*, E.T. Withington (tr.), London and New York, 1927, III, 53, p. 321. He also specifies that the greatest damage to a dislocated body happens when this occurs *in utero*. Ibid., 319. Laes, "Raising a Disabled Child," p. 128: "Hippocratic theory referred to deficiency of the womb, constriction of the fetus by the womb, or weak sperm coming from weaker parts of the body. Aristotle (384–322 BC), basing himself on direct observation, disputes the assumption that "mutilated parents produce mutilated offspring." Aristotle, *Generation of Animals*, Cambridge, MA, and London, 1990 [orig. 1942], 721b–722a, pp. 51–53. Pliny echoes this concept in *Natural History*, VIII, 45, p. 539: "It is also well known that sound parents may have deformed children and deformed parents sound children or children with the same deformity, as the case may be."

34 *Letter to Diognetus*, V, 6, dated to the second century AD. See William A. Jurgens, *The Faith of the Early Fathers*, Collegeville, Minnesota, 1970: "The difference between Christians and the rest of men is neither in country, nor in language, nor in customs .... Like all others, they marry and beget children; but they do not expose their offspring." Laes, "Raising a Disabled Child," p. 139, citing Vuolanto, "Infant Abandonment and the Christianization of Medieval Europe," states that, "The condemnation of exposure seems to have been more a product of self-definition, opposing Christian practice to pagan custom."

35 Amundsen, pp. 62–65, nn. 37 and 38, p. 69.

36 Lactantius, *The Divine Institutes*, William Fletcher (tr.), Edinburgh, 1871, V.9, p. 312. Idem, VI.20, pp. 407–408. For a more recent recap and evaluation of the whole problem connected with infant abandonment in antiquity, see Judith Evans Grubbs, "The Dynamics of Infant Abandonment: Motives, Attitudes and (Unintended) Consequences," in *The Dark Side of Childhood in Late Antiquity and the Middle Ages*, Mustakallio and Laes (eds.), pp. 21–36.

37 Rose, p. 46.

38 Jean-Pierre Vernant, "From Oedipus to Periander: Lameness, Tyranny, Incest in Legend and History," *Arethusa*, 15:I (1982): 19–38. Stiker, p. 58, paraphrasing Vernant, states: "Disability defies order, and order is prey to disorder, which has a primordial and radical character."

39 Stiker, p. 72. The same author poignantly declares: "A society reveals itself by the way in which it treats certain significant phenomena. The problem of disability is one such phenomenon. To speak at all pertinently of disabled people is to disclose a society's depths" (p. 14), and "the social imagination is also social reality" (p. 46).

40 Plato, *Lesser Hippias*, in *The Collected Dialogues of Plato*, Hamilton and Cairns (eds.), 374d.

41 Plato, *Sophist*, in *The Collected Dialogues of Plato*, Hamilton and Cairns (eds.), 228a.

42 *Iliad*, Richard Lattimore (tr.), Chicago and London, 1970, 2, 216–219.

43 See *Lexicon Iconographicum Mythologiae Classicae* (hereafter *LIMC*), Zürich and Düsseldorf, 1981–1999, VIII, 1, 1207–1209, and for images, *LIMC*, VIII, 2, 829, *Thersites 3*, or *LIMC*, I, 2, *Agamemnon 81*.

44 Garland, *The Eye of the Beholder*, figs. 20 and 22 show details from black- and red-figure vases dating from the sixth to the fourth century BC with depictions of a clubfooted dancer and an actor playing an amputee. Fig. 32, possibly depicting Aesop, shows no real deformity of the legs, only a crutch, and fig. 35 is unconvincingly interpreted as the depiction of a cripple. Fig. 60 is the one startling, outstanding image: a statuette from Sicily of a "grossly deformed or disabled man" (ca. 600 BC). Hans Otto Dustmann, "Das Bildnis des Amputierten in der Kunst," in *Der Körperbehinderte in Mythologie und Kunst*, Kark Friedrich Schlegel (ed.), Stuttgart and New York, 1983, p. 58, fig. 2, reproduces the image of a limping *satyr*, with right shin and foot wrapped

around a cane (and a large phallus), from a second-century BC vase at the Louvre. It is obviously a "caricature" of an orthopedic human condition, which reinforces the argument that lameness of human beings was typically not portrayed in Classical art.

45 Hesiod, *Theogony*, Glen W. Most (tr.), Cambridge and London, 2006, 945, p. 79.

46 For Hephaistos, see *The Oxford Classical Dictionary*, N.G.B. Hammond and H.H. Scullard (eds.), Oxford, 1984, 497, and Bonnefoy, I, pp. 384–386. For a full investigation of the literary sources pertaining to Hephaistos and his Etruscan counterpart, Sethlans, along with the various iconographic solutions to distinguish him in Classical art, see *LIMC*, IV, 1, 627–659 and IV, 2, figs. 18a, 103a, 129, 198. On congenital physical impairment, it was clear to the Greeks that the children of crippled parents were primarily sound and that physical defects for the most part were not passed on from parent to child (Aristotle, *History of Animals*, in *The Complete Works of Aristotle*, Barnes (ed.), VII, 6, 585b–586a). However, common belief ran to the contrary (Aristotle, *Generation of Animals*, in *The Complete Works of Aristotle*, Barnes (ed.), 721b–722a). A case in point was the lame Spartan ruler, Agesilaus, whose father had married a little woman and for doing so had been fined by the euphors, since, according to them, she would bear "not kings, but kinglets." See *Plutarch's Lives, Agesilaus*, Perrin (tr.), V, ii, 2–3, p. 5.

47 Hesiod, *The Homeric Hymns and Homerica*, Hugh G. Evelyn-White (tr.), London and Cambridge, 1977, III, 347. See also *Iliad*, Augustus Taber Murray (tr.), London and New York, 1925, XVIII, 394–397, p. 317: "She [Thetis] that saved me when pain was come upon me after I had fallen afar through the will of my shameless mother, that was fain to hide me away by reason of my lameness." Earlier in the same epic, I, 590–593, it was Zeus who cast Hephaistos down from the sky because he took his mother's side. However, the infirmity of the god of the "crook-foot" (*Iliad*, XXI, 331, p. 433) had its socio-anthropological raison d'être in the Greeks' aristocratic contempt for manual labor: as the only craftsman among the Olympian gods, his lameness would be the physical stigma that attached to the less noble artisanal existence.

48 Mitchell and Snyder, *Narrative Prosthesis*, pp. 42–43: "Whereas the ancient Athenians' belief in the perfectibility of the physical body produced a mythology that proffered only one disabled God (Hephaistus), Lois Bragg has argued that the pantheon of Gods with disabilities in ancient Norse myths demonstrates a popular emphasis upon the value of personal sacrifice for one's community."

49 Pausanias, *Guide to Greece*, 2 vols., Peter Levi (tr.), Harmondsworth, 1985, I.14.6.

50 Cicero, *De Natura Deorum*, H. Rackham (tr.), Cambridge, MA, and London, 1979, I, 83. For Vulcanus, see *LIMC*, VIII, 1, pp. 283–298. The representation of this impairment, so indecorous for Classical viewers as to necessitate dissimulation, is further reiterated by Valerius Maximus, who claimed that Alcamenes's statue displayed "a slight trace of lameness indicated under the drapery." Valerius Maximus, *Facta et Dicta Memorabilia*, 2 vols., D.R. Shackleton Bailey (tr.), Cambridge, MA, and London, 2000, VIII, xi, 3. Evelyn B. Harrison, "Alkamenes' Sculptures for the Hephaisteion: Part I, The Cult Statues," *American Journal of Archaeology*, 81:2 (1977): 147, points out that this phrase may be simply Valerius Maximus's own embellishment or interpretation since for the rest he merely reiterates Cicero's statement. The statue of the god may have looked the way it is depicted on a lamp in the Athens National Museum: ibid., p. 147, fig. 3.

51 *Iliad*, χυλλοποδιων, "the crook-foot" (XVIII, 371); χωλός, "lame" (XVIII, 397); ἀμφιγυήεις, a term of difficult interpretation but which seems to imply that his feet were turned backwards (XVIII, 607). See *LIMC*, IV, 1, p. 628.

52 John Boardman, *Athenian Black Figure Vases*, Singapore, 1980, pp. 33–34, 218, fig. 46.7.

53 *LIMC*, IV, 1, p. 646, no. 198, and IV, 2, p. 402, fig. 198.

54 *LIMC*, IV, 1, p. 637, fig. 103a.

55 John Boardman, *Intaglios and Rings: Greek, Etruscan and Eastern from a Private Collection*, London, 1975, p. 38, pl. 121.

56 For extensive reproductions of Vulcan in antiquity, see *LIMC*, VIII, 1, pp. 283–297, and VIII, 2, figs. 1–140.

57 See note 44.

58 Edward Allen Sydenham, *The Coinage of the Roman Republic*, London, 1952, pl. XVIII, no. 14, p. 117, no. 735. Also quoted by Garland, *The Eye of the Beholder*, p. 79, where, however, no reference is given. My thanks to Annie Ravenhill-Johnson for having brought this passage to my attention.

59 Cicero, *Tusculan Disputations*, John Edward King (tr.), London and New York, 1927, IV, 29, xiii, p. 357: "*vitium*, cum partes corporis inter se dissident, ex quo pravitas membrorum, distortio, deformitas."

60 For the humorous, derisory treatment of otherness, especially of dwarfs, see Mitchell, p. 301: "The fear of disease, disability, and especially deformity produces yet another type of warped humour – caricature and mockery of dwarfs, especially in the face of the beautiful youth."

61 Peter Brown, *Poverty and Leadership in the Later Roman Empire*, Hanover and London, 2002, esp. pp. 1–44. One of the signal ways in which one witnesses a change from the pagan to the Christian civilization is in the rapport the upper classes had with the poor. In the Classical world it was civic benefaction that prevailed – that is, the recipient of gifts was the *city*, or the *demos/populus* – whereas in the Christian communities benefaction was focused on the poor. Ibid., pp. 4–5: "A rich man was praised for being *philopatris*, or 'lover of his home-city,' never for being a *philoptôchos*, a 'lover of the poor.'" See later in this chapter.

62 Brian Edward Daley, *Gregory Nazianzus*, London, 2006, Oration 14, "On the Love of the Poor," p. 83: "They are heirs with us of the life to come, even if they have missed out on a great deal of life here on earth; they have been buried together with Christ, and have risen with him; if they suffer with him, it is so they may share in his glory." Although Gregory is talking specifically about the victims of leprosy, the ideology is pertinent to all of the disabled. Howard Clark Kee, *Miracle in the Early Christian World: A Study in Social Historical Method*, New Haven, 1983, p. 159: "For the Q tradition [the scattered literary material found in the gospels of Matthew and Luke but not found in Mark], therefore, miracle is the assuring sign of faith in eschatological vindication."

63 Mitchell and Snyder, "Introduction: Disability Studies and the Double Bind of Representation," in *The Body and Physical Difference*, pp. 3–4.

64 Mitchell and Snyder, *Narrative Prosthesis*, p. 183.

65 For the "Miracle of the Paralytic," see note 60. See also Matthew 9:6, Mark 2:21, Luke 5:25, John 5:5. For other miracles, see further in this chapter.

66 Kee, p. 159, refers to this reparation for physical ailments and suffering as "the assuring sign of faith in eschatological vindication." See note 62.

67 Ibid., p. 82. Cornelia B. Horn, "A Nexus of Disability in Ancient Greek Miracle Stories: A Comparison of Accounts of Blindness from the Asklepieion in Epidaurus and the Shrine of Thecla in Seleucia," in *Disabilities in Roman Antiquity: Disparate Bodies a capite ad calcem*, C. Laes, C.F. Goodey and C.L. Rose (eds.), Leiden and Boston, 2013, p. 118, takes issue with Robert Garland's perspective on miracles in Epidaurus as formulated in *The Eye of the Beholder*, as he claimed that "these 'healings' would wear off, not changing 'the underlying pathological condition.'" For Horn, these sanctuaries "never intended to be institutions of healing. Rather, they provided multi-layered experiences of rituals, and the evidence must be seen within this context" and even encompassed explanations for the failure to hear, namely the lack of faith on the part of the individual.

68 Kee, p. 82.

69 Ibid., p. 87. Horn, p. 124, notes that the vision often took place during *incubation*, "the ritual that constituted the regular and customary cultic practice at this [Epidaurus] and other healing shrines in the ancient world."

70 Suetonious, *Lives of the Caesars*, II, 7, p. 299.

71 Kee, p. 131. The quotation in Kee is from Diodorus Siculus, *Library* 1.25.5.

72 Robin Margaret Jensen, *Understanding Early Christian Art*, London and New York, 2000, p. 123.

73 The healing of Tobias's blindness (Tobit 11–12), perhaps the most widely known miracle from the Old Testament, is executed through the intervention of a supernatural agent, the angel Raphael, which places it in a different category from those miracles in which healing is carried out through the agency of a human being or his relics.

74 See note 60.

75 See *The New Strong's Exhaustive Concordance of the Bible*, James Strong (ed.), Nashville, 1990, under each heading.

76 Stiker, pp. 25, 27 and 33.

77 Diego Gracia, "The Ethics of Diagnosis in Early Christianity and the Middle Ages," in *The Ethics of Diagnosis*, J.L. Peset and D. Gracia (eds.), Dordrecht, 1992, p. 20. For evidence of Christ's novel approach to the topic, Gracia quotes from John 9:1–3, where, in answer to his disciples, who question him as to who sinned, the blind man or his parents, Jesus replies: "Neither hath this man sinned, nor his parents; but that the works of God should be made manifest in him."

78 Gracia, p. 21.

79 Stiker, as in note 76. See also Bryon Grigsby, "Medical Misconceptions," in *Misconceptions about the Middle Ages*, Stephen J. Harris and Bryon L. Grinsby (eds.), New York, 2008, pp. 142–150.

80 Kurt Weitzmann, *Age of Spirituality: Late Antique and Early Christian Art, Third to Seventh Century*, Princeton, 1979, pp. 442–443, nos. 401–402.

81 Ibid., pp. 446–448, no. 407.

82 For the frescoes in San Saba, see Francesco Gandolfo, "Gli affreschi di San Saba," in *Fragmenta picta: affreschi e mosaici staccati del medioevo romano*, Rome, 1989, and Richard Krautheimer, Spencer Corbett and Wolfgang Frankl, *Corpus Basilicarum Christianarum Romae*, IV, Vatican City, 1970, pp. 51–71.

83 For the periodization of Early Christian art, see Jensen, *Understanding Early Christian Art*, pp. 15–20; idem, *The Early Christian World*, 2 vols., London and New York, 2000, II, pp. 750–751.

84 Weitzmann, *Age of Spirituality*, nos. 401–402, 405 and 407. On the "extreme abridgment" or "almost hierographic imagery" of Early Christian art, see André Grabar, *The Beginnings of Christian Art 200–395*, London, 1967, p. 68.

85 On the problems that Christ's miracles posed to the early Christians, see Thomas F. Mathews, *The Clash of Gods: A Reinterpretation of Early Christian Art*, Princeton, 1993, pp. 54–91; Anton Fridrichsen, *The Problem of Miracle in Primitive Christianity*, Roy A. Harrisville and John S. Hanson (trs.), Minneapolis, 1972, as well as Morton Smith, *Jesus the Magician*, New York, 1978. See also Jensen, *Understanding Early Christian Art*, pp. 120–124.

86 Herbert L. Kessler, "The Christian Realm: Narrative Representations," in Weitzmann (ed.), *Age of Spirituality*, p. 449: "Whereas the Greeks and Romans possessed no all-embracing text, Christians had a scripture that recorded man's tenure on earth and established the nature of his relation to God and the tenets of his faith. Inevitably, therefore, Christian art emerged as a book art."

87 On the shift from "image-sign" to "descriptive image" and the desire for greater realism in the second phase of Early Christian art, see André Grabar, *Christian Iconography: A Study of Its Origins*, Princeton, 1968, pp. 92–101.

88 *The Old Testament Pseudepigrapha*, James H. Charlesworth (ed.), New York, 1983, pp. 487–490. See Livio Pestilli, "Blindness, Lameness and Mendicancy in Italy (from the 14th to the 18th Centuries)," in *Others and Outcasts in Early Modern Europe: Picturing the Social Margins*, Tom Nichols (ed.), Aldershot, 2007, pp. 107–129.

89 See also Fridrichsen, p. 71.

90 For the Rabbula Gospels, see Massimo Bernabò (ed.), *Il Tetravangelo di Rabbula*, Florence, 2008, pl. XXI. For the *Parisinus Graecus* 923, see Kurt Weitzmann, *The Miniatures of the Sacra Parallela Parisinus Graecus 923*, Princeton, 1979, fig. 425. For the *Parisinus Graecus* 74, Henri A. Omont (ed.), *Évangiles avec peintures byzantines du XIe siècle*, 2 vols., Paris, 1908, II, p. 6 and pl. 35. For the Laurentian Library Tetra-Gospel, see Tania Velmans, *Le Tétraévangile de la Laurentienne*, Paris, 1971, p. 28, and fig. 65.

91 Kessler, "The Christian Realm," p. 455: "Narrative cycles migrated widely."

92 It is irrelevant in this context whether the illuminated manuscripts reflect the more official art that would have decorated the walls of churches or vice versa. The fact is that with more space available to illustrate the life of Christ, the artists could now afford to be less "stenographic" in their works. See Grabar, *Christian Iconography*, p. 100: "Designed for a very great and largely illiterate public, these images, when they were on church walls or on liturgical furniture, could evoke the gospel passages read during the offices; and when they were represented on various small objects, they served prophylactic ends."

93 On the stylistic affinity between the frescoes at San Saba and Palestinian art of the seventh century, see Gandolfo, "Gli affreschi," p. 186.

94 For the mosaics in the cathedral of Monreale, see Ernst Kitzinger, *The Mosaics of Monreale*, Palermo, 1960. For the drawing, from the *Meditations on the Life of Christ*, Francis X. Taney (tr.), Asheville, NC, 2000, figs. 143–144 and 189.

95 Peter Brown, *Through the Eye of a Needle: Wealth, the Fall of Rome, and the Making of Christianity in the West, 350–550*, Princeton and Oxford, 2012, pp. 61 and 59.

96 Ibid., p. 59.

97 Ibid., p. 61.

98 Ibid., p. 61.

99 Ibid., p. 62.

100 Brown, *Through the Eye of a Needle*, p. 86, states that Christian preachers and writers "constantly repeated Christ's promise of heaven to those who gave 'even a cup of water' to the poor and to his wandering disciples (Matt. 10:42). A gift of copper coins and of basic food and clothing to a beggar reverberated with a sense of their exact opposite – the off-scale quality of the reward in heaven that awaited these small acts."

101 Ibid., p. 85.

102 Ibid., p. 83.

103 A glimpse of what the Greeks thought of wanderers and inactive philosophers may be gleaned from Aristophanes' *Clouds*, Jeffrey Henderson (tr.), Cambridge and London, 1998, p. 21: "'Yuk! That scum. I know them: you mean the charlatans, the pasty-faced, the unshod, like the miserable Socrates, and Chaerephon'" (102–104, p. 21); "'long-haired idlers … whom they [the "heavenly Clouds," actually the Athenians] maintain as do-nothings'" (331–334, p. 53); "'men so frugal that not one of them has ever cut his hair or anointed himself or gone to the bath house to wash'" (834–837, p. 123). Also referred to by Mitchell, *Greek Vase-Painting*, p. 245. For the Christians in late antiquity, see Daniel Caner, *Wandering, Begging Monks: Spiritual Authority and the Promotion of Monasticism in Late Antiquity*, Berkeley, Los Angeles and London, 2002, p. 168.

104 Plato, *Laws*, in *The Collected Dialogues of Plato*, Hamilton and Cairns (eds.), XI, p. 1486.

105 Richard Finn, *Almsgiving in the Later Roman Empire: Christian Promotion and Practice (313–450)*, Oxford, 2006, p. 183.

106 *The Code of Justinian*, in *The Civil Law*, 16 vols., S.P. Scott (tr.), Cincinnati, 1932, XV, Title XXV, p. 185: "Given on the twelfth of the *Kalends* of July, during the Consulate of Antonius and Syagrius, 382."

107 Wendy Mayer, "John Chrysostom: Extraordinary Preacher, Ordinary Audience," in *Preacher and Audience: Studies in Early Christian and Byzantine Homiletics*, Pauline Allen and Mary B. Cunningham (eds.), Leiden, 1998, pp. 123–129.

108 St. John Chrysostom, *On Repentance and Almsgiving*, Gus George Christo (tr.), Washington, 1998, p. 78.

109 Ibid., p. 131.

110 Daley, *Gregory of Nazianzus*, p. 80. Although Gregory is talking specifically about the victims of an outbreak of leprosy, the oration is to be understood within the context of the Church Fathers' attempt to organize relief for the destitute and the infirm. Gregory's oration was probably delivered in Cesaraea around 369–371. See Daley's comments in *Gregory of Nazianzus*, pp. 75–76.

111 St. John Chrysostom, *On Repentance and Almsgiving*, p. 146.

112 John Chrysostom, in *Agostino, Giovanni Crisostomo, Gregorio di Nazianzo, Gregorio di Nissa, Servire i poveri gioiosamente*, Luigi Rosadoni (tr.), Turin, 1971, p. 66 (from Migne, P.G. 48, 974–992). My translation from the Italian.

113 Stiker, p. 35: "[In the Gospels] [t]here is no other sacred than the relations to one's fellows …. The only sacred thing is man and woman."

114 Stahl, p. 729: "But, generally speaking, the disabled person was entirely reliant on his or her family if he or she was to survive. Only the coming of Christianity brought about the notion that helping those in need was somehow a communal responsibility."

115 *The Treatises of Cyprian*, in *The Ante-Nicene Fathers*, 10 vols., A. Cleveland Coxe (comp.), A. Roberts, J. Donaldson, P. Schaff and H. Wace (eds.), Grand Rapids, 1990, V, 8.23, p. 483.
116 Matthew 20:16.
117 *The Treatises of Cyprian*, V, 8.23, p. 483.

2 *Imago Christi*

> They have been made in the image of God in the same way you and I have, and perhaps preserve that image better than we, even if their bodies are corrupted.
>
> (Gregory of Nazianzus, "On the Love of the Poor," 14:14)

Just as slavery did not come to an end with the advent of Christianity, since enslaved manpower was perfectly supported by an "economic system dominated by the ecclesiastical aristocracy,"[1] and just as religious intolerance did not cease once Christianity replaced paganism as the official state religion,[2] so too the general attitude of the able-bodied members of society towards disabled individuals did not change immediately because of the Early Christian Fathers' sermons on the love of the poor and the infirm. Despite Christianity's more empathetic teachings, many people continued to believe that the physically impaired bore their ailments as the visible sign of divine discontent. Thus, Bishop Fulgentius of Ruspe in North Africa (ca. 462–533) did not refrain from declaring that the blind and other disabled persons were being punished for their sins or those of their parents.[3] Similarly, common folk who generated a deformed child could not avoid feeling they had been punished because they had conceived on a Sunday night, contravening Christian homiletics.[4] As in antiquity, Gregory of Tours (ca. 538–594) attests that a child with severe birth defects was "viewed by most people with derision" and admonishes that the errors of one night could lead to the sufferings of a lifetime.[5] Indeed, as late as 1215, in the decrees of the Fourth Lateran Council the Church declared that "sickness of the body may sometimes be the result of sin" and urged the physicians of the body to call in first the physicians of the soul, "so that after their spiritual health has been seen to, they may respond better to medicine for their bodies; for when the cause ceases so does the effect."[6]

Nonetheless, although the Early Christians' attitude towards the disabled did not vary at once, the role the physically impaired played in the spread of the cult of the martyrs and saints cannot be underestimated. The attention they received by the late fourth century was perhaps most tangibly witnessed at the site of the graves of the saints to which the sick and the infirm flocked in the hope of receiving a miraculous cure.[7] It was here that the Christians' belief in an afterlife evinced a new conceptual framework that redefined the individual's rapport with God and the dead[8] since, while the belief in the next world where body and soul would reunite was at the core of Christianity's eschatological message, the link between the Divine and living humans was now provided by the Christian martyrs, who had become the true intermediaries between men and their Creator. However, unlike their predecessors, the pagan *daimones* and *genii* or the Judaic guardian angels, these early Christian intercessors were men themselves who through their martyrdom had become the true servants of God and, thanks to their mediation, brought their fellow men closer to the Creator,[9] thus helping them obtain, as it were, "celestial citizenship."[10] Therefore, when the power to perform miracles – initially carried out by Jesus the "magician"[11] and subsequently by his disciples – was transferred to the earthly remains of the Christian martyrs, who according to Augustine "were the *membra Christi* par excellence,"[12] the disabled began playing a fundamental part as the supporting cast in the many *passiones* – the deeds of the martyrs – read to the Early Christian communities as well as in the *Lives* of the saints written in later centuries. For the miraculous cure of the disabled represented literally and figuratively humanity's physical and spiritual healing, the "reintegration into the community"[13] of the physically impaired, as well as a tangible proof of the saints' thaumaturgic powers.

Among the early sources testifying to miraculous cures at the site of the martyrs' graves is St. Augustine's *City of God*. The reason for including these eyewitness reports was ostensibly to prove that miracles occurred not only in the earliest phase of Christianity but also in contemporary times. In his words: "The accounts [of miracles] are read among the nations, so that the people may believe; but they would never have been read, had they not been believed. And in fact, even now miracles are being performed in Christ's name either by his sacrament, or by the prayers or the memorials of his saints, but they do not enjoy the blaze of publicity which would spread their fame with a glory to equal those earlier marvels."[14]

The problem, according to St. Augustine, was that when these extraordinary events occurred in large cities, they remained known only to a particular neighborhood; when they happened in the country, they were not supported by authoritative individuals who could "ensure ready or even hesitating acceptance."[15] Thus he gives an account of twenty-one miracles garnished with phrases such as "I was there,"[16] "I was present as an eye-witness,"[17] "the scene can be better imagined than described,"[18] "as it happened, I was in the neighbourhood"[19] and "to my certain knowledge,"[20] to shore up public belief in these events with his intellectual, religious and social authority. Nevertheless, while news of the healing miracles at the site of Christian martyrs' and saints' graves spread far and wide, and the cult of their bodily remains (corporeal relics) or their contact relics (*brandea*, *sanctuaria*, *benedictiones*)[21] – such as blood-soaked cloths, oil from lamps, or dust that had been in touch with the saints or in the proximity of their tombs – developed all over Christendom,[22] the commemorative images of the saints or martyrs did not reflect the wondrous effects their miraculous cures had on the disabled. Rather, their representations portrayed the saints as living intermediaries of the faithful, such as the sixth-century mosaic on the entry wall of the church of Saint Demetrius at Thessaloniki (Figure 2.1).[23]

As in the East, in the West, too, the cult of saints was intimately connected with their earthly remains.[24] In fact, one of the earliest instances of this phenomenon as reflected in Roman wall painting occurred around the year 400 beneath the church of Santi Giovanni e Paolo where the relics of the martyrs Cyprian, Justina and Theoctistus were probably venerated.[25] Here, in a fresco on the wall of a chamber (*confessio*) that is connected to the tomb of saints, drawn painted curtains allow view of a standing, praying saint flanked by two prostrated individuals who display their reverence for the holy spiritual mediator (*proskynesis*)

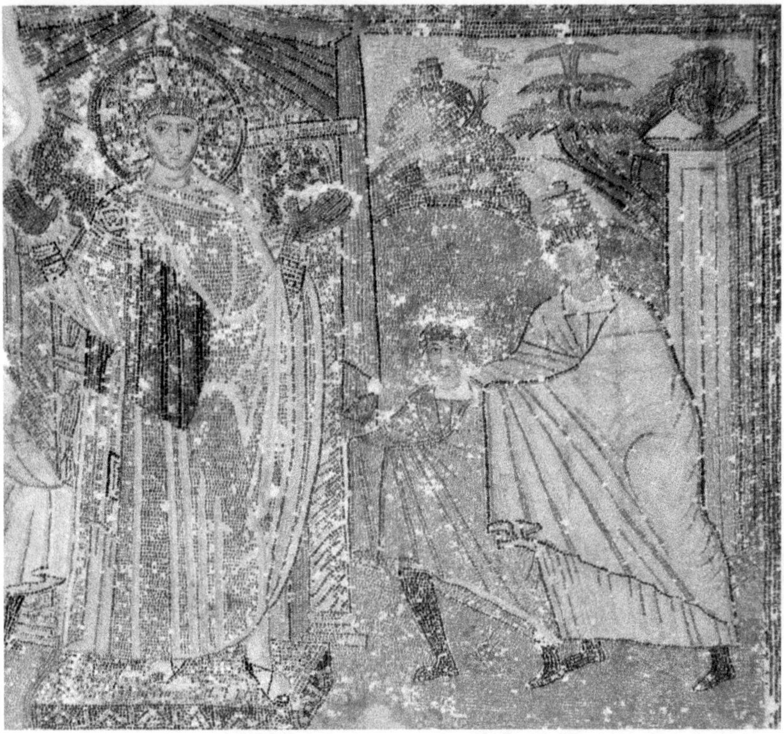

Figure 2.1 St. Demetrius and Faithful, sixth century, church of St. Demetrius, Thessaloniki. Photo: in the public domain

(see Plate 6). According to a legend, the Greek matron Ruffina received the relics of the Eastern saints and, subsequently, her brother-in-law Pammachius built a basilica on the site of the titular church.[26] As Hans Belting points out, "Ruffina's cult of relics, the first of its kind inside the city walls of Rome, not only involved the veneration of Eastern saints but was a practice itself originating in the East."[27]

Despite its Eastern origins, as the cult of relics spread throughout the West – especially given the growing practice of translating the bodies of saints[28] – Rome eventually became the only proper place from which to obtain sacred vestiges and it emerged "as a leading distributor of holy relics *per omnem terram*,"[29] a fact that was reinforced by the synod of Frankfurt in 794 when Charlemagne, in his attempt to harness this phenomenon and sustain his theocratic idea of government, decreed that no new saints were to be venerated and that all altars contain relics "from long-dead saints, preferably martyrs."[30]

Still, as an investigation of the art produced in the East or the West between the fourth and the tenth centuries will evince, frescoes, mosaics, paintings, illuminated manuscripts and reliefs that depict scenes in which humans are healed of their physical ailments were drawn from stories of the New Testament in which Christ or one of his apostles was the protagonist.[31] Even when depicting the martyrs themselves, as in the ninth-century *Homilies of Gregory of Nazianzus*,[32] the images focused on the actual execution of the saintly protagonists rather than their healing powers (Figure 2.2).[33] Indeed, in instances when the tomb of a martyr was illustrated, as in the eleventh-century *Menologion of Basil II*, the image depicted the invention (the discovery) or the veneration of the sarcophagus that contained the relics of the saint and not the ailing, supplicating humanity at the site described in the literary accounts (Figure 2.3).[34] This, of course, is understandable since the Greek word itself *martureo* meant to "bear witness … in favor of another" – that is, of Christ – and to depict their martyrdom was to provide evidence of their "unshakable faith."[35] As to why the phenomenon at the grave sites described by St. Augustine failed to generate comparable visual evidence, one must assume it was at least in part because "the alliance of image and relic was limited by the fact that the cult of saints was secondary to that of Christ and the Virgin."[36] In fact, with regard to the disabled, in Rome there is little evidence of what happened at the tomb of the saints since here the sites were not, overall, "the scene of highly charged miracles of healing"

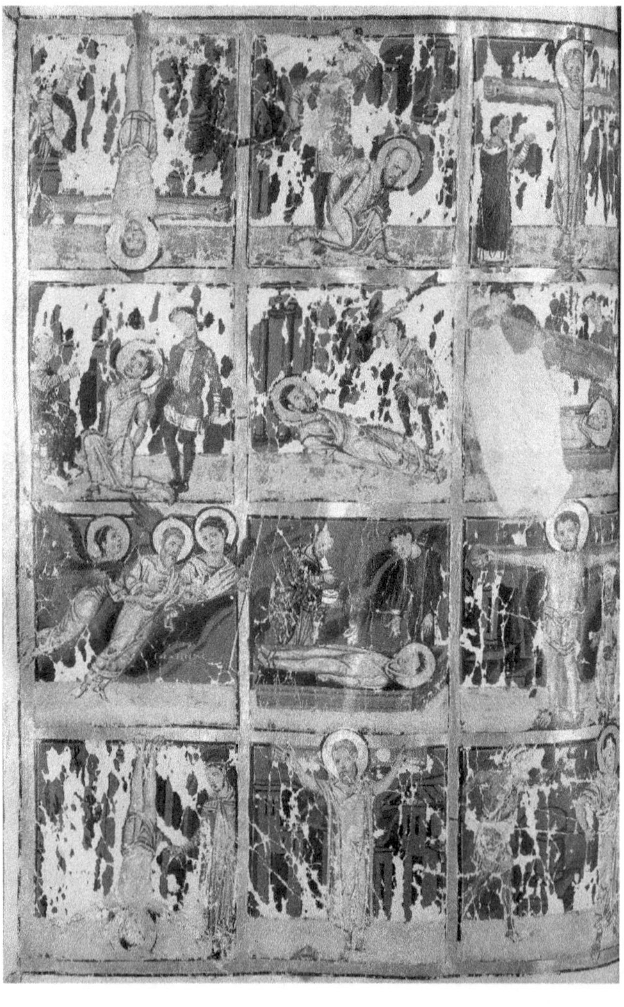

Figure 2.2 Twelve scenes of martyrdom, Homilies of Gregory of Nazianzus made for Basil I, 879–883. Photo: Bibliothèque nationale de France

and Pope Gregory the Great, as a matter of fact, "disapproved of popular manifestations of piety in such environments."[37]

Although a disease and not strictly a disability, the gout is the subject of one of the memorable early images that focuses on impaired locomotion (Figure 2.4). In the ninth-century golden altar retable in the church of Sant'Ambrogio, in Milan, one finds the representation of the miraculous cure of Nicetius, a man of the tribune class, as narrated by Paulinus in the life of St. Ambrose and embossed by Wolvinus. Paulinus informs us that Nicetius was cured of his gout when St. Ambrose stepped on his foot as he approached the altar to receive the host.[38] To understand this image, however, the viewer needs to be privy to the saint's biography, for the only indication of Nicetius's orthopedic ailment is a bandaged left leg whose foot is depicted beneath that of the saint with no recognizable sign of orthopedic impairment represented, such as a cane, crutches, trestles or twisted limbs.

In truth, the paucity of images of the orthopedically impaired during these centuries corresponds to the scarcity of cycles of non-biblical saints that have come down to us.[39] In Italy it was not until the seventh and eighth centuries that many popes of Greek-speaking origin fostered an increment in the depiction of non-biblical hagiographical cycles.[40] In Rome, in fact, there are traces of only five such cycles representing Saints Quiricus and Julitta, the Forty Martyrs of Sebaste, Saint Erasmus, Saints Paul and Anastasius, and Saint Callixtus.[41] Nevertheless, in none of these does one find the representation of the lame. Of course, there may have been a number of exceptions that have not survived the passage of time. Still, the mere difficulty in finding such images produced in those centuries is a probable indication of their near inexistence. Thus, the visual documentation that has reached modernity seems to indicate that for centuries the representation of those whose mobility was impaired was rather limited or totally lacking.

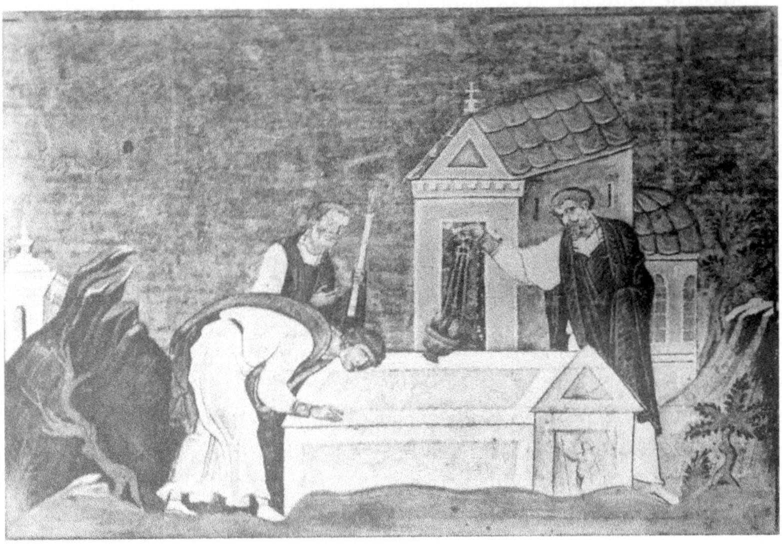

Figure 2.3 Discovery of the Relics of St. Zacchariah, Menologion of Basil II, eleventh century, from *Il menologio di Basilio II. Cod. Vaticano greco 1613*, 2 vols., Turin, 1907, II, p. 391

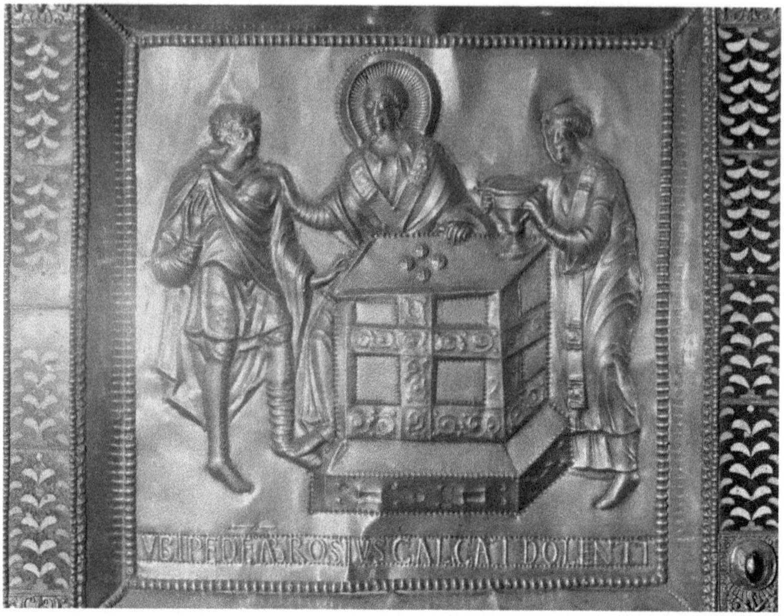

Figure 2.4 *St. Ambrose Steps on Nicetius's Foot and Heals It Miraculously*, Sant'Ambrogio, Milan. Photo: © Bildarchiv Foto Marburg/Rosenberg

This trend changed around the end of the first millennium, when especially pictorial hagiographies produced in monastic institutions began to proliferate.[42] While there is some evidence that in the West images of healings performed by saints or holy persons begin to appear by the end of the tenth and the beginning of the eleventh century, as in the *Healing of St. Agatha by St. Peter*[43] or *St. George Healing the Infirm* at Saint-Martin in Tours,[44] the phenomenon became a common motif by the beginning of the twelfth century, as may be seen in images such as *Bishop Liudger Curing the Blind Bernlef* in the *Life of Liudger of Münster*, Werden, ca. 1100 (Figure 2.5),[45] *Bishop Albinus Cures a Blind Woman* in the *Life of Aubin (Albinus)*, Angers, Saint-Aubin, late eleventh century[46] and *St. Martin Revives a Dead Slave*, in the *Life of Martin of Tours*, ca. 1100.[47]

It was at this time that representations including persons with impaired motor skills begin to emerge more frequently. Among these is the *St. Lucy Giving Away Her Possessions to the Poor* in the *Passion of Lucy* produced in Metz, St. Vincent, ca. 1130 (Figure 2.6).[48] Precariously balanced on crutches, with right foot twisted backwards, a young man is the first in line among a number of needy people to whom Saint Lucy is making a charitable donation.[49] At approximately the same date, *The Charity of Edmund*, from the *Passion of Edmund, King and Martyr*, Bury St. Edmunds,[50] also includes a number of indigent, unshod individuals among whom is a lame, bearded older man who is leaning on a crutch and resting his left knee on a wooden prop or brace.

In all likelihood, this change in attitude on the part of patrons and artists towards the inclusion of the indigent and the infirm in scenes from the lives of the saints reflects a major shift in society that occurred at the beginning of the new era. In André Vauchez's informed view:

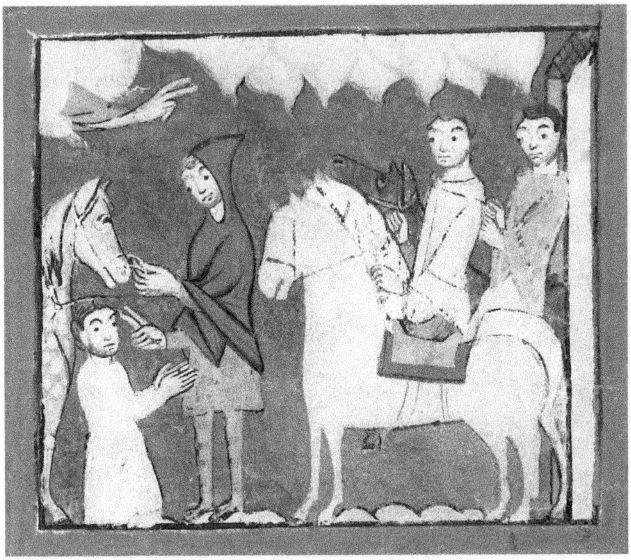

Figure 2.5 *Bishop Liudger Cures the Blind Bernlef*, Life of Liudger of Münster, Werden, ca. 1100. Photo: Staatsbibliothek zu Berlin – Preußischer Kulturbesitz, Manuscript Department, Ms. theol. lat. fol. 323, fol. 12r

> Up to the twelfth century, clergy and faithful primarily venerated saints dating from the first centuries of the Church. Later, these devotions lost none of their prestige, and the vitality of the pilgrimages to the main traditional sanctuaries testifies to their permanence. But, after 1150, in many regions, cults accorded to persons who had only recently died proliferated and they often, in the space of a few decades, became as famous and as highly regarded as the Apostles and the martyrs. This development was linked to a change of perspective which is visible in the Church from the time of the Gregorian Reform. Under the influence of a papacy which now aimed to realize *hic et nunc* an ideal Christianity, there was, from the end of the eleventh century, a break with the Christianity of the first millennium.[51]

In fact, with the rise of the monk Hildebrand on the throne of Peter as Gregory VII not only the papacy sought greater independence from the emperor by claiming the exclusive right to judge Christian society but, perhaps more importantly, the former anxious expectation of society for the end of the world was replaced by a desire to create "here and now" the kingdom of God.[52] That is, the anticipation of the end of the world that distinguished Christian faith in the period between the eighth and the tenth centuries was eventually replaced by the belief that the heavenly kingdom could be achieved by following the path indicated by Christ, by returning to the original ideals of early Christianity that reached out to others, and, generally speaking, "by the greater value afforded the New Testament."[53]

While the appearance of the orthopedically impaired in Italian art does not seem to have emerged as early as in Carolingian and Ottonian art north of the Alps, the phenomenon flourished starting in the early thirteenth century.[54] Not surprisingly, among the earliest

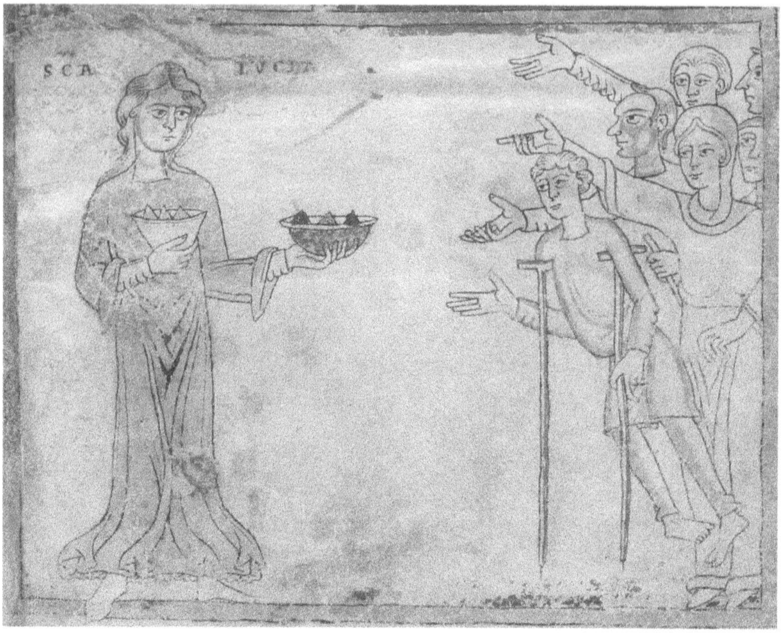

Figure 2.6 Lucy Giving Away Her Possessions to the Poor, *Passion of Lucy*, Metz, St. Vincent, ca. 1130. Photo: Volker-H. Schneider. © 2015. Scala, Firenze/bpk, Bildagentur für Kunst, Kultur und Geschichte, Berlin

occurrences in this evolution one finds images that relate to St. Francis of Assisi, as one of the primary concepts that became fundamental to a contemporary type of sainthood in the Middle Ages was that of "Christo-mimesis."[55] Indeed, Francis's renunciation of his inheritance and embracing of apostolic poverty, his placing himself at the service of the poor, the meek and the infirm, not to mention his vision on Mount La Verna where he received the stigmata, made him the perfect example of the *alter Christus*.[56] In fact, by the early thirteenth century a major change had occurred, for scenes of the life of Christ began to provide the template for the representation of the lives of the saints.[57]

While between the twelfth and fifteenth centuries the majority of those raised to the rank of sainthood in Europe were of aristocratic lineage,[58] quite antithetically in thirteenth-century southern Europe, and especially in Italy, the faithful seem to have shifted their devotion spontaneously towards the less aristocratic sainthood embodied by the poor and those whose lives imitated the suffering of Christ. Although by the end of the twelfth century a sanctity of "charity and labor" had become manifest, with the rise of the mendicant orders in the thirteenth century compassion and charity towards all the suffering and the ill became the evident sign of a holy person.[59] In fact, for the majority of people at the time of Innocent III (r. 1198–1216) sanctity was essentially identified with a number of supernatural powers, chief among them that of healing the sick.[60]

Understandably, at this time the disabled became again the preferred supporting cast for the new "miracle workers," and altarpieces executed soon after St. Francis's death (1226) and canonization (1228) represent the saint exactly as the *alter Christus*,[61] as witness Bonaventura

Berlinghieri's *Saint Francis* (Pescia, 1235) (Plate 7) and the Bardi Dossal in Santa Croce (Florence, ca. 1245–1250) (Figure 2.7).[62] In the subsidiary scenes of these two vita-retables that frame the standing saint, events from the saint's *Life*, such as the *St. Francis Preaching to the Birds* and *St. Francis Receiving the Stigmata*, are inevitably complemented by two depictions of miracles involving the orthopedically impaired: *The Healing of the Cripples by the Tomb of Francis* and *The Healing of Bartolomeo da Narni*.[63] In the first of these scenes (Figure 2.8), the miracle-seeking crippled suppliants are singled out not only by their placement on the ground but also by the hand crutches prominently placed in front of them. However, in the second scene (Plate 8), in the

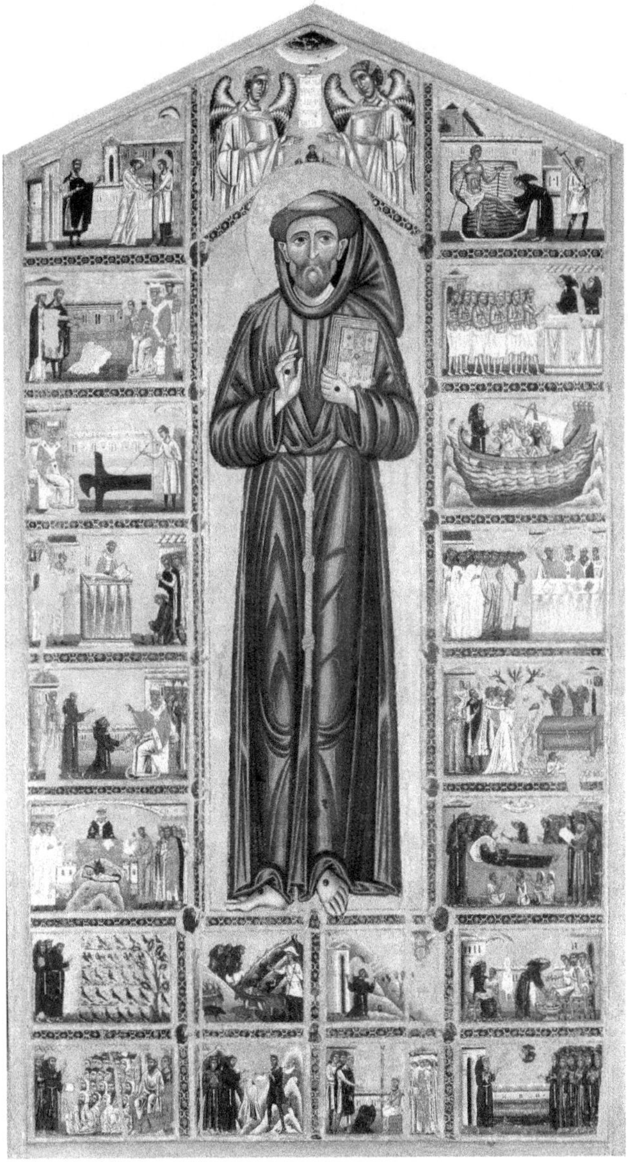

Figure 2.7 Bardi Dossal, *St. Francis and Scenes from His Life*, Santa Croce, Florence, ca. 1245–1250. Photo: © 2015. Scala, Firenze

spirit of earlier depictions of Christ's "Miracle of the Paralytic," Bartolomeo da Narni's paralytic leg is being bathed by Francis, who came to him in a vision, and, concomitantly, within the same frame, Bartolomeo is also shown walking away with crutches on his shoulder signaling his cure.

There were other similar altarpieces, such as the one in the Museo Nazionale di San Matteo in Pisa, but perhaps a clearer example of how significant images of the orthopedically impaired were in shoring belief in the saint's healing powers are the Assisi altar panel (ca. 1253) in the Treasury of the Basilica and its Vatican replica (Figure 2.9).[64] It is of some significance that, out of the four scenes that flank the saint, two are dedicated to the curing of a paralytic and a cripple: Bartolomeo da Narni, on the left, and Nicholas of Foligno, on the right. Unlike the artist in the Bardi altarpiece (Figure 2.7), who had a total of twenty scenes to depict[65] when deciding which events from the saint's life would be most forceful on the viewer, the artist who painted the Assisi panel or his advisor settled on four *posthumous* miracles, two of which focused on the healing of the orthopedically impaired. This was not coincidental since, starting with the canonization of Saint Homobonus in 1199, Innocent III had declared in the bull *Quia pietas* that for the militant Church two things were essential before anyone be declared a saint: "virtue of morals and truth of signs, that is, works of piety in life and evidence of miracles after death."[66] Thus the artist's insistence on depicting posthumous miracles was "proof" of Francis's sanctity; that is, the images were reassuring "evidence" for both the infirm and the Church authorities.[67] Indeed, as the representatives of an ailing humankind, the lame were perhaps the best qualified to act as Francis's co-protagonists. Given the saint's exaltation of poverty, they in fact provided the perfect iconographic counterpoint to the *Poverello*, since those who frequently begged for a living

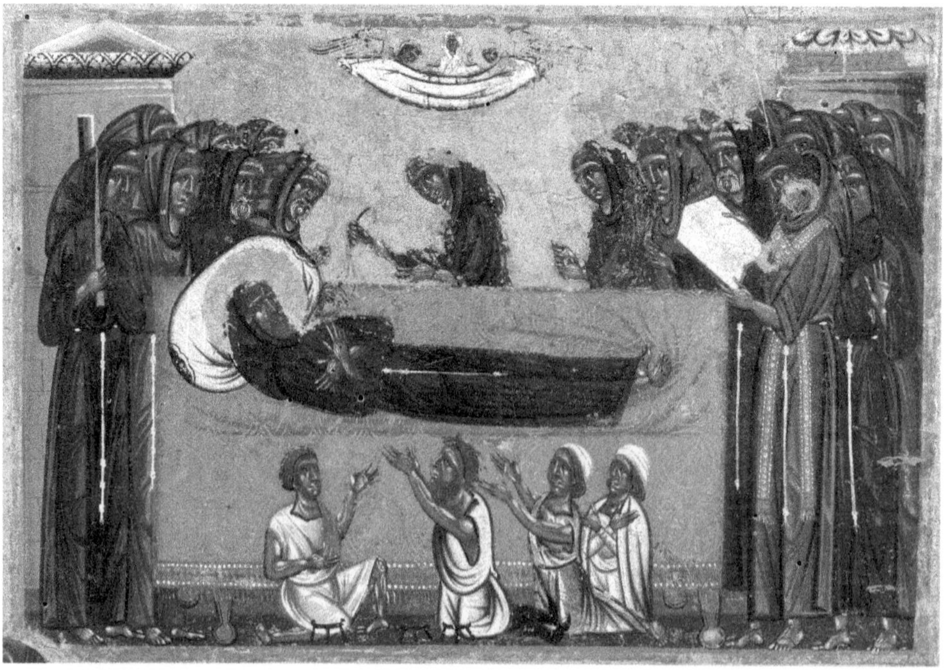

Figure 2.8 Bardi Dossal, *Healing of the Cripples at the Tomb of St. Francis*, detail of Figure 2.7. Photo: © 2015. Scala, Firenze

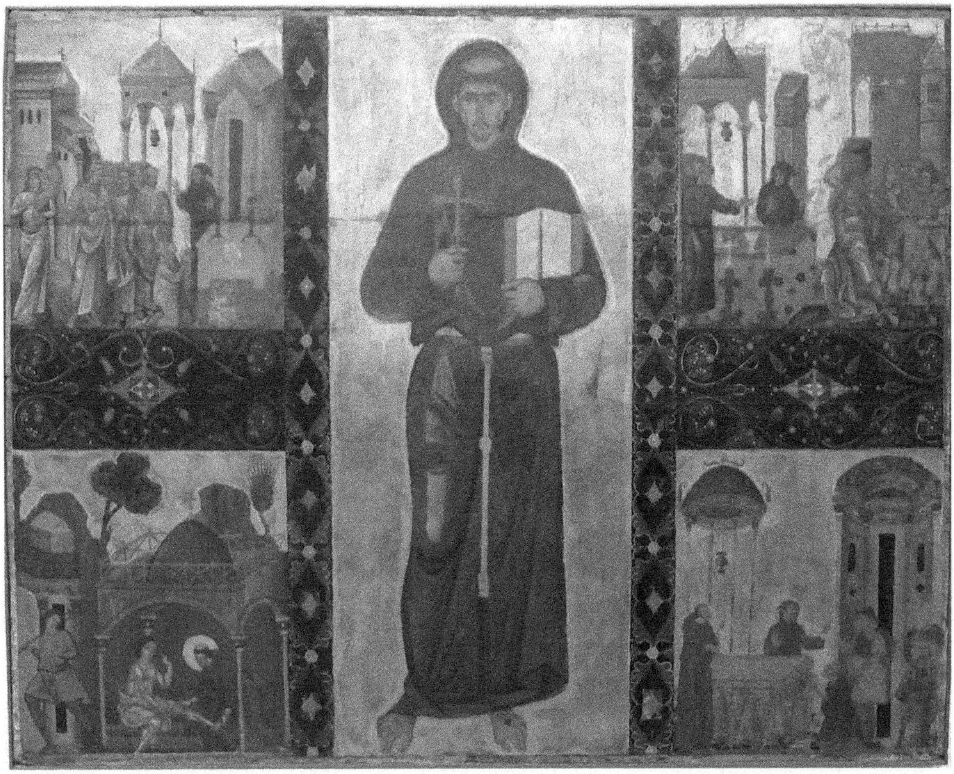

Figure 2.9 Giunta Pisano (attr.), *St. Francis Altarpiece*, Pinacoteca Vaticana. Photo: author

because of their inability to work, like some of the orthopedically impaired, were, in a sense, the "professional poor" of the Middle Ages.[68]

Consequently, there were mainly three contexts in which the disabled were predominantly featured in Italian Medieval and Renaissance art: as the implorers of a miraculous cure at the hands of living saints, as the supplicants of wondrous healing through the posthumous intercession of saints at the site of their grave, and as the recipients of alms in *exempla* of Christian charity.

Adopting George Kaftal's classic iconographic encyclopedia of saints as our *vade mecum*, an example of the first category of images – the disabled as implorers of a miraculous cure at the hands of a living saint – is *St. Anthony of Padua Curing a Lame Man and a Cripple* (Figure 2.10).[69] In all cases such as in this panel, the common denominator is the depiction of a Christ-like saint, who heals bystanders through the means of the sign of the cross. True to their intercessory role and as emissaries of Christ, they re-enact the healing gesture that artists had traditionally reserved for the Messiah. As in the *Parisinus Graecus* 923 (Figure 1.12), the *Parisinus Graecus* 74 manuscript (Figure 1.13) or the *Healing of the Infirm* mosaics in the cathedral of Monreale (Plate 4), these saints, too, are depicted performing a miracle by blessing the limbs of the physically impaired.

Examples of images from the second category – that is, of the disabled seeking a miraculous cure at the site of a saint's tomb – may be subdivided into those that allow view of the corpse of the holy person inside the tomb and those that do not. Those images that do represent the physical presence of the saints provide visual proof of a key feature of sainthood: bodily incorruptibility. In fact, "before being a quality of the soul or a spiritual state, sainthood, in the popular mind, was first an energy (*virtus*) which expressed itself through a body. Its presence was revealed by a number of signs of a physiological order. The first was incorruptibility. It was believed that the mortal remains of the saints could not experience the same lot as those of ordinary mortals."[70] Valid instances of this type of representation are the thirteenth-century fresco in the crypt of the cathedral of Anagni depicting the *Miracles of St. Magnus* (Plate 9) and the fourteenth-century illumination by Pacino di Buonaguida of *The Blessed Gerard of Villamagna* at the J.P. Morgan Library in New York (Plate 10).

The fresco depicting the *Miracles of St. Magnus* (Plate 9) includes an episode in the life of St. Peter bishop of Anagni, who, having left town under the accusation of undue appropriation of funds to build the local church, is persuaded to return thanks to a miracle brought about by St. Magnus. The scene portrays on the left side Andrew ("ANDRE | AS | CLAV | [D] (V) S"), the crippled doorman of the bishop's palace, kneeling by the perfectly preserved body of St. Magnus inside a sarcophagus, while some bystanders gesticulate as the miraculous healing of Andrew is taking place in front of their very eyes. Once healed, St. Magnus ordered Andrew to overtake St. Peter, who was on his way to Rome, and bring him back to Anagni. Accordingly, on the right side of the fresco, the artist depicted the epilogue to the story as the bishop, along with a cleric and others in his retinue, returns to said town.[71]

Pacino di Buonaguida's illumination found at the J.P. Morgan Library (Plate 10) shows a comparable scene with the exposed body of the Blessed Gerard (Tintorio) of Villamagna (died in 1207), also known as Gerard of Monza, who, much like his contemporary St. Francis of Assisi, came from a well-to-do family and, upon reaching adulthood, spent his patrimony building a hospital and taking care of the sick and the poor.[72] Here, too, prominently placed in the foreground, are a supplicating, orthopedically impaired woman in a litter, on the left, and a crippled man leaning on his hand crutches, on the right. High above them, in a casket

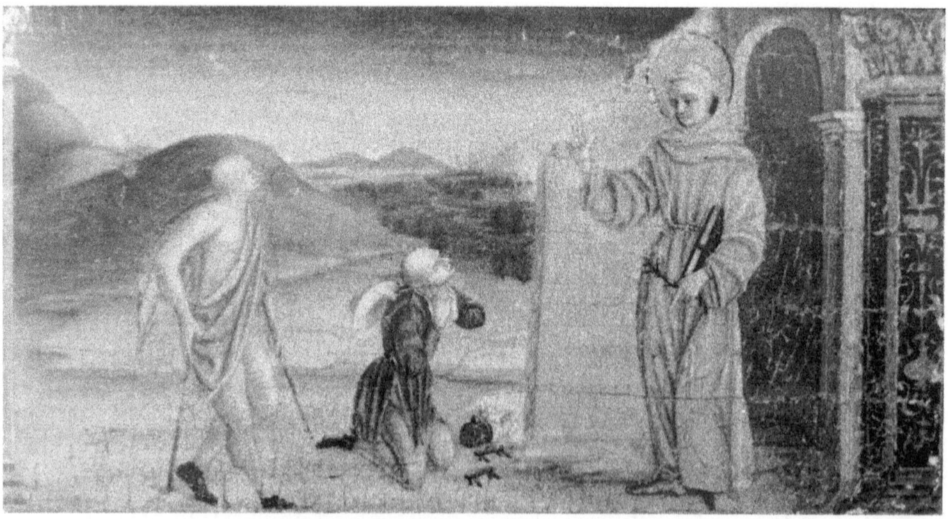

Figure 2.10 St. Anthony of Padua Healing a Lame Man and a Cripple, from George Kaftal, *Iconography of the Saints in Central and South Italian Schools of Painting*, Florence, 1986, fig. 122

placed among the branches of an oak tree as recorded in Gerard's legend,[73] one sees the exposed remains of the patron saint of Monza. At the foot of the tree two armed soldiers protect Gerard's remains from bystanders who might be tempted to obtain the saint's relics.[74] This detail, rather than being a whimsical invention of the artist, was an element of great pertinence to the Medieval viewer, since in the thirteenth and the fourteenth centuries, when it came to saintly bodies, "people waited with unconcealed impatience for the moment of death to take possession of the remains."[75]

An example of an image in which pleading individuals are depicted next to a tomb that conceals the body of the saint is found in the Vanni Altarpiece in the Vatican Museum (Plate 11). Painted in the style of Turino Vanni (ca. 1349–1438), the Vatican panel depicting St. Margaret of Antioch standing on a dragon is an altarpiece flanked by eight scenes from the life of the saint (Figure 2.11).[76] At bottom right (Plate 11), the artist painted a group of suppliants by the saint's sanctuary, two of which are orthopedically impaired: the one at center-left has obvious defective motor skills as he displays a bandaged leg and moves about using a rocking seat made of wood or metal (a sort of *testudo*) strapped to his body

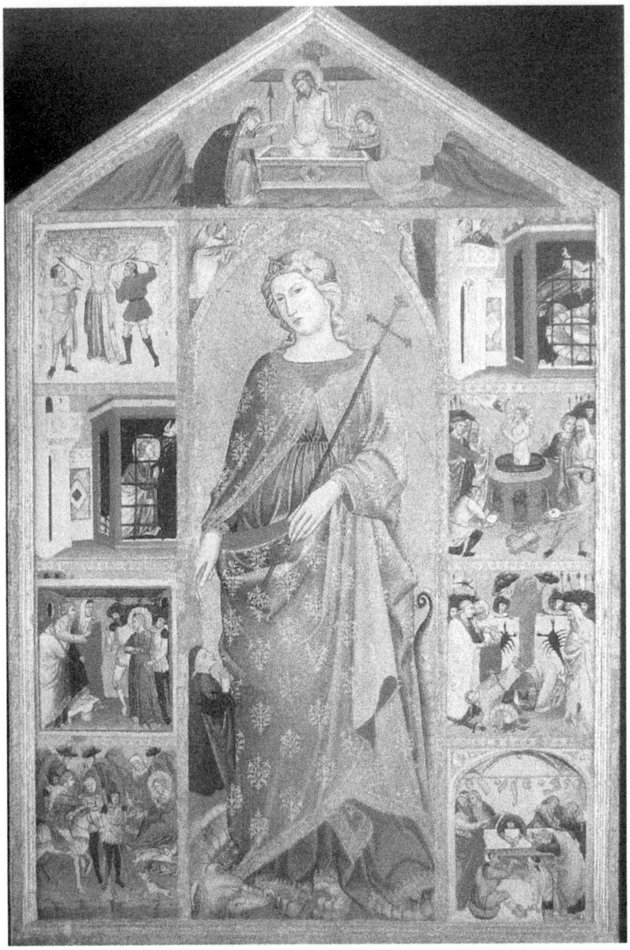

Figure 2.11 School of Turino Vanni, *Vanni Altarpiece*, ca. 1400, Pinacoteca Vaticana. Photo: author

by a seatbelt;[77] the one at center-right is an amputee who, gesticulating with his right hand, implores a cure while he supports his upper body with the aid of hand crutches. This scene is rendered more valuable by the inclusion of an important detail representing casts of parts of the human anatomy hanging from a rod over the sarcophagus. These are indicative of a fundamental aspect of "the rules of intercession" between supplicants and their advocates.[78]

Medieval sources evince that a saint's intercession was contingent on the making of a vow, which, for all intents and purposes, "compare[d] the vow to homage."[79] André Vauchez elucidates the nature of this exchange: "Admittedly, the majority of these commitments were made *ad experimentum*; if they did not get what they wanted after a certain period of time, the supplicants recovered their freedom. But if the request was successful, they must remain faithful to their 'patron' as long as they lived."[80] An important feature of this spiritual contract was that petitioners who did receive a miraculous cure left an ex-voto often representing the diseased or healed part of the body.[81] Thus, the yellowish wax molds of three heads, along with the thigh, foot, leg, arm and hand one sees hanging over St. Margaret's tomb in the Vanni Altarpiece are clear evidence to the pleaders, as well as to the faithful viewing the panel, that her intercession was real and reliable as it had proved successful for other supplicants who had preceded them.[82]

One final example that in a sense combines the first two categories of images just outlined is the *St. Barbara* panel in the Vatican Pinacoteca (Plate 12). This tempera predella, in fact, while displaying the saint's body also included an altar-like stone pedestal that alludes to both the saint's sacrificial martyrdom (if envisioned as an altar) and the shrine that will contain her bodily remains (if taken as a reminder of a sarcophagus). Moreover, this painting is of interest for the different types of disabilities included.

Set in a Classical-looking, colonnaded portico in the middle of a public square rendered in Albertian one-point perspective, the saint is "lying in state" on a thin slab of marble (?) under a baldachin embellished by oil lamps and drawn curtains.[83] Seven men surround the sanctuary: on the left there are a leper (sounding his approach by the clapping of a rattle) and a blind man (making his way with the aid of a cane); to the right of the baldachin, there are a lame on crutches with a brace for his right leg along with a man exhibiting a withered left hand held in a strap; center stage, three cripples look on and implore the saint for relief from their condition. In line with the higher percentages of miracles related to *contracti* – people with motor problems – in processes of canonization between 1201 and 1417, in the painting more than half of the supplicants are orthopedically impaired.[84] The painting tangibly evinces the extent to which people with mobility problems pervaded the Medieval and Renaissance cityscape and how normal or true to life images such as the Santa Barbara panel must have looked to the contemporary viewer.

The third category in which the lame are featured in Italian art is that of destitute recipients of alms in scenes where saintly individuals are portrayed as paragons of Christian charity. These images, as well, may be subdivided into two further categories: those that represent the almsgiving in the form of monetary gifts and those that exemplify the saint's largess through the donation of bread.

An instance of the first type of illustration occurs in a fifteenth-century codex by Bartolomeo or Giovanni Gadio in the Archivio Diocesano di Cremona, a depiction of St. Homobonus, who, "not content with giving his tenths to the distressed members of Christ … seemed to set no bounds to his alms; he sought out the poor in their homes and, whilst he relieved their corporal necessities, he exhorted them to a good life"[85] (Plate 13). Wearing a *lucco* – a long garment in use since the thirteenth century by the noblemen and subsequently by all male citizens who had come of age – the saintly merchant is shown in the act of handing a coin to one of two lame individuals propped on crutches who, synthetically, represent all of the indigent people of Cremona.

Although benefaction in the form of foodstuff probably comprised a much more frequent form of almsgiving in the course of human history, it was much less represented by Italian artists than monetary donations.[86] Among these representations of compassionate treatment of the poor and the infirm is the work of the Sienese painter Andrea di Bartolo (ca. 1360–1428), who depicted *Joachim and the Beggars* (ca. 1400) (Plate 14).[87] Andrea's panel takes its narrative clue from the second-century Greek *Protoevangelium of James* – a work that forms part of the apocryphal *Infancy Gospels*.[88] Conceived as a means of filling the void left by the New Testament with regard to questions the Early Christians had about the infancy of both the Virgin Mary and her Son, this gospel also provides information about Mary's parents: Sts. Joachim and Anne. In a Late Medieval style that fails to unite in one single vanishing point the various elements of the composition, Andrea di Bartolo took his lead from the very opening passage of his source and focuses on Joachim's exemplary enactment of his Christian *caritas*. James declares: "In the histories of the twelve tribes of Israel, Joachim was an extremely rich man. He always brought a double offering to the Lord, telling himself, 'My offering for all the people is from my surplus and my own offering to the Lord God is for forgiveness, to atone for my sins.'"[89] True to the *Protoevangelium*, on the left side of the lovely painting Andrea depicted Joachim standing in a portico holding a basket of buns with his left forearm and, reaching towards the imploring hands of a woman, a lame man with crutches, and a cripple, hands them their ration of *bucella* – a poor people's bread that formed the most frequent type of public assistance given to the poor.[90]

Two final categories in which the orthopedically impaired were prominently featured, deserve to be treated independently: allegories depicting the *Triumph of Death*[91] and images of victims of venereal disease.

Originating in Tuscany around 1340, thus even before the devastating impact that the Black Death of 1348 had on Europe,[92] scenes depicting the *Triumph of Death* are typically set in a cataclysmic landscape in which all of humanity's differences between rich and poor, aristocrats and peons, monarchs and subjects, clergy and laity are soon to be leveled. With a compelling gesture, the weakest members of society are shown reaching out to the terrifying, scythe-wielding figure of Death, "begging" it to put an end to their painful existence. As if to provide a sense of divine justice, these images reify the concept that, despite physical, economic and social shortcomings, one could ultimately envision that in the grand scheme of things there was, indeed, equality among people. These images obviously provided a sobering reminder to the viewer of the common denominator of the human condition.

There are a number of such images from Bolzano to Palermo, Florence, Lucignano and Subiaco, but the one that best captures the spirit of the age and somehow seems to reflect the mindset of the destitute in Medieval societies, is the fresco painted by Buonamico Buffalmacco in the Pisa Camposanto (1326–41) (Figures 2.12 and 2.13).[93] Just right of a group of finely clad lads and young ladies confronted by the unexpected, ghastly sight of decomposing cadavers in their caskets, at center stage eight persons – prominently featuring the blind, lame men, cripples and amputees – vigorously reach out to Death, beseeching it to bring an end to their earthly existence. Lest the viewer miss the point, the artist included an explicative inscription: "Since prosperity has abandoned us, oh Death – cure of all suffering – for pity's sake, come and serve us our last supper."[94] For the destitute and the disabled, who struggled to survive on a daily basis, never knowing from where the next morsel of bread to fill their empty stomachs would come, the ultimate relief from this world's injustices is ironically and metaphorically equated with a final meal. It would be difficult to find a more paradoxical yet eloquent way of expressing their death wish.

A last group of images of individuals whose mobility was seriously curtailed was one representing victims of venereal disease. Having become rampant in Italy in the mid-1490s, syphilis was an illness that had no lineage, with people of one nation blaming another for having brought about this scourge. The Italians called it the "Mal Francese" (French Disease), claiming that it had spread through the country when Charles VIII's troops marched south to Naples. The French, however, maintaining that they had been infected after they got to Naples, named it the "Mal de Naples."[95] Rabelais, giving vent to his usual wit, re-baptized the victims of the disease "les Napleux."[96] However, the *morbus gallicus*, as it was labeled in the medical treatises on the subject – the earliest of which were written by Italian and German doctors – was the term favored by the Italians, Spanish, German, Polish and English.[97] Given human nature and the propensity to blame others when problems arise, it is not surprising to learn that the Catholics in Spain blamed syphilis on the *marranos*, the Muslims and Jews who had converted to Catholicism.[98]

Although no one agreed as to who had fathered the disease, there was a general consensus as to who the mother was: Venus, the goddess of love. It was generally recognized that the disease was transmitted through sexual contact, but the first person to refer to it as a *venereal* disease was Jacques de Béthencourt, a protestant doctor from Rouen, in his 1527 book on ailments and remedies for it.[99] Instead, the person who initially used the word *syphilis* was Girolamo Fracastoro (1476/78–1553), Pope Paul III's (1534–1549) personal doctor, who employed it originally as a fictional, proper noun for the shepherd Syphilis who first contracted the disease and included it in the title of his poem: *Syphilis sive morbus gallicus* (*Syphilis or The French Disease*). It took more than a century before the word *syphilis* was used as a

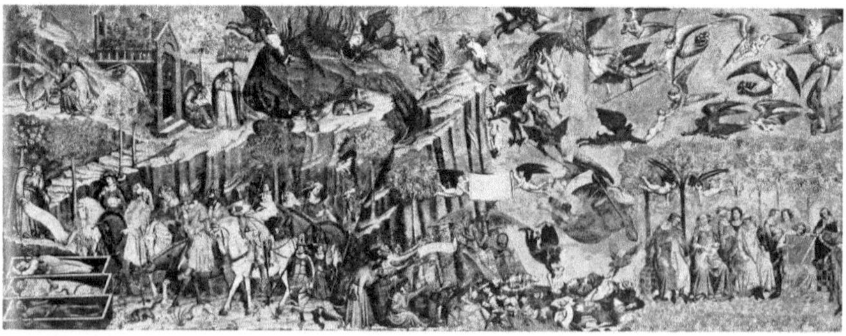

Figure 2.12 Buonamico Buffalmacco, *Triumph of Death,* Camposanto, Pisa. Photo: in the public domain

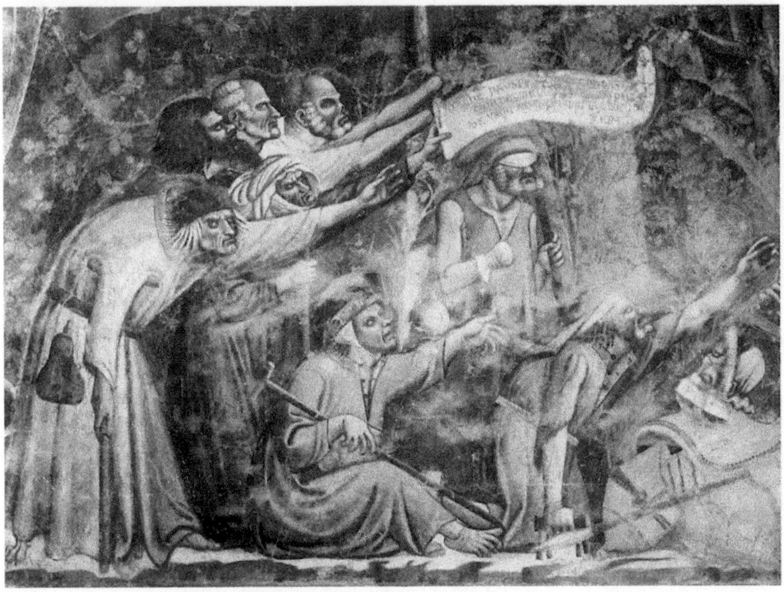

Figure 2.13 Buonamico Buffalmacco, *Triumph of Death*, detail of Figure 2.12, Camposanto, Pisa. Photo: in the public domain

common name and adopted to describe the disease itself, along with the other appellations that were used to refer to it.[100]

The initial symptoms associated with this disease were pustules that developed into "ulcers that dissolved skin, muscle, bone, palate, and tonsils – even lips, noses, eyes and genital organs."[101] Indeed, these patients were covered with boils that emitted a revolting smell and a dark green pus.[102] The papal bull *Salvatoris Nostri* issued in 1515 by Leo X makes specific reference to this problem and adds a detail that allows us to understand the iconographic features artists used to depict the victims of this disease:

> For a number of years large numbers of sick poor have come together in Rome, all infected with incurable diseases. [They have come] in such great numbers that they cannot find shelter in the hospitals of the city for their incurable sicknesses, [which] give annoyance to the sight and sense of smell, so that they are obliged to beg for their living through Rome, *dragging themselves along on little carts*.[103]

By the time the syphilitic patient's illness had progressed into the secondary and tertiary stages,[104] besides the malodorous sores, it also caused baldness and affected the persons' nervous system, making them unable to walk and dependent on little carts to move about.

Thus, when seeing an invalid with a headband covering his hair being carried by a porter in a wheelbarrow at the bottom far right of Annibale Carracci's painting *The Charity of St. Roch* (1587/88–1595) in the Gemäldegalerie Alte Meister, Dresden[105] (Figure 2.14), or the comparable figure propelling himself on a wheelchair in Biagio Falcieri's engraving of *The Charity*

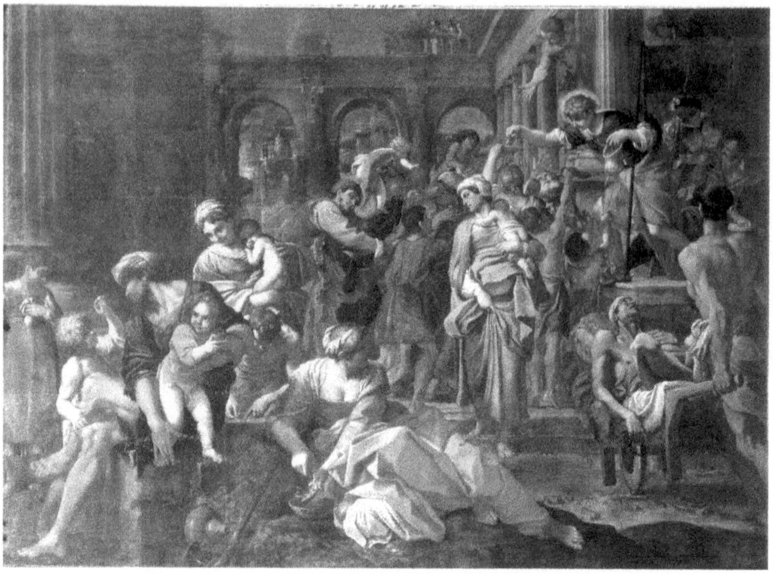

Figure 2.14 Annibale Carracci, *The Charity of St. Roch*, 1594–1595, Dresden, Gemäldegalerie Alte Meister, Staatliche Kunstsammlungen. Photo: Hans-Peter Klut, © 2015. Scala, Firenze/bpk, Bildagentur für Kunst, Kultur und Geschichte, Berlin

of St. Gaetano (1694) (Figure 2.15),[106] the viewer must understand that these individuals, whose ambulatory powers have been totally curtailed, are not paralytics. Rather, they represent the victims of a debilitating disease that seldom allowed individuals to recover. One can only imagine how the Neapolitans must have reacted to the bearded man sitting in a cart with head covered by a cloth and being sustained by a woman in Paolo de Matteis's fresco of *St. Francis Xavier in Glory Protecting the City from Hunger, Plague, and Fire, and the Shipwrecked from Drowning* (1693) (Plate 15) in the church of San Ferdinando.[107] In Naples, where according to some it all began, the sight of such individuals must have conjured up not only a true-to-life daily experience but also the accusation the French had placed at their doorstep as the culprits and initiators of syphilis.

In imitation of a number of institutions called "Incurabili" hospitals that had begun in northern Italy – first among them being the one in Genoa – the Roman Ospedale di San Giacomo degli Incurabili was created in 1515 with the support of Leo X.[108] Located on Via Lata (today's Via del Corso) and stretching all the way back to the Via di Ripetta, this hospital incorporated the small chapel of Santa Maria in Porta Paradisi with its entrance on Via di Ripetta. In the portico of this chapel, as a reminder of the hospital's *raison d'être*, there is a small marble plaque with an opening for depositing alms for the victims of syphilis (Plate 16). A mustached man sitting in a cart with headband and a swath of cloth covering a festering sore on his right shin looks towards the viewers who pass by. Beneath his image the caption reads: "Alms for the poor, sore-ridden [individuals] of the Incurabili [hospital]" (*Elemosina per li poveri impiagati dell'incurabili*). With the praying, supplicating gesture of the hands, the image of this diseased, orthopedically impaired man begs the passersby to pause temporarily and solicits them for both alms and attention.

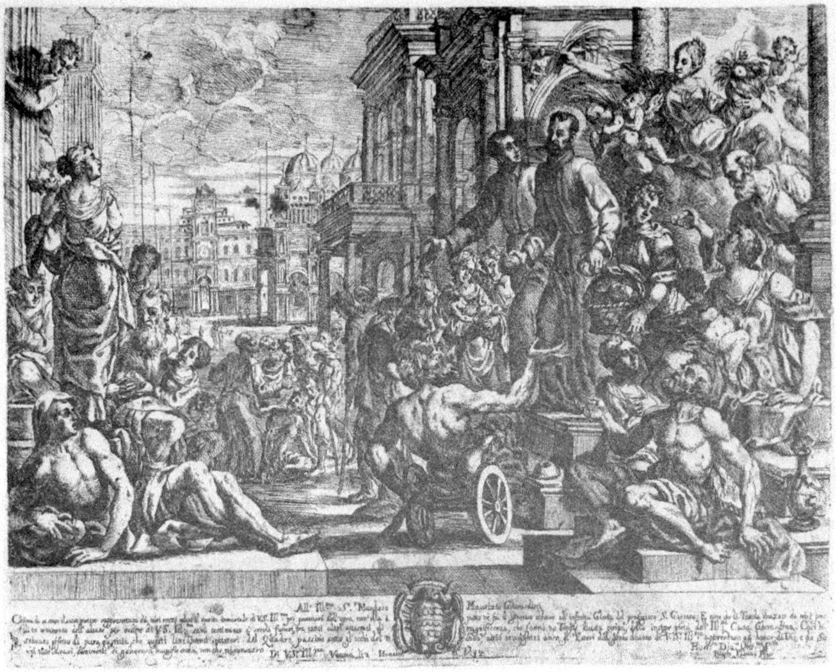

Figure 2.15 Biagio Falcieri, *Charity of St. Gaetano, The Illustrated Bartsch*. Photo: from *The Illustrated Bartsch*, Walter L. Strauss, John T. Spike and Isabelle de Ramaix (eds.), 108 vols., New York, 1978–, XLVII, p. 209, no. 004

As this brief excursus of illustrations depicting the orthopedically impaired has shown, the lame or the destitute were represented, if not in a positive, at least in a neutral light. Although one may sense in these representations all of the distance that separated the "normal," able-bodied society from those members of the community who were less fortunate because of their physical ailments or economic vulnerability, the artists were still able to empathize with their subjects. The major reason for this is that through the Middle Ages and a good part of the Renaissance – at least through the first half of the sixteenth century – the prevailing attitude towards the indigent and the infirm was to identify them with the suffering Christ. Had not Christ promised the kingdom prepared for the virtuous by declaring, "For I was hungry and you gave me food; I was thirsty and you gave me drink; I was a stranger and you made me welcome; naked and you clothed me, sick and you visited me, in prison and you came to see me"? And had he not just as significantly added, "I tell you solemnly, in so far as you did this to one of the least of these brothers of mine, you did it to me"? (Mt 25:35–46). It was in keeping with this evangelical view, as Francis's biographer Thomas of Celano claimed, that the *Poverello* "saw Christ suffer in every wretch he encountered" but also "recognized in all the poor the son of Our Lady, who was poor."[109]

This feature of Francis's religiosity, his divesting himself of his worldly clothes – literally and figuratively – so as to be able to "follow naked the naked Christ,"[110] his exaltation of poverty and empathy with the poor, his equating them with the suffering Christ, was so prominent that it eventually led contemporaries to address the Franciscans as *pauperes Christi* ("Poor of Christ"). However, as if by osmosis, by 1330 the epithet *poveri di Cristo* changed meaning. In relating an extraordinary distribution of alms doled out upon the death of a Florentine merchant, Giovanni Villani penned a list of those who were part of the seventeen thousand beneficiaries: "male and female, young and old, not counting the shamefaced poor and those in the hospitals and prisons, or the mendicant friars, [all of] whom also received their alms, and who added up to [another] four thousand [persons]."[111] Concluding his account of the remarkable event, Villani exhorted his contemporaries to perform comparable acts of mercy and ended his description of the event with a final counsel: "We have chosen to record this deed because of the great esteem in which it was held, and also *so it be of good example to those who, for the benefit of their soul, will want to give alms to the Poor of Christ*."[112] The identification of Francis with Christ, and the appellation *poveri di Cristo* with reference to the Franciscans, by the early fourteenth century was reverting back to the original meaning it had had in 386 for St. Ambrose, who was the first to use such a term to describe the poor themselves.[113]

While it is prudent to underline that with regard to the treatment of the poor in Europe there is more continuity than change between the Middle Ages and the Renaissance[114] and that, if there was a change, "the most striking advance in the sixteenth century lay in the ardour and sophistication of the attempts made, not to reject or punish, but to reclaim the undeserving – not merely to support the virtuous and innocent, but to redeem the habitual sinner,"[115] it is nevertheless true that, starting in the late sixteenth century, images of the lame reflect a greater emphasis on negative connotations than previously observed.[116] In fact, the association between those disabled persons, who because of their physical ailments were unable to work, and the poor, who for comparable reasons depended on alms, did affect negatively the way people looked upon those whose mobility was impaired and the way artists depicted them. In the changing cultural, social and religious climate of the sixteenth and seventeenth centuries the uneven gait of the lame, to remain in the Franciscan context just described, was inevitably stigmatized.[117]

Notes

1 Danièl Alexandre-Bidon and Didier Lett, *Children in the Middle Ages: Fifth–Fifteenth Centuries*, Jody Gladding (tr.), Notre Dame, 1999, p. 37.

2 Geoffrey R. Elton, *Persecution and Toleration: Studies in Church History*, Oxford, 1984, p. xiii: "Among the religious, toleration is demanded by the persecuted who need it if they are to become triumphant, when, all too often, they start to persecute in their turn. A highly unsubtle interplay of persecution and toleration thus conveniently sums up the millennia of religious history and more especially of ecclesiastical history. To say this is not cynicism, but sobriety of judgement." Quoted by Peter Brown, *Authority and the Sacred: Aspects of the Christianisation of the Roman World*, Cambridge, 1997, p. 30.

3 Laes, "Learning from Silence," p. 115. See also Stephen Pender, "In the Bodyshop: Human Exhibition in Early Modern England," in Deutsch and Nussbaum (eds.), *"Defects,"* p. 103.

4 Laes, "Learning from Silence," p. 113.

5 Ibid., p. 115. Gregory of Tours, *De Virtutibus Sancti Martini*, 2,24: "quod una nocte committitur, per multorum annorum spatial perferatur." Quoted by Laes, *The Dark Side of Childhood*, Mustakallio and Laes (eds.), p. 61, n. 96. Laes also points out that the same concept is expressed by Caesarius of Arles in Sermon 44,7.

6 *Decrees of the Ecumenical Councils*, 2 vols., Norman P. Tanner (ed.), London and Washington, 1990, I, decree 22, "That the sick should provide for the soul before the body," pp. 245–246.

7 Peter Brown, *The Cult of the Saints: Its Rise and Function in Latin Christianity*, London, 1981, pp. 6 and 50. Amundsen, p. 9: "Furthermore, it is interesting to note that it is not until the fourth century that reports of miraculous healings are frequently encountered. With the rise of the cult of saints and relics in the later part of that century, they become commonplace." As in Northern Africa, in sixth-century Tours, "the focal point of the entire process of healing was, therefore, somewhat incongruously, the saint's tomb." See Raymond Van Dam, *Saints and their Miracles in Late Antique Gaul*, Princeton, 1993, p. 90.

8 Brown, *The Cult of the Saints*: "Thus, in Christian belief, the grave, the memory of the dead, and the religious ceremonial that might surround this memory were placed within a totally different structure of relations between God, the dead, and the living."

9 Ibid., pp. 51 and 60–61. Brown points out how book 10 of Augustine's *City of God* was "devoted to redefining the nature of the true intermediaries between God and men." See Augustine, *Concerning the City of God Against the Pagans*, Henry Bettenson (tr.), Middlesex, 1972, XXII, 10.

10 Vauchez, *Sainthood*, p. 17.

11 On the adverse effect that Christ's miracles could have on his Messianic reputation see Smith, esp. pp. 81–93, and Fridrichsen.

12 Brown, *The Cult of the Saints*, p. 72.

13 Ibid., p. 100.

14 Augustine, *City of God*, XXII, 8, p. 1034. The initial statement in *The Passion of St. Perpetua* echoes St. Augustine's words: "If ancient examples of faith, both bearing witness to God's grace and teaching man, have been written down, that by their reading, as if by their showing forth, God may be honoured and man comforted; why should not modern and equally relevant documents be set forth?" Francis Wormald, "Some Illustrated Manuscripts of the Lives of the Saints," *Bulletin of the John Rylands Library*, 35 (1952–1953): 248.

15 Augustine, XXII, 8, p. 1034.

16 Ibid.

17 Ibid., XXII, 8, p. 1035.

18 Ibid.

19 Ibid.

20 Ibid., XXII, 8, p. 1043.

21 Alan Thacker, "*Loca Sanctorum*: The Significance of Place in the Study of the Saints," in *Local Saints and Local Churches in the Early Medieval West*, Alan Thacker and Richard Sharpe (eds.), Oxford, 2002, p. 17. See also John M. McCulloh, "The Cult of Relics in the Letters and 'Dialogues' of Pope Gregory the Great: A Lexicographical Study," *Traditio*, 32 (1976): 145–184, where the author gives the various meanings of *reliquiae*, *beneficia*, *sanctuaria*, *brandea* and *benedictio*.

22 Victor Saxer, under "Martirio," in *Dizionario patristico e di antichità cristiane*, 2 vols., Angelo Di Berardino (ed.), Casale Monferrato, 1984, II, p. 2139. Saxer points out that the cult of images that John Damascene (676–749) describes as prevalent in the East (*De fide orthodoxa* 4, 15), had to wait until the Middle Ages to develop analogously in the West. Hippolyte Delehaye, *Les orgines du culte des martyrs*, Paris, 1933, pp. 52–53, points out that while in Rome the integrity of a human's remains was sanctioned by law, and thus developed the concept of contact relics, in the East people were not satisfied with the "fiction" of the healing powers of *brandea* and, when asking for relics, they expected that part of the saint's remains be detached. St. Augustine's *libelli miraculorum* that related of posthumous wonders "helped confirm the process by which portable relics from the site of an *inventio* were assimilated to the body itself and hence believed to share fully in its wonderworking *virtus*." See Thacker, "*Loca Sanctorum*," p. 13.

23 On the development of the cult of relics and the progressive changes in the way the Early Christians portrayed their saints, see André Grabar, *Martyrium: recherches sur le culte des reliques et l'art chrétien antique*, 2 vols., Paris, 1946, esp. II, pp. 25–75. For the image of St. Demetrius, see

Hans Belting, *Likeness and Presence: A History of the Image before the Era of Art*, Chicago and London, 1994, p. 82, fig. 33, p. 86.

24 Among the earliest individuals who were instrumental in the development of relics are Pope Damasus (366–384) in Rome and St. Ambrose in Milan. See Thacker, "*Loca Sanctorum*," pp. 3–12. Alan Thacker, "Rome of the Martyrs: Saints, Cults and Relics, Fourth to Seventh Centuries," in *Roma Felix: Formation and Reflections of Medieval Rome*, Éamonn Ó Carragáin and Carol Neuman de Vegvar (eds.), Aldershot and Burlington, 2007, pp. 13–49, revisits the development of the cult of relics, emphasizing how Damasus – an "impresario of cults" (p. 36) – with the creation of inscriptions "exquisitely carved by his friend Philocalus" (p. 31), appropriated existing *loca santa* or created new ones. After him, Prudentius and Ambrose promoted the cult of *local saints* (p. 38). See also Caroline J. Goodson, "Building for Bodies: The Architecture of Saint Veneration in Early Medieval Rome," in Ó Carragáin and Neuman de Vegvar (eds.), *Roma Felix*, pp. 51–79.

25 Belting, p. 80, fig. 29, p. 82. A contemporary example mentioned by Grabar is the fourth-century fresco in the catacombs of Domitilla, where St. Petronilla leads Veneranda into the garden of Paradise. Grabar, *Martyrium*, pl. XXXIV, 1. See also Cynthia Hahn, "Seeing and Believing: The Construction of Sanctity in Early-Medieval Saints' Shrines," *Speculum*, 72 (1997): 1079–1106.

26 Belting, p. 80.

27 Ibid. See also Delehaye, p. 68.

28 Thacker, "Rome of the Martyrs," p. 16, actually points out that from the sixth through the mid-eighth centuries in Rome there was papal opposition to translation. By preventing "the disturbance of the holy dead" the papacy actually defended themselves against the "importunate demands to share their great heritage of sacred bodies." In his analysis of Pope Gregory's *Dialogues*, McCulloh, p. 153, claims that, indeed, "in most areas of Italy the sixth-century Christians respected the Roman prohibition against moving corpses."

29 This was the case, if not by the sixth, certainly by mid-eighth century. Thacker, "*Loca Sanctorum*," pp. 13, 16 and 43. The phenomenon did not go unchallenged. Idem, pp. 11–12: "In Gaul, in the first years of the fifth century, Vigilantius of Calagurris . . . attacked the cult of the martyrs, condemning observances such as the keeping of vigils or the lighting of candles before the sacred tombs. In particular, he ridiculed the practice of venerating 'a bit of powder wrapped up in a cloth,' 'dust and ashes wrapped in silk in a golden vessel' which were 'kissed and adored' or 'carried about.'" The trend in favor of the translation of relics was given impetus especially after Paschal I (817–824) translated the bodies of over 2,300 martyrs from the catacombs surrounding Rome to his new churches within the city walls. See Caroline Goodson, "The Relic Translations of Paschal I: Transforming City and Cult," in *Roman Bodies*, Hopkins and Wyke (eds.), pp. 123–141.

30 Paul J. Fouracre, "The Origins of the Carolingian Attempt to Regulate the Cult of Saints," in *The Cult of Saints in Late Antiquity and the Middle Ages: Essays on the Contribution of Peter Brown*, A. Howard-Johnston and P.A. Hayward (eds.), Oxford, 1999, pp. 145 and 165. For a useful recap of the cult of the saints see Cynthia Hahn's preface to *Passio Kiliani*, 2 vols., Graz, 1988, II, pp. 1–22.

31 See Cynthia Hahn, "Narrative on the Golden Altar of Sant'Ambrogio in Milan: Presentation and Reception," *Dumbarton Oaks Paper*, 53 (1999): 167–187, fig. 5.

32 Made for Basil I around 879–883: Paris, Bibliothèque Nationale, gr. 510, fol. 32v.

33 For comments and a reproduction of this folio see Lyn Rodley, *Byzantine Art and Architecture: An Introduction*, Cambridge, 1994, pp. 180–182, fig. 141, p. 181.

34 Biblioteca Apostolica Vaticana, *Vaticanus graecus 1613*.

35 Cynthia Hahn, *Portrayed on the Heart: Narrative Effect in Pictorial Lives of Saints from the Tenth through the Thirteenth Century*, Berkeley, 2001, p. 59.

36 Belting, p. 302.

37 Thacker, "*Loca Sanctorum*," pp. 14–15.

38 On the altar in the church of Sant'Ambrogio in Milan, see Victor H. Elbern, *Der karolingische Goldaltar von Mailand*, Bonn, 1952; Carlo Bertelli, "L'altare di Volvinio nella basilica milanese di Sant'Ambrogio," *Rivista dell'Istituto per la Storia dell'Arte Lombarda*, 5 (2012): 41–54; and

Erik Thunø, "The Golden Altar of Sant'Ambrogio in Milan," in *Decorating the Lord's Table*, Søren Kaspersen and Erik Thunø (eds.), Copenhagen, 2006, pp. 63–78.

39 Wormald, p. 252: "It is unfortunate that extremely little is known about any early series of scenes from the lives of the saints in the West. As will be seen none actually exists before the ninth century either on the walls of churches or in objects or manuscripts." As note 41 below specifies, there are actually five such cycles from before the ninth century, but that is still very little. Wormald considers the golden altar in the church of Sant'Ambrogio in Milan as the starting point of this trend of depicting scenes of the lives of the saints.

40 Cynthia Hahn, "Pictorial Cycles of Non-Biblical Saints: The Seventh- and Eighth-Century Mural Cycles in Rome and Contexts for their Use," *Papers of the British School at Rome*, 67 (1999): 234. Wormald, p. 251: "With the growth of large churches on the sites of the burial places of the saints, it is most likely that the walls were decorated scenes from the life of the patron."

41 Wormald, p. 251. They are located in the churches of Santa Maria Antiqua, the first two; Santa Maria in Via Lata, the third; Sant'Adriano, the fourth; and in the catacombs of Calepodius, the last.

42 Barbara Fay Abou-El-Haj, *The Medieval Cult of Saints: Formations and Transformations*, Cambridge, 1997, p. 26: "Most pictorial hagiographies, however, belong to the later Middle Ages not by accident of survival but because they were part of the expansion of the cult of saints, part of the effort to renew and enlarge cults that were put to use in protecting clerical interests, and in competing for pilgrims and their coins in the new exchange economy."

43 Paris Bibliothèque Nationale, MS Lat. 5594, fol. 70r; Hahn, *Portrayed on the Heart*, p. 76, fig. 19.

44 Hahn, *Portrayed on the Heart*, p. 111, fig. 36.

45 Berlin Staatsbibliothek, Cod. Lat. Theol. Fol. 323, fol. 12r; Hahn, *Portrayed on the Heart*, p. 154, fig. 61.

46 Paris Bibliothèque Nationale, MS n.a.l. 1390, fol. 1r; Hahn, *Portrayed on the Heart*, p. 155, fig. 62.

47 Tours, Bibliothèque Municipale, MS 1018, fol. 18r; Hahn, *Portrayed on the Heart*, p. 162, fig. 66.

48 Berlin Staatliche Museen, Kupferstichkabinett 78 A 4, fol. 2r; Hahn, *Portrayed on the Heart*, p. 110, fig. 35.

49 Hahn's comment on the type of donation being made ("The bowls hold blue cones, but since bread was at times represented in this conical shape, one must surmise that the colorist used his imagination") is not convincing. More research is needed to fully understand what the indigent and the infirm are actually receiving from the saint. Hahn, *Portrayed on the Heart*, p. 369, n. 57.

50 Pierpont Morgan Library, MS M. 736, fol. 9r. Hahn, *Portrayed on the Heart*, pl. 6.

51 Vauchez, *Sainthood*, p. 106.

52 André Vauchez, *The Spirituality of the Medieval West: The Eighth to the Twelfth Century*, Colette Friedlander (tr.), Kalamazoo, MI, 1993, p. 67.

53 Ibid., p. 33 and Chapter 3, esp. pp. 75–88.

54 The reason for the earlier appearance of the orthopedically impaired north of the Alps may have been the need on the part of the northern hagiographers, in their desire to have their "own" saints (as opposed to those "imported" from south of the Alps) recognized by the religious authorities. It would have been an attempt by them to align the miracles of the new saints with the biblical miracles performed by Christ. For this Christo-mimesis, see further in this chapter. The more frequent presence of the orthopedically disabled from Medieval to Renaissance Italian art may be ascertained by consulting George Kaftal's classic compendium of *Saints in Italian Art*. This fundamental iconographic study of paintings in which saints were held responsible for miracles involving individuals with impaired mobility lists a total sixty-two works of art. To be precise, there are twenty-five images in vol. I (*Iconography of the Saints in Tuscan Painting*, Florence, 1986), twenty in vol. II (*Iconography of the Saints in Central and South Italian Schools of Painting*, Florence, 1986), twelve in vol. III (*Iconography of the Saints in the Painting of North East Italy*, Florence, 1978) and five in vol. IV (*Iconography of the Saints in the Painting of North West Italy*, Florence, 1985).

55 Hahn, *Passio Kiliani*, p. 10. Abou-El-Haj, p. 43: "Healings modeled on Christ's miracles tend to reproduce essentially Gospel iconographies."

56 For the life of St. Francis see Thomas of Celano's *First Life* (ms. ca. 1228 discovered again only in 1768), *Second Life* (ms. ca. 1247 recuperated in 1806) and *Treatise of his Miracles* (ms. ca. 1245–1247

rediscovered in 1899), in addition to St. Bonaventure's *Legenda Maior* (1263). In an attempt to quell the strong divisions that arose within the Franciscan Order after the saint's death about the interpretation of his "message" and his rule, at the Chapter General held in 1266 in Paris, St. Bonaventure issued the order that from that time on only his version of the saint's biography be considered official. Consequently almost all of the earlier biographies by Thomas of Celano were destroyed. See Chiara Frugoni, *Francesco: un'altra storia*, Florence, 1988, pp. 8–9. For the treatment of the early images of St. Francis and the ideological implications they carried, see also Rona Goffen, *Spirituality in Conflict: Saint Francis and Giotto's Bardi Chapel*, University Park and London, 1988, and Rosalind B. Brooke, *The Images of St. Francis: Responses to Sainthood in the Thirteenth Century*, Cambridge, 2006, especially p. 401ff.

57 Émile Mâle, *The Gothic Image: Religious Art in France of the Thirteenth Century*, New York, 1972, p. 176. Cynthia Hahn, "Picturing the Text: Narrative in the *Life* of the Saints," *Art History*, 13 (1990): 6: "The true subject of the saint's life is not the saint himself but Christ. Both the origin for hagiographic structure and the ultimate intent of saints' lives is the imitation of Christ."

58 Vauchez, *Sainthood*, p. 158. See also Donald Weinstein and Rudolph M. Bell, *Saints and Society: The Two Worlds of Western Christendom, 1000–1700*, Chicago and London, 1982, pp. 194–204, and André Vauchez, *Saints, prophètes et visionnaires: le pouvoir surnaturel au Moyen Âge*, Paris, 1999, pp. 67–78.

59 Vauchez, *Sainthood*, esp. pp. 141–144, 157–158, 197, 199, 342, n. 293.

60 Ibid., p. 36.

61 Goffen, p. 31. The classic accounts are Klaus Kruger, *Der Frühe Bildkult des Franziskus in Italien: Gestalt- und Funktionswandel des Tafelbildes im 13. und 14. Jahrhundert*, Berlin, 1992, and Chiara Frugoni, *Francesco e l'invenzione delle stimmate*, Turin, 1993, esp. pp. 325–334. For the visual arts see Mario Alberto Pavone, *Iconologia francescana: il Quattrocento*, Todi, 1988, and Simonetta Prosperi Valenti Rodinò and Claudio Strinati (eds.), *L'immagine di San Francesco nella Controriforma*, Rome, 1983, p. 74, cat. 8. For the Roman context see William Cook, "Early Images of St. Francis of Assisi in Rome," in *"Exegisti Monumentum Aere Perennius": Essays in Honor of John Frederick Charles*, Bruce Baker and John Fischer (eds.), Indianapolis, 1994, pp. 19–34, esp. pp. 21–22; William Cook, *Images of Saint Francis of Assisi in Painting, Stone and Glass from the Earliest Images to c. 1320 in Italy: A Catalogue*, Florence, 1999, pp. 183–196; Gregory W. Ahlquist and William R. Cook, "The Representation of the Posthumous Miracles of St. Francis of Assisi in Thirteenth-Century Italian Painting," in *The Art of the Franciscan Order in Italy*, William Robert Cook (ed.), Leiden, 2005, pp. 211–256; Brooke, esp. pp. 160–217.

62 See Hendrik W. van Os, "St. Francis of Assisi as a Second Christ in Early Italian Painting," *Simiolus*, 7 (1974): 115–132, who in turn refers to Stanislao da Campagnola, *L'angelo del sesto sigillo e l'"alter Christus": genesi e sviluppo di due temi francescani nei secoli XII–XIV*, Rome, 1971.

63 Ruth Wolff, *Der Heilige Franziskus in Schriften und Bildern des 13. Jahrhunderts*, Berlin 1996, pp. 141–200, esp. p. 186 and pl. 38.

64 The Assisi panel in the Treasury of the Sacro Convento, tempera on wood, 96 × 138 cm, was painted either by Giunta Pisano or by one of his associates. The four stories are: upper left, the cure of the girl with a twisted neck on the day of the saint's death; lower left, the paralytic Bartolomeo da Narni is cured; upper right, a possessed woman is exorcised; bottom right, a cripple and a leper at St. Francis's tomb, with the cripple walking away cured at right. The close replica of this panel, executed around 1255 and now in the Vatican Pinacoteca (67 × 86.5), was probably commissioned by a pope who had seen the panel in Assisi. See Cook, *Images of St Francis of Assisi in Painting*, pp. 62–63 and 192–193.

65 For the Bardi panel see Chiara Frugoni, *Francesco, un'altra storia*, Genoa, 1988.

66 Vauchez, *Sainthood*, p. 36, who quoted from Othmar Hageneder and Anton Haidacher, *Das Register Innocenz' III*, I, Graz and Cologne, 1964, pp. 761–764. See also André Vauchez, *Omobono di Cremona (1197): laico e santo, profilo storico*, Cremona, 2001. Adelaide Ricci, "'Nel catalogo dei santi': riflessioni sulla santità di Omobono," in *Strenna dell'ADAFA*, new series, I, 2001, Cremona, p. 81: "Duo tamen virtus [vierures] videlicet morum et vivus signorum, opera scilicet pietatis in vita et miraculorum signa post mortem, ut quis reputetur sanctus in militanti Ecclesia, requiruntur."

67 On the "proof" images provided for the faithful in the Middle Ages, Herbert Kessler pointedly declares, "words are uncertain, seeing is believing." See Herbert L. Kessler, "Pictorial Narrative and Church Mission in Sixth-Century Gaul," *Studies in the History of Art*, 16 (1985): 75–91. See also Ahlquist and Cook, esp. 250–256.

68 Bronislaw Geremek, *Poverty: A History*, Oxford, 1994, esp. p. 169. The literature on the subject of poverty is extensive. For the lack of rigor attached to the word "poverty," its equation with "indigence," and for the use and understanding of the word "poor" by the rich and the clergy, on the one hand, and the indigent wage-earners, on the other hand, in fourteenth-century Florence, see Charles-M. de la Roncière, "Pauvres et pauvreté à Florence au XIVe siècle," in *Études sur l'histoire de la pauvreté (Moyen Âge–XVIe siècle)*, Michel Mollat (ed.), Paris, II, 1974, pp. 661–745. See also Bronislaw Geremek, *The Margins of Society in Late Medieval Paris*, Cambridge, 1987; Michel Mollat, *The Poor in the Middle Ages: An Essay in Social History*, Arthur Goldhammer (tr.), New Haven and London, 1986; John Henderson, *Piety and Charity in Late Medieval Florence*, Oxford, 1994.

69 See Kaftal, II, pp. 109–110, fig. 122. Comparable examples are *St. Vigilius Healing the Infirm* and *Blessed Philip Ciardella of Castelli Miraculously Healing the Ulcerous Leg of a Man*, for which see Kaftal, III, pp. 1057–1058, fig. 1363, and Kaftal, I, pp. 849–850, fig. 961, respectively. See note 54.

70 Vauchez, *Sainthood*, p. 427.

71 See Martina Bagnoli, "Fonti per la storia delle pitture della cripta," in *Il restauro della cripta di Anagni*, Alessandro Bianchi (ed.), Rome, 2003, pp. 77–78, and Alessandro Bianchi, "I dipinti," in idem, p. 110.

72 *Butler's Lives of the Saints*, 4 vols., Westminster, Maryland, 1990, II, p. 491.

73 Kaftal, I, p. 448. See Giuseppe Maria Brocchi, *Vita di S. Gherardo*, Lucca, 1750, pp. 22–23: "Divulgatasi pertanto la morte di S. Gherardo, concorse un'infinità ... di popolo a Villamagna per venerare il di Lui sacro Corpo bramando ciascheduno di prendere di Esso qualche Reliquia onde essendo già stati fatti in pezzi, per sodisfare alla comune divozione, i suoi vestimenti, si correva risico, che non fosse guastato ancora il medesimo santo Corpo; perciò fu stimato bene il porlo, come fu fatto, in una Cassa, e collocarlo sopra una quercia fintantoché ... [e] per maggior sicurtà di quella sacra Reliquia, furono mandati dalla Repubblica Fiorentina ... alcuni soldati." ("As soon as the news of St. Gherardo's death spread, innumerable people traveled to Villamagna to venerate his holy Body, each of them desiring to take from him a relic. Consequently, having already cut his garments into pieces to satisfy their common devotion, his very holy Body ran the risk of being violated. Therefore, it was deemed best to place it, as was ultimately done, in a casket and placed in an oak tree ... and, for the greater protection of that holy Relic, some soldiers were sent [to Villamagna] from the Florentine Republic.")

74 For the traditional Western objection to the dismembering of corpses see Delehaye, pp. 52–53, as in note 22. On the related issue of the translation of bodies and the opposition to it see Thacker, "*Loca Sanctorum*," p. 16. For the Medieval practice of the division of the body north of the Alps, especially that of separating the flesh from the bones, and the interdiction in Italy by Boniface VIII in 1299 (*Corpus iuris canonici* II, cols. 12713; *Registres de Boniface* VIII, no. 3209), see Agostino Paravicini Bagliani, "The Corpse in the Middle Ages: The Problem of the Division of the Body," in *The Medieval World*, Peter Linehan and Janet L. Nelson (eds.), London and New York, 2001, pp. 327–341, esp. pp. 333–334. Godfrey of Fontaines, master of the Faculty of Theology in Paris, equally in favor of the integrity of the body, in 1291 claimed that "only the bodies of saints could be divided 'for the common good.'"

75 Vauchez, *Sainthood*, p. 430. Idem, no. 15, p. 430: "When the inhabitants of Assisi heard that the 'Poverello' was seriously ill, they despatched [*sic*] an armed escort to Bagnara, near Nocera, where he then was, with orders to bring him back, dead or alive, to his native town. When this had been done, the commune posted guards in front of the episcopal palace until his death, for fear the Franciscans would seize the body secretly and take it away: *Legenda antiqua Perusiana*, c. LXIV, Desbonnets and Vorreux (eds.), p. 937."

76 Leanne Gilbertson, "The Vanni Altarpiece and the Relic Cult of Saint Margaret: Considering a Female Audience," in *Decorations for the Holy Dead: Visual Embellishments on Tombs and Shrines of Saints*, Stephen Lamia and Elizabeth Valdez del Álamo (eds.), Turnhout, 2002, pp. 179–190.

77 In Angelo Decembrio's Latin panegyric ("Vergiliana panaegyris") for Prince Carlos de Viana (1441–61), recited in 1463, there is a long list of disabled people who are healed at the passage of Carlos's bier with a description of the many apparatuses used by the disabled to get around. The kind of rocking seat depicted in the Vatican panel is described in verse 168 as "qui testudineo perreptant corpora gyro," which may be translated as, "those who drag their body on a shell in the shape of a tortoise" or "those who drag their body on a tortoise's shell." My thanks to Silvia Rizzo for this information and the reference to the text where the panegyric was published, Michael D. Reeve, "The Rediscovery of Classical Text in the Renaissance," in *Itinerari dei testi antichi*, Oronzo Pecere (ed.), Rome, 1991, pp. 115–157, esp. pp. 148 ff., verses 149–169.

78 Vauchez, *Sainthood*, pp. 444–477.

79 Ibid., p. 453.

80 Ibid., pp. 453–454.

81 Ibid., p. 456. Vauchez lists the offerings found at the tomb of St. Thomas Cantilupe in Hereford Cathedral during an investigation initiated by Clement V to learn what miracles had been performed. The list included: 170 silver ships (that had been saved from a storm), 41 wax ships, 129 silver images of a person or of human limbs, 1,424 wax images of a person or of human limbs, 77 animal figures, 108 crutches, 3 wooden vehicles. See Vauchez, *Sainthood*, pp. 456–457.

82 The significant reassuring sign of the regained ambulatory powers of formerly disabled individuals represented by the painted votive tablets depicting the miracle or cure brought about by saintly or divine intercession has a long history. The tradition goes back to antiquity, when such painted tablets were left in temples, as attested by Cicero's comments in *De Natura Deorum*, p. 375. The tradition of painted votive tablets presented by supplicants at the temples is also corroborated by Tibullus in *Elegies* (I, 3, 27–28). Cited by Stefano Papetti, "Gli ex voto: la 'Sistina dei poveri,'" in *Per grazia ricevuta: gli ex voto del Museo di San Nicola a Tolentino*, Tolentino, 2005, p. 7. On the Vanni Altarpiece see Fredrika H. Jacobs, *Votive Panels and Popular Piety in Early Modern Italy*, New York, 2013, p. 156: "Although not visibly present, the martyred saint possesses a vital presence that at once refers to the *praesentia* documented by her *eikōn* [the central image of the saint in the altarpiece] and the *potentia* of her relics avowed by the pilgrims gathered around her tomb and the testaments to her postmortem interventions suspended from a tie rod above it – *immagini* of arms, heads, hands, breast, and thighs." According to Jacobs, although votive tablets were used in the Classical period, these all but disappeared in the West during the Middle Ages. Their resurgence occurred around 1470, while their disappearance took place around 1610.

83 On Leon Battista Alberti's treatise *De pictura*, published in 1435 in Latin and, for the benefit of artists, in Italian in 1436, see *On Painting*, Rocco Sinisgalli (tr.), Cambridge, 2011.

84 Although between 1201 and 1300 miracles involving people with motor problems accounted for the highest percentage (28.8), followed by individuals with contagious and organic illnesses (28.6), between 1301 and 1417 these two types of miracles took on an inverted trend, with those involving illnesses reaching 31.2 percent and those pertaining to the orthopedically impaired dropping to a surprising 12.5 percent. On the possible explanations for this statistical inversion, see Vauchez, *Sainthood*, pp. 468–470.

85 *Butler's Lives of the Saints*, IV, pp. 334–335. My thanks to Monsignor Achille Bonazzi at the Ufficio Beni Culturali Ecclesiastici-Diocesi di Cremona and Dr. Francesca Campana for their help in tracking down the Codex IX, procuring the image and giving permission to reproduce the illumination on folio 224.

86 Robert Davidsohn, *Storia di Firenze*, 3 vols., orig. title *Geschicte von Florenz*, Florence, 1957, III, pp. 323–324: "Sfugge a ogni valutazione quello che facevano i privati, mentre abbiamo un punto di riferimento per calcolare quello che i monasteri facevano per i poveri, attraverso le loro somministrazioni di pane. Infatti apprendiamo che a volte le case dei religiosi assorbivano un buon quinto di tutto

il frumento che entrava in città; e poiché la popolazione monastica assommava solo all'1% di tutta la fiorentina, se ne deduce (e la notizia ci è tramandata proprio a questo proposito) che erano i frati e le monache che davano agli affamati quel tozzo di pane che valeva a sottrarli alla morte per inedia." ("There is no way of knowing what private citizens did, while one may gather what the monasteries did for the poor through their donation of bread. In fact we learn that at times the religious orders received well over a fifth of all the wheat that was brought into the city. And since the monastic community amounted to only 1% of the Florentine population, one may surmise (and the information has been handed down to posterity exactly for this reason) that it was the friars and the nuns who gave to starving individuals that crust of bread that saved them from dying of starvation.") Paolo Liverani, "Saint Peter's and the City of Rome between Late Antiquity and the early Middle Ages," in *Old Saint Peter's, Rome*, Rosamond McKitterick, John Osborne, Carol M. Richardson and Joanna Story (eds.), Cambridge, 2013, p. 27: "If alms giving to the indigent took place in the form of distributions of bread – as was normal for the *annona* at least since the time of Aurelian – we ought not to think that near the basilica of the apostle Saint Peter there existed only one structure for distribution."

87 Andrea di Bartolo's tempera painting measures 44.2 × 32.6 cm. See http://www.nga.gov/content/ngaweb/Collection/art-object-page.184.html (last accessed July 23, 2014). Another example of alms being doled out in the form of bread is Domenico di Bartolo's fresco depicting the *Reception of Pilgrims and Distribution of Alms* (1442) in the Pellegrinaio of the Ospedale di Santa Maria della Scala in Siena, for which see S. Roettgen, *Italian Frescoes: The Early Renaissance 1400–1470*, New York, 1996, pp. 186–203.

88 The text was discovered by the French humanist Guillaume Postel (died in 1582). The author, however, was not James the Great, son of Zebedee and brother of John the Evangelist; rather, James the Less, "brother of the Lord." See Luigi Moraldi (ed.), *Apocrifi del Nuovo Testamento*, Turin, 1971, p. 61.

89 The text here reproduced is taken from Shelley Matthews's translation based on the Greek text printed in Ronald F. Hock's *The Infancy Gospels of James and Thomas*, found on the web at http://www.earlychristianwritings.com/text/infancyjames-hock.html (last accessed on July 14, 2014). For information on the Andrea di Bartolo image in the National Gallery, see note 87.

90 Piero Camporesi, *Il libro dei vagabondi*, Milan, 2003, p. 377. Robert Davidsohn, *Storia di Firenze*, 3 vols., Florence, 1957, III, pp. 323–324.

91 Lilian Brion-Guerry, *Le thème du "Triomphe de la Mort" dans la peinture italienne*, Paris, 1950. See also Thomas Riis, "I poveri nell'arte italiana (secoli XV–XVIII)," in *Timore e carità: i poveri nell'Italia moderna*, Giorgio Politi, Mario Rosa and Franco della Peruta (eds.), Cremona, 1982, pp. 45–58, esp. pp. 54–55.

92 Traditionally believed to have developed *after* the Black Death of 1348, the theme is now seen as having come about before or slightly after 1340. See Antonio Caleca, "Costruzione e decorazione dalle origini al secolo XV," in *Il Camposanto di Pisa*, Clara Baracchini and Enrico Castelnuovo (eds.), Turin, 1996, pp. 13–48. My thanks to Jean Cadogan for pointing out this article to me. For a reference to the traditional interpretation see Riis, p. 55, quoting Brion-Guerry, p. 129.

93 Ibid. Brion-Guerry, p. 120, cites Vasari, who had stated that the version in Santa Croce in Florence was similar to the one in Pisa but of better artistic quality.

94 Ibid.: "Poi che prosperitade ci à llasciati,/o Morte, medicina di ongi [*sic*] pena,/dè vienci a dare ormai l'ultima cena." Brion-Guerry, p. 120: "Dacché prosperitade ci ha lasciati/Ho morte, medicina d'ogni pena, deh, vien/Ci dare omai l'ultima cena."

95 John Henderson, "'Mal Francese' in Sixteenth-Century Rome: The Ospedale di San Giacomo in Augusta and the 'Incurabili,'" in *Popolazione e società a Roma dal medioevo all'età contemporanea*, Eugenio Sonnino (ed.), Rome, 1998, p. 483.

96 Jérôme Fracastor, *La syphilis ou le mal français*, Jacqueline Vons (ed.), Paris, 2011, p. XVII.

97 Ibid.

98 Ibid., p. XX.

99 Ibid., pp. XXII–XXIII. The full title of the medical tract is, *Nova poenitentialis Quadragesima necnon purgatorium in morbum gallicum sive venereum una cum Dialogo aquae argenti ac ligni guaiaci colluctantium*

super dicti morbis curationis praelatura, opus fructiferum, a Jacobo Abethencourt [...] nuper editum [...], Paris, 1527.

100 Fracastor, p. XXXV. Ibid., p. 81, Book III, vv. 331–332: "Insomnes primus noctes conuulsaque membra/sensit, et a primo traxit cognomina morbus,/Syphilidenque ab eo labem dixere coloni." ("The first to witness the sleepless nights and the pain that torments the body, and it is from him, as he was the first to fall ill, that the disease derives its name: the peasants called it *syphilis*, from the name Syphilis.")

101 Peter Lewis Allen, *The Wages of Sin: Sex and Disease, Past and Present*, Chicago and London, 2000, p. 41.

102 Ibid.

103 Quoted by Henderson, "'Mal Francese,'" p. 484. My italics.

104 Lewis Allen, p. 52. See also Franz Swediaur, *Complete Treatise on the Symptoms, Effects, Nature and Treatment of Syphilis*, Thomas T. Hewson (tr.), Philadelphia, 1815, esp. chapter 16.

105 See Daniele Benati, "Annibale Carracci e il vero," in *Annibale Carracci*, Daniele Benati and Eugenio Riccòmini (eds.), Milan, 2006, pp. 27–29, and Ulrich Pfisterer, "*L'Elemosina di san Rocco* di Annibale Carracci e l'innovazione della *historia* cristiana," in *Programme et invention dans l'art de la Renaissance*, Michel Hochmann (ed.), Rome, 2008, pp. 247–269. See also Claire Robertson, *The Invention of Annibale Carracci*, Cinisello Balsamo, 2008, pp. 96 and 198, pl. 82a. For a description of the "invalid" in the painting see Giovan Pietro Bellori, *The Lives of the Modern Painters, Sculptors and Architects*, Alice Sedgwick Wohl (tr.), Cambridge, 2005, pp. 75–76.

106 *The Illustrated Bartsch*, Walter L. Strauss, John T. Spike and Isabelle de Ramaix (eds.), 108 vols., New York, 1978–, XLVII, part 1, p. 209, no. 004.

107 For this fresco and Paolo de Matteis in general see Livio Pestilli, *Paolo de Matteis: Neapolitan Painting and Cultural History in Baroque Europe*, Farnham, 2013, p. 177 and pl. 52.

108 Henderson, "'Mal Francese,'" pp. 486 and 490.

109 Quoted by Vauchez, *Sainthood*, p. 390.

110 Mollat, p. 23: "It was Jerome who issued the famous invitation to 'follow naked the naked Christ' (*Nudus nudm Christum sequi*)."

111 See Giovanni Villani, *Cronica*, 3 vols., Florence, 1847, III, X:162, p. 150; pp. 149–150: "Per lo gran fatto che allora fu tenuto n'avemo fatta memoria, e per dare buono esempio a chi per l'anima sua vorrà fare limosina a' poveri di Cristo." Also cited by Henderson, *Piety and Charity in Late Medieval Florence*, p. 258.

112 My italics. According to Samuel K. Cohn, Jr., *Death and Prosperity in Siena, 1205–1800: Strategies for the Afterlife*, Baltimore and London, 1988, p. 27, who quotes from Richard C. Trexler, "The Bishop's Portion: Generic Pious Legacies in the Late Middle Ages in Italy," *Traditio*, 28 (1972): 433–436, "to identify 'the poor,' notaries in the testaments before the Black Death of 1348 instead usually labeled them *pauperes cristi*."

113 The term *pauperes Christi* was first used by St. Ambrose in *Ep.* 21.33. See Giles Constable, *The Reformation of the Twelfth Century*, Cambridge, 1996, p. 148, n. 103.

114 Brian Pullan, "Support and Redeem: Charity and Poor Relief in Italian Cities from the Fourteenth to the Seventeenth Century," in *Poverty and Charity: Europe, Italy, Venice, 1400–1700*, Aldershot, 1994, p. 201.

115 Ibid., p. 202.

116 Of course, in the artistic world lameness continued to maintain the negative connotation of imperfection it had had since antiquity, for causes that were quite separate from the sociological reasons here adduced. Writing about which of the two arts of painting and sculpture is superior and of the necessity of mastering both theory and practice, Benedetto Varchi stressed that "e sempre che vi manchi o l'una o l'altra di queste, è necessario che l'arte zoppichi" ("and should you fail to master one or the other of these two, [your] art will inevitably be lame"), Benedetto Varchi, "Della maggioranza delle arti," in *Scritti d'arte del Cinquecento*, 3 vols., Paola Barocchi (ed.), Milan and Naples, 1971, I, p. 14. Responding to Varchi about this very topic of the *paragone* between painting and sculpture, Tribolo answered, "perchè la natura non inganna l'uomini: s'è uno zoppo,

lo mostra, se è bello, bello ve lo mostra" ("because Nature does not fool humanity: if one is lame, it will reveal him so; if handsome, handsome will he appear"), ibid., I, p. 518. Vasari, in his life of Michelangelo, referring to the giant marble block that was to become the *David*, claims that the *Gigante*, which had been begun and then discontinued by two other artists, had been ruined, "storpiato" ("crippled").

117 To this day the epithet "un povero cristo" is used in Italian to refer to a poor man, a poor beggar, a poor wretch, a down-and-outer. Mollat, p. 226: "By the end of the fourteenth century the idea of the poor as a 'dangerous class' had come close to supplanting the image of the pauper as God's chosen and a symbol of Christ."

3 Parasites

> The parasite, however, thinking that everything is all right and thoroughly convinced it would not be any better if it were other than it is, eats and sleeps in great peace and comfort, with nothing of that sort annoying him, flat on his back, with his arms and legs flung out, like Odysseus sailing home from Scheria.
>
> (Lucian, *The Parasite. Parasitic an Art*[1])

Societies may comprise progressive and conservative people, the former aiming for an inclusive and the latter for a more exclusive community; the first group of individuals more willing to help those members who have been less fortunate by birth or chance to improve their lot in life, the second more prone to protect its privileges and less inclined to change the status quo. However, the one thing both, reformists and traditionalists, have in common is a mistrust of "spongers," who, like Terence's (195/185–159 BC) Gnatho in *The Eunuch*, made it a profession to live a life of ease at the expense of others – so much so in the case of Gnatho that he could envision having a school named after him: "When that wretched starveling saw me complimented in this way and getting a living so easily, the fellow at once fell to begging me give him lessons in the business. I told him to become my disciple in the hope that, as schools of philosophers have their names from their masters, so hangers-on may be called Gnathonists."[2] Memorably captured also by Lucian (ca. AD 125 to after 180) in the character of Simon the "Parasitic," Classical authors satirized individuals who shirked work while expecting others to provide for them.[3] The problem is a recurring one in the history of humankind and the way societies have responded to the real or perceived threat posed by those considered to be freeloaders to the more industrious members of their community is a captivating story that is reflected in Italian art of the sixteenth and seventeenth centuries.

As mentioned in Chapter 1, envisioning a Utopia rid of all undesirable features that real societies face, Plato (ca. 429–347 BC) suggested that legislators enact a strict statute that would eliminate all forms of begging.[4] Plato's summon did not make any allowance for situations when such comportment may be not only justified but also endorsed by a community that attempts to leave no one behind. Centuries later, *The Code of Justinian* focused more realistically on the crux of the matter.[5] Unlike Plato's design for a perfect society, Roman legislation differentiated between those individuals who begged out of necessity, because they had been afflicted by disease, and those who were brought to this condition out of laziness. In the eyes of many, this was probably a just ruling, for, while everyone could empathize with people whose inactivity was dictated by physical incapacity, this might not happen in instances when the beggar chose, out of sheer indolence, to live off "the fat of the land."

That this was a widespread sentiment, not limited to the pagan Greeks and Romans but equally shared by the Christian communities, one may gather from Paul's second letter to the Thessalonians, where he warns:

> In the name of the Lord Jesus Christ, we urge you, brothers, to keep away from any of the brothers who refuses to work or to live according to the tradition we passed on to you. You know how you are supposed to imitate us: now we were not idle when we were with you, nor did we ever have our meals at anyone's table without paying for them; no, we worked night and day, slaving and straining, so as not to be a burden on any of you. This was not because we had no right to be, but in order to make ourselves an example for you to follow. We gave you a rule when we were with you: not to let anyone have any food if he refused to do any work. Now we hear that there are some of you who are living in idleness, doing no work themselves but interfering with everyone else's. In the Lord Jesus Christ, we order and call on people of this kind to go on quietly working and earning the food that they eat.[6]

Indeed, concomitantly with the Early Church Fathers discussed earlier in this book, whose homiletics stressed that the character of the beggar did not matter since alms given to the destitute were actually being given to God,[7] some representatives of the Christian community associated able-bodied beggars with indolence and were thus less prone to justify their way of life. More skeptical than the likes of John Chrysostom and Gregory of Nazianzus, as we saw in Chapter 1, Epiphanius of Salamis (ca. 315–403), for example, already in the fourth century attacked the Messalian vagrants for begging on the streets of Antioch.[8] These ascetics, who pursued an apostolic model of monastic life that focused on prayer, did not engage in work and depended on material support from others. Thus, by embracing voluntary poverty these Syrian monks were creating a dangerous precedent for society and the established Church at large.[9]

By the early fifth century Nilus of Ancyra (ca. 390–430) similarly followed the Pauline approach to human inactivity in his *On Voluntary Poverty* by prescribing a moderate regimen of manual labor for the indolent members of the Christian community, as he was especially concerned by the impact that "pseudo-monks," who had abandoned the austere life in the country monasteries and adopted a life of ascetic vagrancy in the cities, might have on others.[10]

> The cities are being overwhelmed by those who wander around them at random. People in their houses are being mobbed and look in disgust at the very sight of them planted at their gates, begging utterly without shame. Many even gain entry into houses where they feign piety for a while. Cloaking their mischief with the mask of hypocrisy, they later go away after defrauding their hosts.[11]

Not surprisingly, this ambivalent attitude towards beggars in the Christian world – to condone or to condemn their *modus vivendi* – resurged in the Middle Ages and, as evident from Gratian's *Decrees* and the twelfth-century Decretists, beggars were now seen to fall into two categories:

the "honest" and "dishonest."[12] Among these authors, Stephen of Tournai was to distinguish the difference between *hospitalitas* and *liberalitas*, that is, between almsgiving and welfare.[13] As Bronislaw Geremek elucidates: "*hospitalitas* is unconditional: its principle is that 'we provide for all those for whom it is in our power to provide' .... *Liberalitas*, on the other hand, must distinguish between the 'honest' and the 'dishonest', 'kin' and 'strangers', old and young, humble and arrogant, and provide aid to the first in each of these categories"[14] – a differentiation that by the fifteenth century acquired a definite class distinction in the theory and practice of charity that privileged the "shame-faced" poor (*pauperes verecundi* in Latin or *poveri vergognosi* in Italian) – that is, those whose ill fortune had brought them to a lower social status and were ashamed to stoop so low as to go begging in the streets.[15] The Decretists' attitude towards beggars could oscillate between the more discriminating approach, represented in late antiquity by St. Ambrose and St. Augustine, to the more inclusive attitude of St. John Chrysostom.[16] Their common sentiment, however, was not to consider the state of poverty a moral defect.[17]

Regardless of these distinctions, problems arose for the Church when the mendicant orders in the twelfth and thirteenth centuries also attempted a return to the Early Christian roots and adopted begging as their sole means of sustainment. In fact, this caused sufficient preoccupation for the Church to induce Pope Innocent III to approve St. Francis's *Rule* and sanction his order, thus making sure that these mendicant friars would keep operating within the Church's parameters.[18]

Although in the Medieval period voluntary poverty was considered praiseworthy, by the early fourteenth century pontifical documents cease to refer to poverty as the greatest of virtues.[19] Perhaps in response to the conflict that arose within the bosom of the mendicant order over the interpretation of St. Francis's prohibition against money and property, saints were now officially praised more for their piety and obedience to the Church than for their indigence.[20] This attitude is understandable, as the excessive exaltation of poverty reflected adversely on the papacy and its curia.[21] As the thirteenth-century evangelical ideal represented by the mendicant orders was superseded in the fourteenth century by the Church's valorization of culture and orthodoxy, the realistic character of evangelical poverty was replaced by the vaguer concept of "spiritual poverty." In fact, indigence was now seen as a distraction to the contemplative man.[22]

It is against this background that one must view the resurgence of literary interest in beggars and the concomitant artistic response to the phenomenon in fifteenth- and sixteenth-century Europe. Works such as Leon Battista Alberti's *Momus* (written between 1443 and 1450 and circulated in manuscript form before being published in 1520), Erasmus's colloquy *Beggar Talk* (1524) and Cornelius Agrippa's *De incertitudine et vanitate scientiarum et artium* (ca. 1530) were obviously inspired by the rediscovery and translation of Classical precedents, their satirical or critical comments about beggars being clearly indebted to authors such as Terence and Lucian.[23]

The literary sketches these authors painted of their idle protagonists revolve around their freedom from worldly care, the life of ease that they lead and their ability to procure their necessities from others without lifting a finger. Thus, in Momus's view, "a beggar grazes on the sweat and hard work of others, he misuses his leisure as he pleases, he asks freely, says no with impunity, and takes from everyone, because the wretched give voluntarily and the fortunate won't refuse."[24] Indeed, from the beggars' perspective, at least as interpreted by the intellectuals and the ruling class, they were better off than monarchs, as Irides explains to Misoponus in Erasmus's colloquy:

> I wouldn't trade this 'misery' even for kings' wealth .... The freedom, than which nothing is sweeter, belongs to no king more than it does to us. I don't doubt there are many kings who envy us. Whether there's war or peace, we're safe. We're not drafted for the army; we're not called to public offices; we're not taxed when the public is plundered by levies .... Neither in peace nor in war may kings enjoy themselves, and the mightier they are the more men they fear. The common people have a superstitious dread of harming us, as though we were under God's protection.[25]

With Gutenberg's introduction of movable type (ca. 1439) and the greater dissemination of literary works to a wider public than preceding generations, the seminal mistrust for freeloaders expressed in antiquity and in the Middle Ages by the late sixteenth- and the beginning of the seventeenth century acquired greater currency and found ancillary support in the visual arts, primarily in prints. Actually, although by this time in "high" art destined for public and religious venues beggars were represented as "ideal" or deserving, in woodcuts, engravings and etchings they tended to be portrayed as false, while the orthopedically impaired, so often used compassionately to extol Christian *caritas* and as evidence of a saint's healing power of body and soul, were now being used to stigmatize beggars as rogues and swindlers; parasites who made it their profession to beguile and deceive able-bodied, industrious citizens.[26] This dichotomy in beggar imagery may have various reasons for being, but one is certainly that in works of public and religious import the artifacts were undoubtedly seen as reflecting the patrons' social status and decorum was an essential element of "serious" art. In popular prints, however, artists and their clientele would have no such qualms in depicting able-bodied or lame mendicants as they were perceived by mainstream society: intrusive and pestering individuals.[27]

In fact, simulating a disability so as to procure alms has never been seen in a favorable light. If the infirmity flaunted also happens to be among the easiest to enact and the simplest to unmask, then it is inevitable that this particular form of incapacity could represent the very symbol of deceit. Such became lameness or halting as it gave rise to the Italian proverb "più tosto si arriva a un bugiardo, che uno zoppo" ("a liar is sooner caught than a cripple"),[28] with the explicit reference to the disability paraded by the pseudo-lame individual who, when necessary, could "miraculously" regain the use of the affected member so as to avoid being caught by someone in their pursuit.[29] Actually, this proverb reflects anecdotes present throughout Europe about pseudo-cripples who wondrously regain their ambulatory powers. One of these stories refers to two "paralytics" who learn of the miracles that took place during the transfer of St. Martin's relics from Auxerre to Tours. In one version of the story, "the two paralytics therefore decide to flee and, in their haste, throw the crutches on which they leaned while begging over their shoulders: thus the miracle was accomplished nonetheless."[30] Another version was widely disseminated because it was included in the *Life* of St. Martin as told by Jacobus de Voragine (1230–1298) in his *Golden Legend*, one of the most widely read works that had an impact on people from the Middle Ages well into the modern era. It involves a blind man and a cripple, with the former hauling the latter in a cart: "by begging this way they made a good living."[31] When they heard that the body of St. Martin during its translation might come too close to the house where they lived and that they "by chance might be made whole – which they did not want to happen, because it would deprive them of their income – they moved to another abode." At this point Jacobus de Voragine does not resist including the pernicious punch line that tainted the impression many able-bodied people had of the disabled: "But just as they were moving, they met the body being carried in procession, and since God bestows blessings even on those who do not ask for them, the two partners found themselves completely cured against their will and were sorely aggrieved at this turn of fortune."[32] Even if it had been a true story, it is difficult to invoke a more cynical interpretation of an incident whereby the disabled benefitting from the miraculous intervention wish it had not occurred.[33] To be sure, the impression that behind a beggar's halting gait there might be an impostor is a recurring motif, especially in a period of increasing, widespread poverty that refined human wits and the art of survival. "Inexhaustible, too, were the techniques and subtle tactics triggered by hunger. The school of poverty was indeed the mother of invention. Then as never before was the truth of the proverb felt: "*sola est paupertas, artes quae suscitat omnes* [poverty is one, the arts it engenders are innumerable]."[34]

Emblematic of the cultural and social change in the perception of the lame in Renaissance and Baroque Italy, is a booklet entitled *L'arte della forfanteria cantata da Gian Pitocco Fornaro alla sua amata Signora* (*The Art of Roguery Sung by John the Beggar Baker to his Beloved Lady*) published in 1618 (Figure 3.1).[35] In this work, dedicated to the swindlers (*baroni*) in Rome's Piazza di Campo de' Fiori, the author found no better image to capture the spirit of the pamphlet than to publish on its frontispiece the print of a fake lame who proceeds through the street with the aid of a cane, crutch and a cup for collecting alms.[36] Equally indicative of this mindset is a 1675 print by Giuseppe Maria Mitelli (1634–1718) of a vendor of ribbons, lace and needles ("Venditore di fiocchi, merletti ed aghi) (Figure 3.2). Beneath the image a clear message is sent to all those women who might buy these items from such a vendor: "Abhor this man, ladies – I'll set it down in writing – because you'll fall into some trap. Even a righteous [male] purchaser will fear frequenting a lame vendor." ("Aborrite costui vel lascio scritto/Donne, ch'inciamperete in qualche intoppo./Che teme insino un comprator diritto/Il praticar un venditor, ch'è Zoppo.")[37]

There were certainly individuals in the middle of the sixteenth century who, like Domingo de Soto in his *In causa pauperum deliberatio* published initially in Salamanca in 1545 in Spanish and Latin, with a second Latin edition appearing in Venice in 1547,[38] still paraphrased authors such as Maximus the Confessor (ca. 580–662) who had claimed, "He that [*sic*] in imitation of God does almsdeeds knows no difference between evil and good, just and unjust, in regard to the needs of the body, but distributes equally to all according to their need, even though for his good intention he prefers the virtuous to the bad."[39] However, to better understand representations such as the frontispiece of *L'arte della forfanteria*, one must take a closer look at how secular and religious authorities responded to the growing problem of poverty and how they attempted to eradicate begging.[40]

It has been noted that in sixteenth-century urban centers people tolerated the poor and their cost to the community in the form of assistance so long as the number of the poor did not exceed 3–4 percent of the overall population.[41] If one considers that in times of famine, such as during the serious agrarian crises between 1586 and 1590,[42] the level of the poor

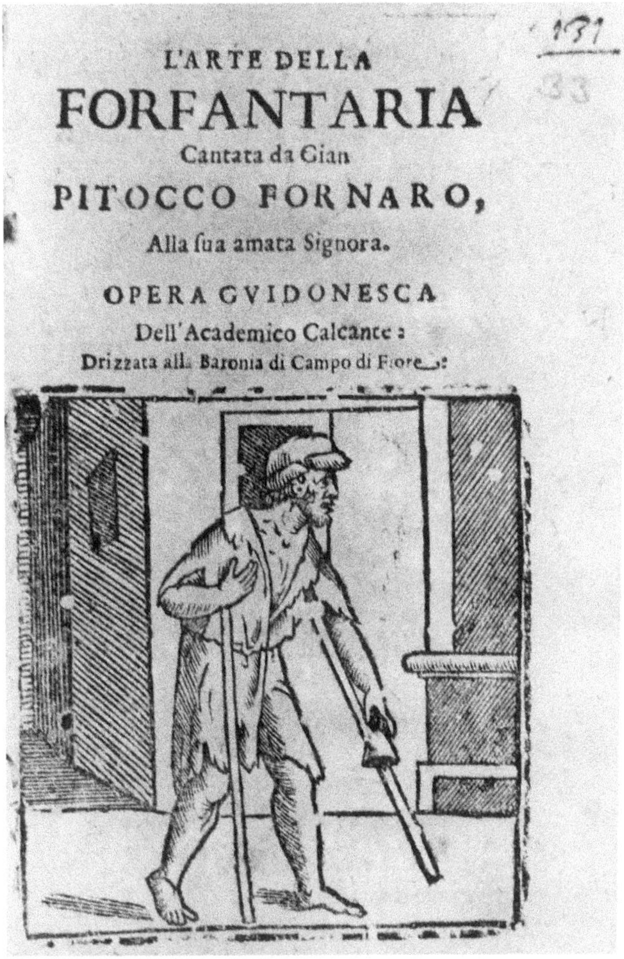

L'ARTE DELLA

FORFANTARIA

Cantata da Gian

PITOCCO FORNARO,

Alla ſua amata Signora.

OPERA GVIDONESCA

Dell'Academico Calcante:

Drizzata alla Baronia di Campo di Fiore.

Figure 3.1 *L'arte della forfanteria*, Biblioteca Apostolica Vaticana, 1618. Photo: Biblioteca Apostolica Vaticana

reached even 20 percent of the population, it was inevitable that the rest of society would feel imperiled and that conceptually it lumped the idle, the vagrant, the mendicant and the peasants, who invaded the cities in search of some means of nourishment, into a single threatening group.[43] On an ethical level, of course, the menace was not posed by the truly disabled, since many of them were really unable to earn a living. Rather, the problem was mostly raised by vagabonds – those whom the Franciscan Berthold of Regensburg in the thirteenth century placed, along with the Jews and strolling jongleurs, in the "family of the devil"[44] – for, by moving from place to place with no permanent abode, they were frequently suspected of being disease carriers and, even more, because, being unknown to the local prospective benefactor, they would often be seen as impostors whose laziness prompted them to obtain alms by faking ailments or physical infirmities.[45]

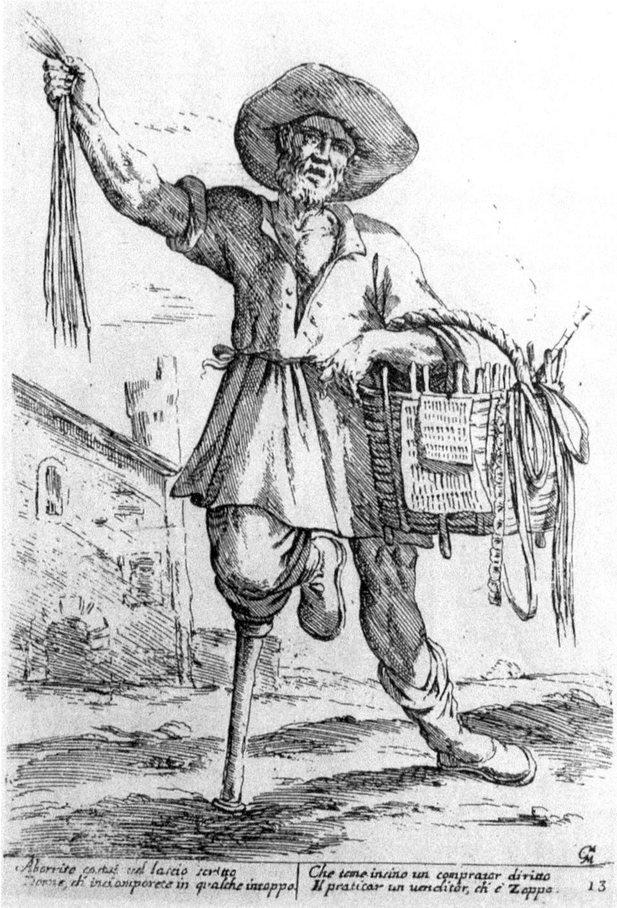
Che teme insino un comprator diritto
Il praticar un uenditor, ch' è Zoppo.
13

Figure 3.2 Giuseppe Maria Mitelli, *Vendor of Ribbons, Lace and Needles*, 1675. Photo: *The Illustrated Bartsch*, XLII, p. 427

On a moral level, these simulators not only deprived the truly poor local mendicants of their means of sustenance but also deceived the charitable donor. As Sharon Farmer poignantly elucidates: "Just like the man who gave money to a prostitute, the almsgiver expected an intimate favor in return: the beggar, whom the almsgiver believed to be both needy and unable to work, was supposed to say prayers for the soul of the one from whom he, or she, accepted alms. If the beggar was not truly disabled, then the one giving alms was 'buying' prayers, in a sense, from the wrong person."[46] Actually, in early modern Europe the poor had ironically come to represent "an 'order' or estate in the economy of salvation,"[47] for almsgiving had become a way for individuals to redeem their sins and thus was "a natural part of God's plan of salvation."[48] The poor, in other words, came to be part of an "economics of salvation" as poverty acquired a spiritual function: through charity, the rich were given the possibility of buying their salvation and the poor, whose primary function was to receive, found their justification in the divine plan.[49] Nevertheless, one might add, what this state of affairs indicates is that all of the emphasis on charity was just a reflection of a bad social conscience.[50]

The myriad guises under which a begging impostor might hide may be gathered from a manuscript in the Estense Library in Modena, where a total of forty-one *trionfi* or *rase* (frauds) by swindlers are listed. Among these are the following: the *rase delle sossolle*, that is, to deceive someone by simulating lameness with the aid of crutches; the *rasa di moscardino*, to fraud an individual by pretending the loss of one or both arms; the *rasa di mandragolla*, to cheat one by faking the amputation of one's feet; and the *rasa di desteso*, to beguile a donor by lying prostrate in front of a church.[51] This world of cheats is corroborated by two young Roman mendicants who, interrogated by the pontifical police in 1595, enumerated a total of thirty *compagnie* of swindlers operating in Rome.[52] These *compagnie* were a common phenomenon present in all of Europe that saw as protagonists groups of destitute vagrants who tried to survive the hardships of life by using their wits. These mendicants not only operated in groups but also developed their own language, or cant, that gave them a sense of communal bond.[53] Paradoxically, paraphrasing and simplifying Northrop Frye's differentiation between tragedy and comedy – the former being characterized by the isolation of a leader from his society, the latter, reversing this process, by a central figure who creates his or her own society "in the teeth of strong opposition"[54] – one might say that by creating their own impenetrable jargon these mendicants were "comically" excluding from their underworld the very members of society whose probity and prevailing mores had marginalized them. In this upside-down world the outcasts formed a subculture or brotherhood that, in the face of adversity, did what it could to survive.

Thus, in Rome there were, among others, the *Compagnia delli Baroni*, that is, those individuals who were healthy but lazy and did not want to work; the *Compagnia delli Rabrunati*, mendicants who, pretending to be afflicted by a mental disorder, fell to the ground emitting foam from their mouth duly produced by a soapy mixture previously ingested; the *Compagnia delli Trabocchi*, comprising individuals who made believe they were lame by leaning on crutches; and the *Compagnia delli Abbici*, the poor blind or those feigning blindness who begged for a living.

The person most responsible for popularizing the notion that mendicants were to be mistrusted was Teseo Pini in a treatise written around 1485. This work remained in manuscript form until 1621 when it was "updated" by the Dominican Giacinto Nobili, who published it under the pseudonym Rafaele Frianoro by the title *Il Vagabondo, overo Sferza de' bianti e vagabondi* (*The Vagabond, or The Chastening of Vagrants and Vagabonds*).[55] The forty-three types of vagrants, charlatans, swindlers and downright cheats Teseo Pini had described in *De cerretanorum origine eorumque fallaciis*[56] (1485) in Rafaele Frianoro's text are trimmed down to thirty-four.[57] From the *pitocchi* or *bianti*[58] (that is, vagabonds who frequently falsified and sold papal bulls promising their naïve customers redemption not only from purgatory but also from hell itself) to the *falsi bordoni* or "false pilgrims" (who roved about begging and claiming it had been their vow to undertake their pilgrimage by sustaining themselves strictly by collecting alms[59]), the *accapponi* (who, "with the aid of a powder derived from burnt feathers, hare's blood and other substances, exposed large, repulsive pseudo-sores on their legs"[60]) and the *accadenti* (who "fall down pretending to be afflicted by epilepsy"[61]), the world the author describes is one of a social order mined by fraudulent appearances. Although Frianoro claims that his intention in writing the pamphlet was to protect the readers from the subtle crafts and maliciousness of those who practiced said arts, he paradoxically concludes his work by admonishing: "However, without judging others, and having always a good opinion of everyone, you will keep distant from all and trust few people."[62]

Against this backdrop of social mistrust, a decisive step towards the elimination of mendicancy and its deceitful exponents was taken in the early sixteenth century with the publication of *De subventione pauperum* (*On Assistance to the Poor*) written by the Spanish Juan Luis Vivès and published in Italian in Venice in 1545.[63] In this work the old Franciscan ideal of aiding the Poor of Christ was totally abandoned. Indeed, for Vivès, Christ's praise for the poor was not to be taken literally: "[He] does not call 'blessed' those who are monetarily poor; rather, those are spiritually so" ("non pauperes pecuniae pronuntiat beatos, sed spiritu").[64] For Vivès, in fact, the Medieval concept of individual and indiscriminate almsgiving should be replaced by a more farsighted, state-funded assistance that, while not denying aid to the truly disabled, would force all able-bodied beggars to find a job.[65] Quoting St. Paul's *Second Letter to the Thessalonians* (3:6–16), he warned against idleness among the poor and feeding those who refused to work. According to Vivès, like Leon Battista Alberti before and Giovanni Botero after him, even the blind should be made to work.[66] Their inactivity, he claimed, was not justified by their disability: theirs was just laziness. In the city where his social experiment might take place, the abolition of mendicancy could be achieved by confining all the really poor to hospices, and by expelling all vagrant, non-native beggars. No doubt, Plato's proscription must have been vividly present in Vivès's mind: "There shall be no begging in the state . . . that our land [may] be entirely cleaned of such creatures."[67]

The scenario delineated helps to better appreciate images such as *Landscape with Five Beggars* (Figure 3.3) derived from a drawing by either Agostino or Annibale Carracci and the print of a *Birbante* or "Rascal" by Giuseppe Maria Mitelli (Figure 3.4).[68] The first engraving depicts five vagrant *monelli* (that is, rascals or thieves), marching across a landscape. In no uncertain terms the couplets at the bottom of the print explain that these individuals, while claiming to be affected by false ailments, roamed about in search of "prey" to defraud. The Latin version of the print states:

> We live by robbery; for our clever hand seeks to gain/secretly the riches, which Fortune has denied./He who pretends to be blind, when fate has offered him something,/sees with sharp-sighted eyes the things that have to be taken./He who staggers with limping step, when he brings back the things that are stolen,/you would believe him, while running, to have winged feet./Let fools labor in finding nourishment for themselves through working./No art is better than the thievish hand.[69]

Moreover, the Italian edition of the print (Figure 3.5) ends with a couplet that fully explains one of the basic reasons why these paupers were so disliked: "*Il calcante ultimo è raro: Che di tutte le feste hà il calendaro*" ("The last beggar is unique, as he has a calendar of all the fairs").[70] By wandering from place to place, following a master plan based on a calendar of all the town fairs where the gathering of large crowds made the collection of alms an easy affair and fraudulent activity an effortless pursuit, these vagabonds became the ultimate symbol of the social parasite.[71]

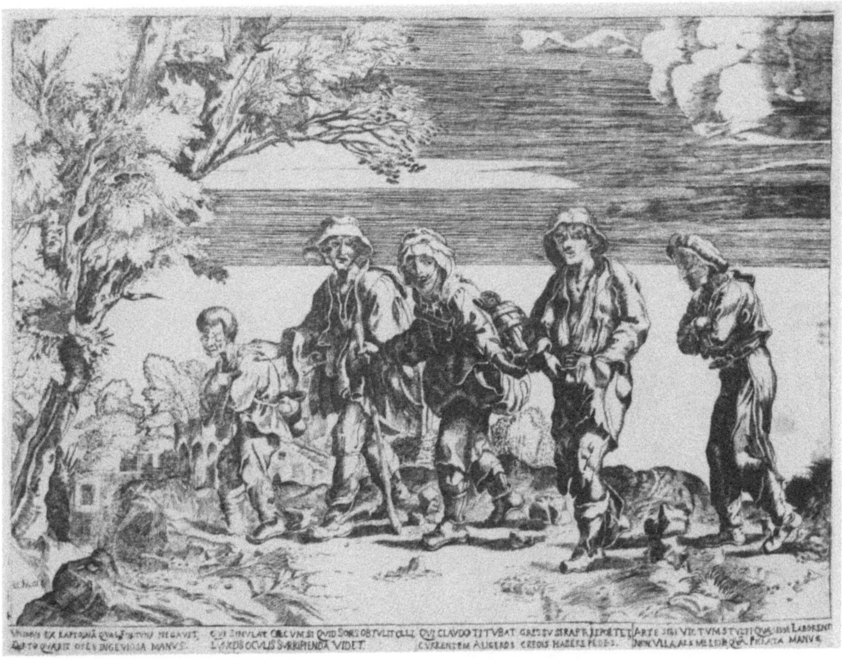

Figure 3.3 Agostino or Annibale Carracci, *Landscape with Five Beggars*. Photo: *The Illustrated Bartsch*, XL, p. 265

Equally condemning of the false lame is Mitelli's print (Figure 3.4) of a rascal who claims, like Erasmus's Irides, he could not be happier than he is with his life of mendicancy: "*Più pitocco, che Ré d'esser mi piace/Poiche senza timor trionfo in terra,/Mi dà tributo ogn'un senza far guerra/E la maggior disgratia è andarne in pace.*" ("I'd rather be a beggar than a king/since in this world I triumph without fear./All pay tribute to me without my waging war/and to be left alone is the worst that can befall.")[72] Of course, the successful reading of the couplets lies in the double meaning of the word *trionfo*, which in the jargon of the underworld meant to "enjoy oneself at table eating and drinking."[73] In other words, this swindler would not trade places with a king since his fraudulent lifestyle assures him a more peaceful and joyful life than could real triumphs to a king. Echoing Leon Battista Alberti's sentiments, in Italy this view of the mendicants was eventually "codified" by Tommaso Garzoni in his *La Piazza Universale di tutte le Professioni del Mondo* where, in discussing cheats ("De' Guidoni, O Furfanti, O Calchi"), he glosses:

> There are some individuals who not as much for want or indigence as out of mere laziness, craftily indulge in a life of sloth and negligence, and cherish no greater happiness than to fraudulently beg for food and alms. This they deem the sweetest and most blessed lifestyle possible .... Now, their swindling profession has no other aim than to cheat the world and furtively enjoy themselves at other people's expense.[74]

Emblematic of able-bodied, bourgeois communities in which social success and financial gain are achieved through diligence and industry, these prints and Garzoni's proclamation make

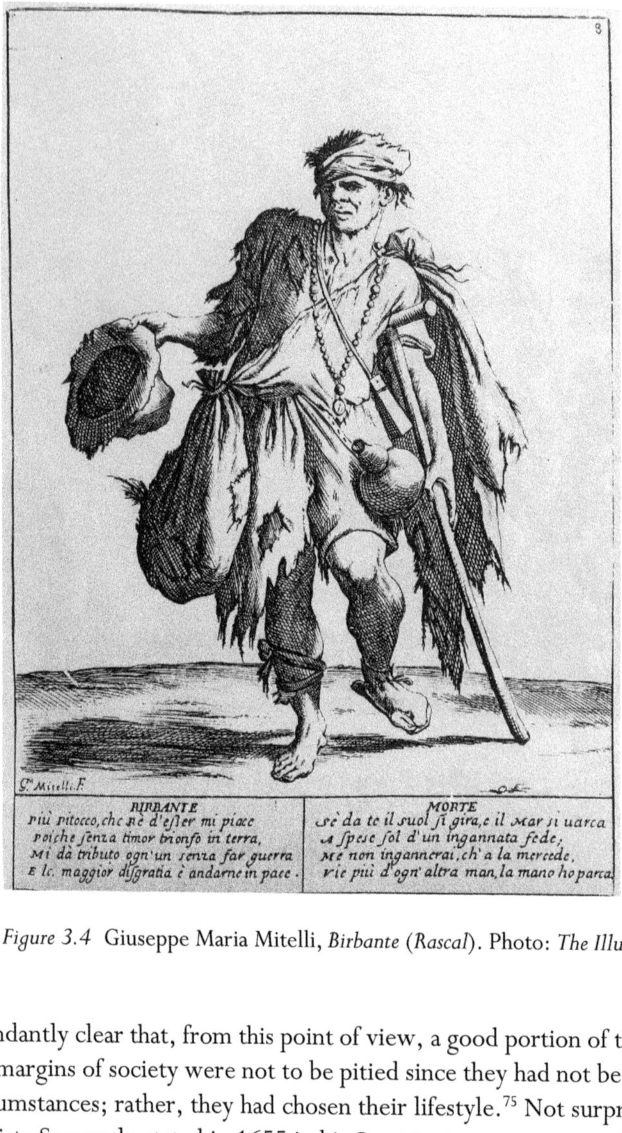
G.M. Mitelli.F.
BIRBANTE
più pitocco, che rè d'esser mi piace
poiche senza timor trionfo in terra,
Mi dà tributo ogn'un senza far guerra
E la maggior disgratia è andarne in pace.
MORTE
Sè da te il suol si gira, e il Mar si varca
A spese sol d'un ingannata fede;
Me non ingannerai, ch'a la mercede,
Vie più d'ogn'altra man, la mano ho parca.

Figure 3.4 Giuseppe Maria Mitelli, *Birbante* (*Rascal*). Photo: *The Illustrated Bartsch*, XIX, p. 449

abundantly clear that, from this point of view, a good portion of the poor and those living on the margins of society were not to be pitied since they had not been forced there by external circumstances; rather, they had chosen their lifestyle.[75] Not surprisingly, as Cardinal Giovan Battista Scanarolo stated in 1655 in his *De visitatione carceratorum* (*On Visiting the Incarcerated*), by this time poverty was seen "no longer [as] the 'bride' of Christ and the saints; rather, the worst ill after death."[76]

Clearly telling of the changing climate and the obdurate, cynical view "normal" society had of mendicants, in general, and of those who exhibited disabilities, in particular, is the broadsheet *Le barrarie del mondo* (*The Swindles of the World*) printed in Rome by Giovanni Antonio de' Pauli around 1590 (Figure 3.6). Out of the sixty-eight figures that populate this microcosm of swindlers and cheats, eleven are individuals whose ambulatory capacity is partially or totally inhibited. Lest the viewer misunderstand the gist of the images, apposite captions are placed beneath the representations of the many crooks infesting the world, who are ready to fraud the first "babe in the woods" they encounter.[77]

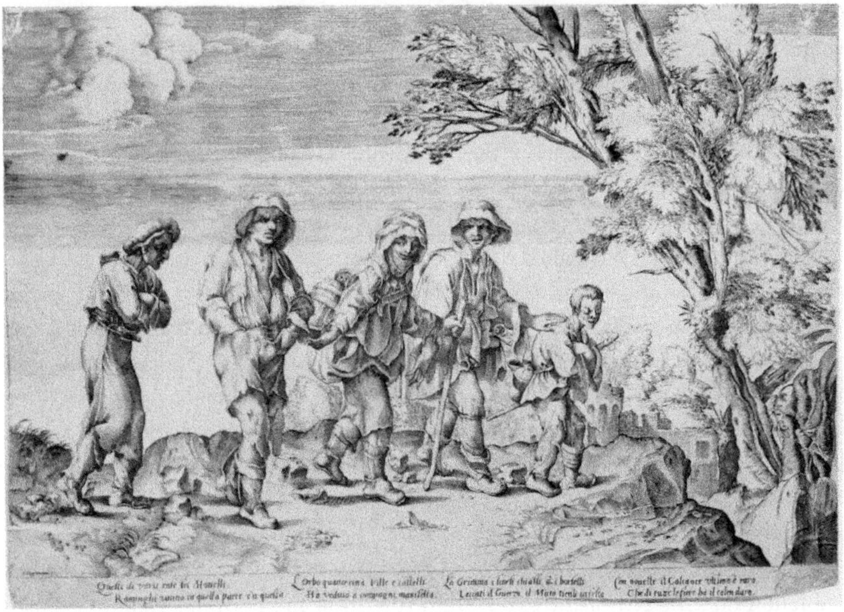

Figure 3.5 Francesco Brizio, Pietro Stephanoni or Pietro Faccini, *Landscape with Five Beggars*. Photo: *The Illustrated Bartsch*, XVIII, p. 143

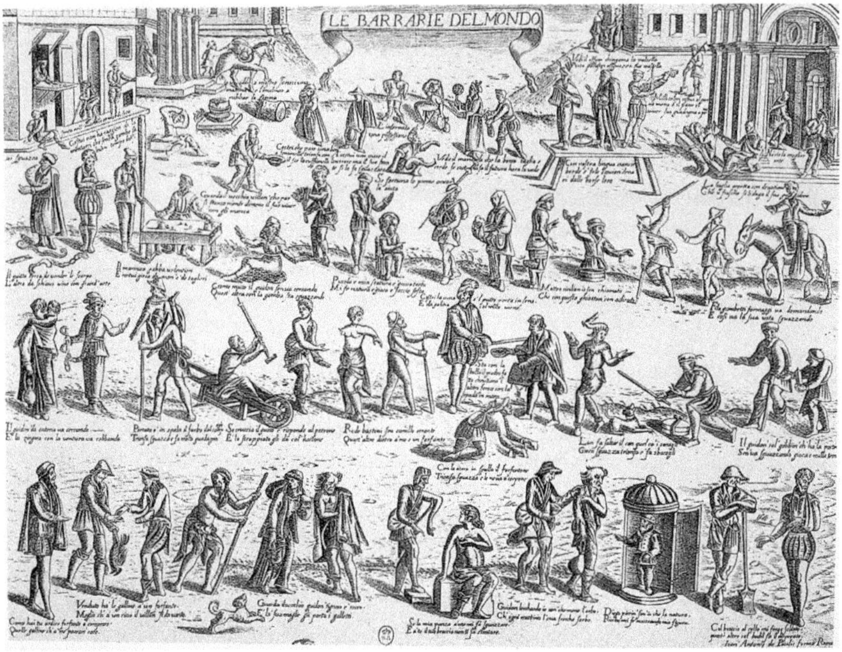

Figure 3.6 Giovanni Antonio de' Pauli, *Le barrarie del mondo*, ca. 1590. Photo: from Helen Langdon, "Bari, zingari e venditori ambulanti," in *Il genio di Roma, 1592–1623,* Beverly L. Brown (ed.), Milan, 2001, p. 46, fig. 12

In the upper left corner of the sheet, next to the entrance to a building, an amputee stands by supporting himself on stilts. Beneath him a gloss explains: "This one has no reason to complain, who, [although] legless, is able to keep himself amused" ("Costui non ha ragion di lamentarsi che senza gambe sa buon tempo darsi"). Further down, at center stage, so to speak, another amputee is shown crawling on the ground with shin pads, hand crutches and an instrument on his back. In this instance the comment is even more caustic: "With a cittern on his back, this rogue swindles, enjoys himself and goes on all his fours" ("Con la citara in spalla il forfantone/Trionfa sguazza e le na va carpone").[78]

The wide diffusion and adaptability such broadsheets had may be gathered by a specular engraving with images flipped left to right and published with a slightly different spelling (*Le bararie del mondo*) (Figure 3.7). This version was executed by A. Ronco, and today it is found in the Achille Bertarelli Collection in Milan.[79] Although the people who populate this print are almost exactly like the ones in Giovanni Antonio de' Pauli's – the major difference is that the man with a club approaching the gentleman with sword and cap in the middle of the second row from the bottom in de Pauli's engraving, in Ronco's is replaced by a small tree with the drum of a column at its base – and despite the fact that all captions are different in the two engravings, what does not change is the overall essence of the artifact. Typically revealing of the intentions of the producers of such engravings is the caption beneath the group of three orthopedically impaired fellows on the left of the sheet, third row from the bottom: "Ring of cripples and rascals/superb pranksters and swindlers" ("Circa delli stropiati e de forfanti/superbi giocatori

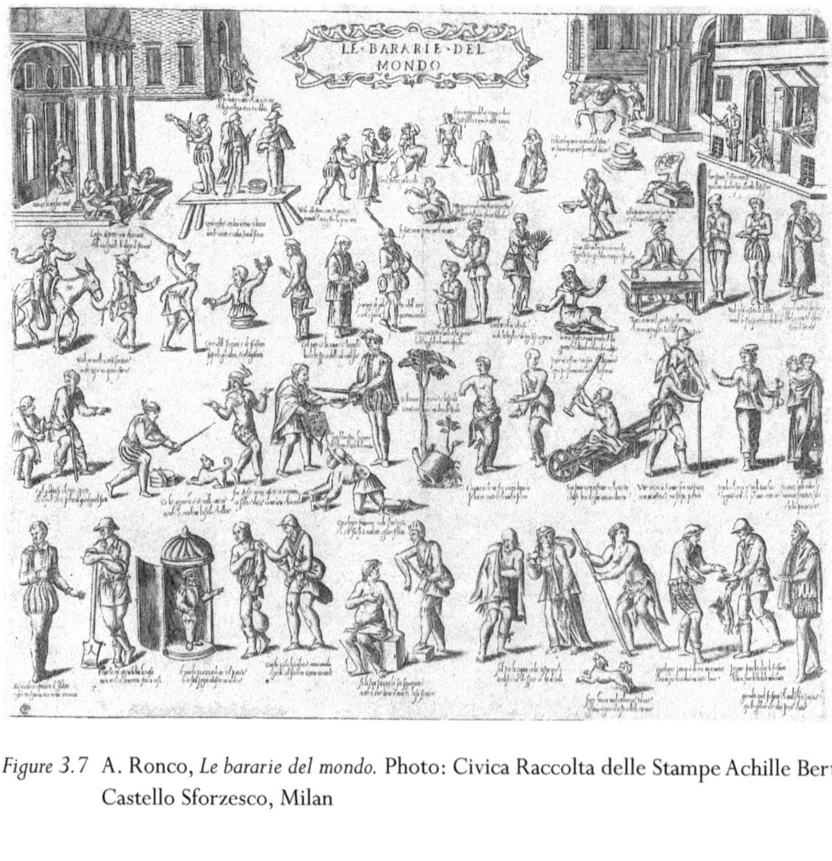

Figure 3.7 A. Ronco, *Le bararie del mondo.* Photo: Civica Raccolta delle Stampe Achille Bertarelli, Castello Sforzesco, Milan

e calcagnanti"). This triad comprises amputees only: one, missing the right foot, is leaning on a crutch while flinging the other crutch at his friend; the second, whose lower body has been truncated below the crotch, is hurling one of his hand trestles towards the first; a third amputee, with missing left foot and leg supported by a peg, seems to be admonishing moderation.[80]

Despite the obviously hyperbolic captions that, one must assume, tickled the fancy of the able-bodied bourgeoisie as well as the gentry that could afford to purchase these prints,[81] the fact remains that such an attitude towards "otherness," especially when faced with amputees, reflects a change in the predisposition on a part of society that had come a long way from identifying these less fortunate members of the community with the suffering Christ. Produced in different parts of the country, surely these popular prints must have played a definite role in consolidating negative commonplaces about the disabled mendicants.[82]

Executed by the French artist Jacques Callot, but derived from a series of drawings he had done during his Florentine sojourn from circa 1612 through to 1621, where he possibly studied with Antonio Tempesta,[83] the famous print *Captain of Rogues* (1622–1623) (Figure 3.8) also exhibits, if not the typical "bourgeois ferocity" mentioned by Fernand Braudel, the less-than-sympathetic view towards the marginalized members of society.[84] While sporting a dubiously distorted leg and a concealed hand – a symbol of idleness[85] – Callot's *Captain of Rogues* condenses in a single image the world of cheats whose members are to be avoided.[86] While seemingly objective in his recording of the social drama that came across his visual field, through his drawings and subsequent prints, this artist compiled a catalogue of stock characters comparable to that described to the papal police by two Roman youths previously mentioned.[87]

As to how successful Callot's prints were in contemporary society, one may surmise by the impact they had on the Genoese painter Giovanni Battista Carlone (1603–1683/4), who, about a generation later, adopted six different prints out of the twenty-five that Callot had engraved for his *La compagnia di baroni* (*Band of Rogues*) to create his own mélange of such characters (Figure 3.9).[88] However, the difference in Carlone's painting is that on the one hand the very large, monumental dimensions of the canvas (196 × 342 cm) take a low genre scene, typically treated in small works of art, and elevate it physically and ideologically to a grand, noble scale normally reserved for religious and historical subjects, and, on the other hand, the painting presents a subject, normally rendered by artists with supercilious superiority, with a seemingly detached, impassive objectivity.[89] Admittedly, it is difficult to discern whether the painter here has represented with subtle irony a group of beggars in front of a "locanda baronorum" ("tavern of rogues") or is giving us pause to reflect on the serious condition and fate of the indigent in society.[90]

Another indication of how orthopedic impairment could be manipulated to underscore devious human attitudes may be ascertained by two images from the first half of the seventeenth century. The first was included in what was to become the most popular handbook of graphic personifications to be utilized by artists in their allegorical composition: Cesare Ripa's *Iconologia*. Initially published in 1593 without illustrations, in 1603 this "bestseller" was enriched by images for the most part derived from drawings by Giuseppe Cesari, also known as Cavalier d'Arpino (1568–1640).[91] Under the heading "Lie" ("Bugia"), Ripa included a print that reified the personification of the concept by using the image of a woman with a wooden leg (Figure 3.10). As the gloss clarifies:

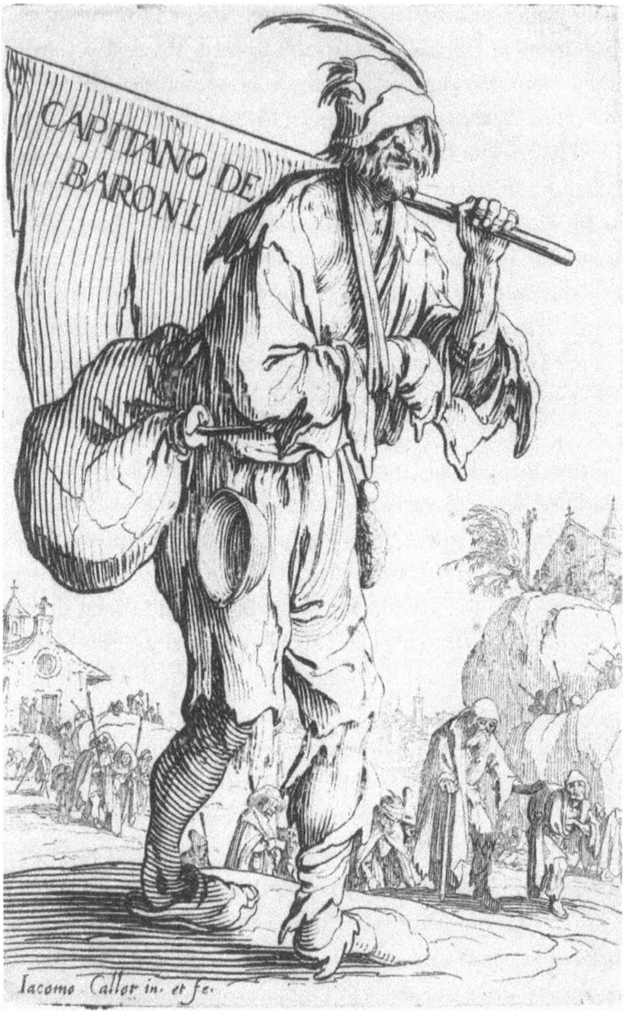

Figure 3.8 Jacques Callot, *Captain of Rogues*, 1622–1623, National Gallery of Art, Washington, Rosenwald Collection, 1949.5.282. Photo: Open Access

[*Lie* is to be represented by] an ugly young woman artfully dressed in an iridescent garb covered with different types of masks and many tongues. [She] will be [represented as] lame, that is, with a wooden leg, holding a burning bundle of straw and artfully dressed because with her art she craftily makes believe things that are not. Her iridescent dress is covered with masks and tongues to indicate the fickleness of a liar, whose speech diverges from the truth and gives a different appearance to everything, thus giving rise to the proverb: *Mendacem oportet esse memorem* [a liar should have a good memory].[92] The burning bundle of straw means nothing more than, just as a flame is quickly ignited and quickly goes out, so does a lie quickly come about and quickly dies out. Her lameness represents that which people commonly say, that is, lies have short legs.[93]

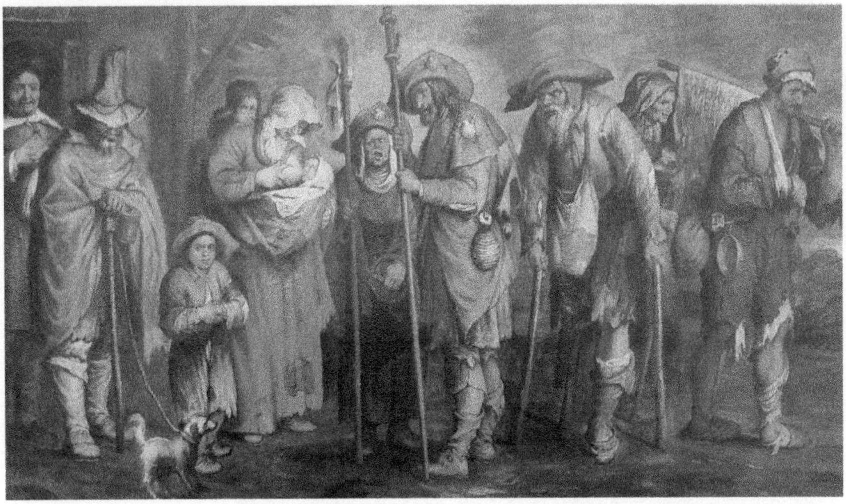

Figure 3.9 Giovanni Battista Carlone, *Band of Rogues,* private collection. Photo: from *Da Caravaggio a Ceruti: la scena di genere e l'immagine dei pitocchi nella pittura italiana,* Francesco Porzio (ed.), Milan, 1998, p. 199

Thus, this image gave visual substance to the Italian idiom, "la bugia ha le gambe corte" – that is, because of their "faulty gait," lies do not get too far and are quickly unmasked. Quite typical of mainstream society, the inability of a liar to get too far without being discovered and exposed in the Italian popular imagination could not be better expressed than by referring to the lame man's inability to walk speedily.

In a similar vein, when Annibale Carracci's drawings depicting *Le arti di Bologna* (*The Crafts of Bologna*) were posthumously engraved in 1646, among the eighty figures included in the booklet there was one representing "a famous spy" whose body is depicted bent over, with the right hand leaning on his knee and his lame stride supported by a cane (Figure 3.11). In the contemporaries' mentality, apparently, the odious character of an unreliable individual who might snitch on another and betray that person's trust could be best rendered by an orthopedically impaired informant.[94]

Comparable negative connotations are attached to the lame in images related to emblematic figures, such as Baccio Baldini's (1436–ca. 1487) engraving representing *Saturn* (Figure 3.12)[95] and Enea Vico's (1523–1567) *Old Age* (Figure 3.13).[96] In the former engraving, Baldini represents the world over which the planet Saturn presides. Besides the agricultural, autumnal activities – as specified in the inscription – of men plowing a field, a woodman chopping down a tree, and men butchering hogs, in keeping with Saturn's dark, melancholic nature, in the upper left or "sinister" corner of the image the artist places a man hanging from the gallows, a prison in the left middle-ground, and, immediately in front of it, a man restrained in stocks, while beggars leaning on crutches and a cripple with hand trestles progress from left to right. In other words, "Saturn's children ... are often condemned to a miserable fate and generally belong to the lowest estate of mankind."[97]

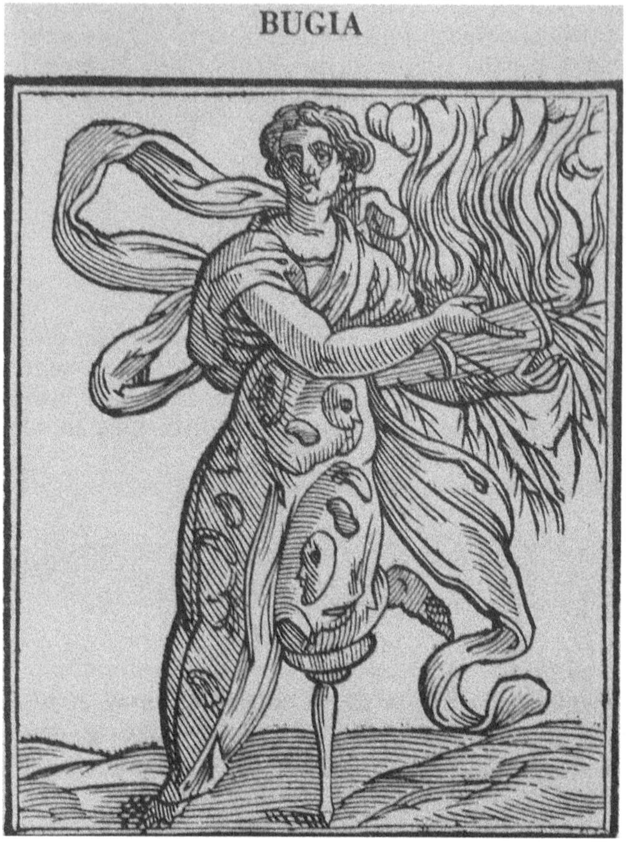

Figure 3.10 Cesare Ripa, "Bugia," *Iconologia*, Piero Buscaroli (ed.), Milan, 1992, p. 45

In the second engraving, Enea Vico admonishes all youth about the ailing condition that awaits those who reach old age. *Senectus* is represented by a hunchbacked, bald, bearded man whose right leg is bandaged, with shin strapped to his thigh and waist. He supports his impaired leg with a wooden prosthesis, while the upper part of the body is sustained by two crutches. Unlike Seneca, who in his letters to Lucilius was wont to emphasize the pleasures of old age ("life is most delightful when it is on the downward slope, but has not yet reached the abrupt decline"[98]), or Cicero, who found solace in the immortality of the soul ("for death is so pleasant, that the nearer I approach death the more I feel like one who is in sight of land and is about to anchor in his home port after a long voyage"[99]), perhaps reflecting more closely common opinion, Enea Vico chose to bring to the viewer's attention the aches and pains that inevitably accompany the descending curve of human existence. Yet, in the context of this study, it is significant that the prevalent feature of the emblem should be lameness.

Of course, not all members of society chose to focus on the predominant misanthropic views of beggars, be they honest or dishonest, disabled individuals, truly or falsely claiming to

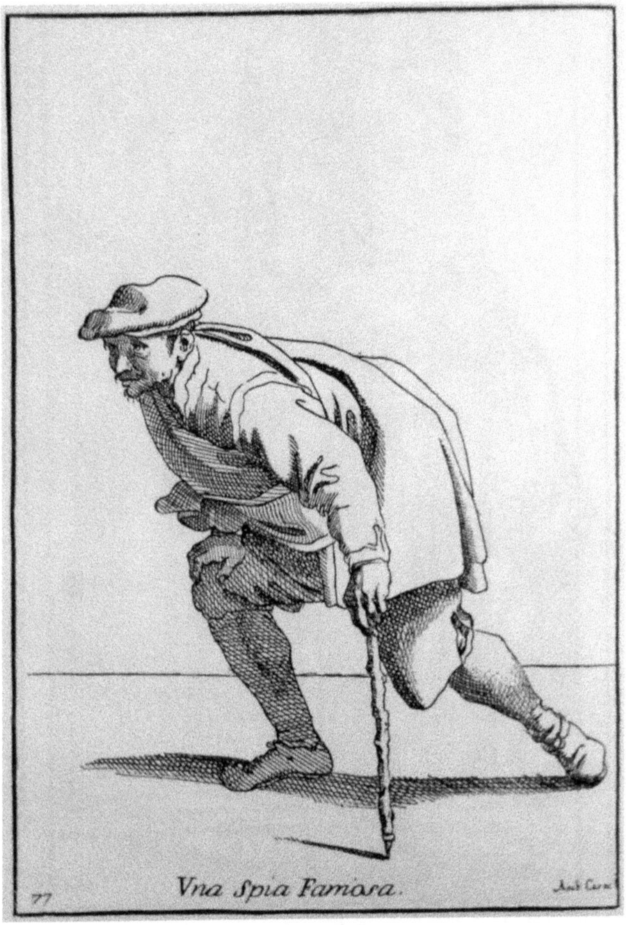

Figure 3.11 Annibale Carracci, *A Famous Spy*. Photo: from Annibale Carracci, *Le arti di Bologna di Annibale Carracci*, Alessandro Marabottini (ed.), Rome, 1966, fig. 77

be such, or any outcast altogether. Annibal Caro's translation for Cardinal Cervini, director of the Vatican Library and future Pope Marcellus II (1555), of Gregory of Nazianzus's oration *On Love for the Poor* as well as his rendition of Cecil Ciprian's first sermon in praise of almsgiving, for example, must not have fallen on deaf ears and there are certainly enough images that argue in favor of a more charitable, Christian attitude towards the needy.[100] In fact, the same Mitelli who executed the lame *Birbante* who would not trade places with a king, in a series of illustrated proverbs also engraved, in which a print praising almsgiving reminded the reader, "no one ever became poor through almsgiving" (Figure 3.14).[101] Similarly, in a series of forty-two prints illustrating *The Life of St. Philip Neri*, Ludovico Ciamberlano exalted this saint's philanthropy by commemorating an event that occurred in 1537 when he sold his books and gave the money to the poor: he designed an engraving that, once again, features prominently a lame man in the foreground (Figure 3.15).[102]

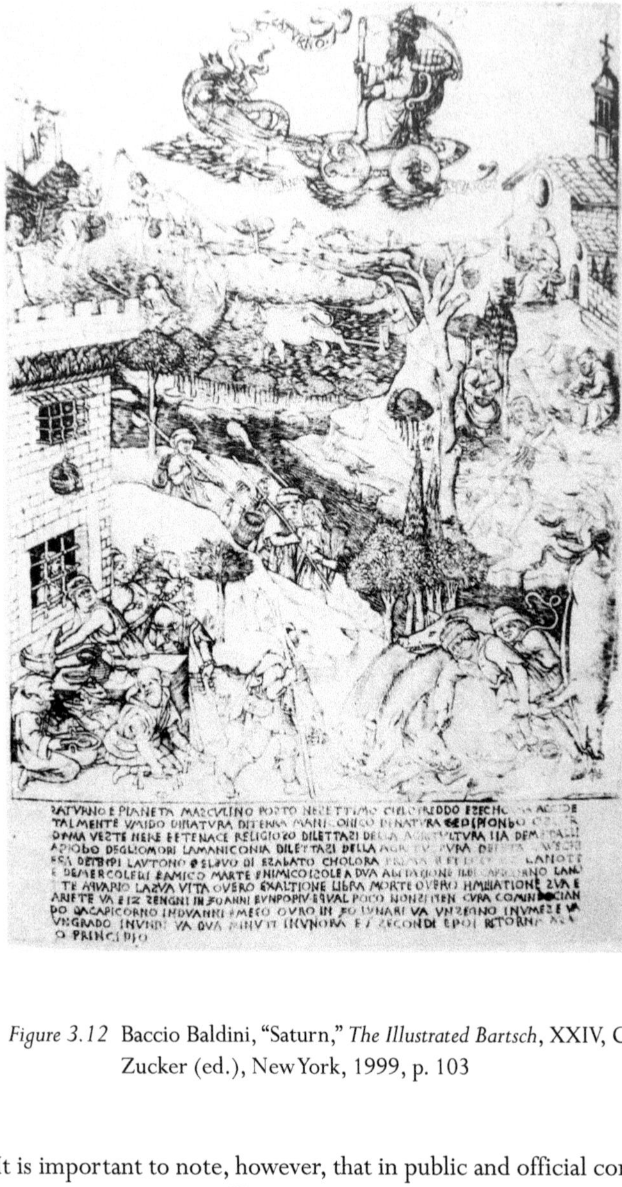

Figure 3.12 Baccio Baldini, "Saturn," *The Illustrated Bartsch*, XXIV, Commentary, Part 1, Mark J. Zucker (ed.), New York, 1999, p. 103

It is important to note, however, that in public and official commissions, but especially in the context of sacred art,[103] as opposed to prints and broadsheets, the interest that patrons and artists showed for a more benevolent approach to the indigent and the disabled was also a reflection of the post-Tridentine reaction to the Protestants' emphasis on "justification by faith alone."[104] In fact, in an attempt to rationalize his inadequacy in justifying himself before God through the traditional means of sacraments and good works, Luther believed that man's basic sin was exactly his attempt to justify himself, and not "accept that his future rests alone in the gratuitous act of God."[105] After much soul searching, Luther had arrived at this understanding by turning to St. Paul's second letter to the Ephesians, in which the evangelist had stated, "because it is by grace that you have been saved, through faith; not by

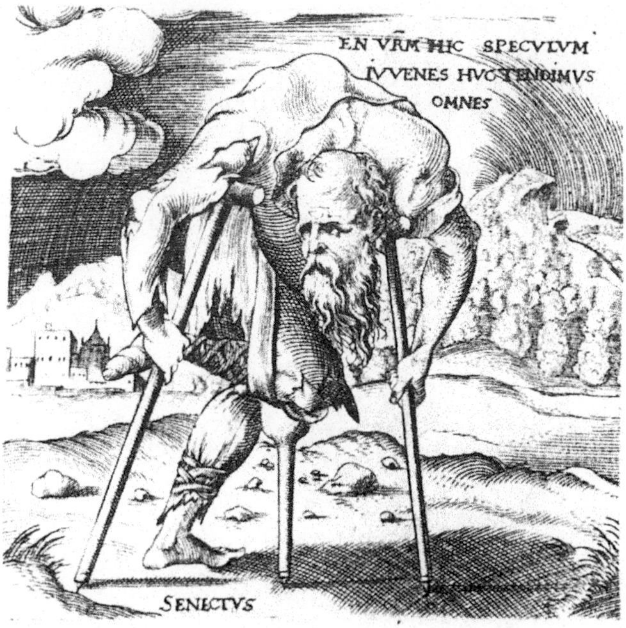

Figure 3.13 Enea Vico, "Old Age," *The Illustrated Bartsch*, XXX, John Spike (ed.), New York, 1985, p. 79

anything of your own, but by a gift from God; not by anything that you have done, so that nobody can claim the credit" (Ep 2:8).[106] In man's rapport with God, in other words, good works are not fundamental since Divine grace is all encompassing and good works follow from it. As Luther emphasized in *The Freedom of a Christian*, "Good works do not make a good man, but a good man does good works; evil works do not make a wicked man, but a wicked man does evil works."[107] For the Protestants, human redemption was achieved solely through the sacrifice of Christ and merciful acts merely showed that a person was doing God's will. Charitable works were not meritorious in themselves, but they could be seen as the "fruits and signs of salvation."[108]

While the most threatening aspect of Luther's theology, as seen from south of the Alps, was his claim that the Christian religion meant first and foremost freedom from any authority such as the pope,[109] justification by faith alone became one of the most memorable issues that encapsulate Luther's position on religious matters that were strongly opposed by the Church of Rome. And for good reason, since, if humanity's salvation depended totally on God's grace and nothing that humans did could truly gain them salvation, then the whole edifice on which Christianity was founded, the Mass, the sacraments, Church hierarchy, penance, and prayer itself, was "a needless empty show."[110]

In a letter of 1539 addressed to the Senate and the people of Geneva who had fallen under the spell of John Calvin and his views on justification by faith, Cardinal Jacopo Sadoleto had already amicably refuted the Protestant stance.[111] However, when the Council of Trent (1545–1563)

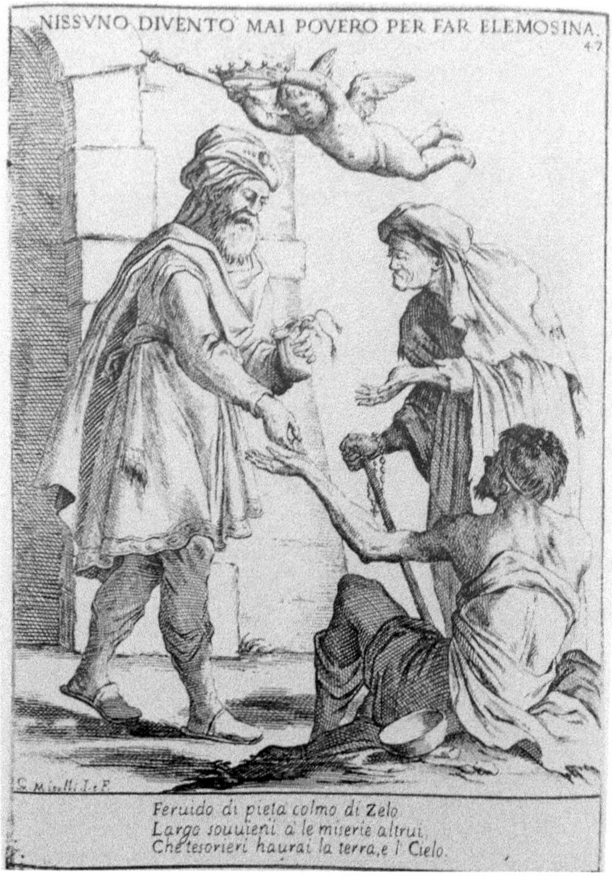
NISSVNO DIVENTO MAI POVERO PER FAR ELEMOSINA.
47
Feruido di pieta colmo di Zelo
Largo souuieni à le miserie altrui,
Che tesorieri haurai la terra, e l' Cielo.

Figure 3.14 Giuseppe Maria Mitelli, "Almsgiving," *The Illustrated Bartsch*, XLII, John Spike (ed.), New York, 1981, p. 39

met for its sixth session on January 13, 1547 and issued the *Decree on Justification*, the Catholic position became dogma. It did so "by imposing a strict check on anyone who dares to believe, preach or teach otherwise than is defined and declared in the present decree" and specified that, "for faith, unless hope is added to it and charity too, neither unites him perfectly with Christ nor makes him a living member of his body. Hence it is very truly said that faith without works is dead and barren."[112]

Although Tridentine concepts had less of an impact in Venice than in other parts of Italy,[113] the Counter-Reformation stance on the issue of good works, for instance, lends additional significance and a deeper understanding of paintings such as Giampietro Silvio's *Marriage of the Virgin* and the *Annunciation* by Girolamo Dente in the Venetian Scuola Grande della Carità (now incorporated in the Gallerie dell'Accademia), in which a lame mendicant (Figure 3.16) and an amputee beggar (Figure 3.17) are prominently placed in the foreground. The paintings reflect not only the specific raison d'être of this charitable confraternity, as its name implies, but also provide an indication of the greater accent Catholics placed on good works.[114]

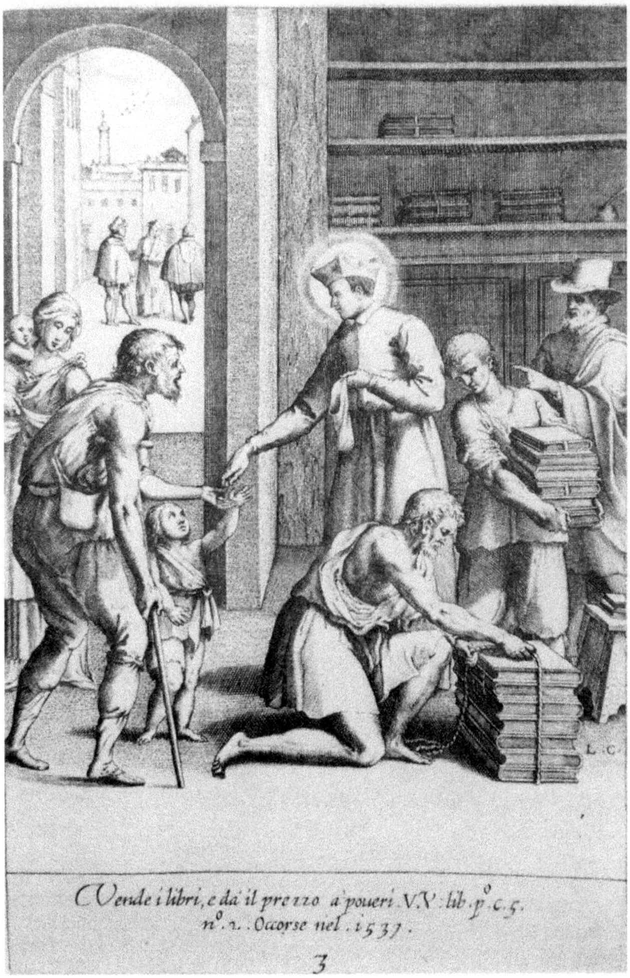
Vende i libri, e da' il prezzo a' poueri. V.X: lib. p°. c. 5.
n°. 2. Occorse nel. 1537.
3
L.C.

Figure 3.15 Ludovico Ciamberlano, "St. Philip Neri Selling His Books and Donating the Money to the Poor," *The Illustrated Bartsch*, XLIV, Paolo Bellini and Mark Carter Leach (eds.), New York, 1983, p. 89

It is probably coincidental, but certainly no less meaningful, that while the stock figure of the mendicant painted by Giampietro Silvio between 1543 and 1545 (Figure 3.16) – ennobled by a clear reference to the Hellenistic statue of the *Laocoön* (Figure 3.18)[115] – simply gestures for alms, in Girolamo Dente's painting (Figure 3.17) the beggar obtains a more active reminder of the importance that good works had for the members of the Scuola Grande della Carità and Christians at large. Executed in 1557–1558, a full decade after the sixth session of the Council of Trent that had stipulated that "faith without works is dead and barren," Dente's *Annunciation* may be taken as a valid representation of the Catholic belief that salvation was not only possible thanks to the mystery of the *Incarnation*, the intercession of the sacred vessel that carried God made man – that is, the Virgin Mary – but also a definite reminder that active

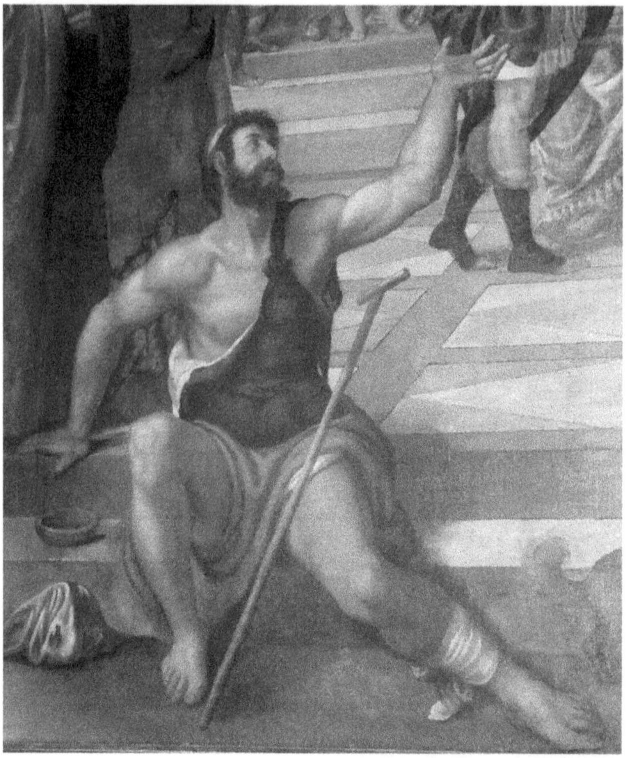

Figure 3.16 Giampietro Silvio, *Marriage of the Virgin*, 1543–1545, Gallerie dell'Accademia, Venice. Photo: author

acts of charity truly facilitated human redemption. Although Girolamo Dente's amputee is also beholden to a Classical work of art – the *Falling Gaul* of ca. 200 (Figure 3.19)[116] – in this detail of the painting the artist ably evokes an "incitement to piety"[117] through the greater sympathetic, realistic depiction[118] of an orthopedically impaired mendicant and the active dispensation of monetary donations and victuals (the girl handing a coin to the beggar and the loaf of bread next to him).

At the social level, however, by the seventeenth century these images only reinforced an attitude that was convenient for the leading members of society who ultimately, while praising charity, used it as a way of not confronting with resolution the issues posed by poverty and mendicancy. As Brian Pullan has pointed out, the problem of mendicancy was never really solved since both the state and private philanthropists "did not attempt to reconstruct the social edifice; they merely shored it up."[119] The same historian pointedly concludes: "Despair could lead to violence, but uncertainty – the basic characteristic of poverty – could lead to submission and docility. Charity was a stabilizing agent not only because it averted despair but also because, while rewarding the humble, it instilled in them an attitude of acceptance and resignation."[120] As Giuseppe Palmieri perspicaciously remarked in 1761, the problem lay elsewhere. His laconic statement limpidly went to the heart of the matter: "manca più tosto

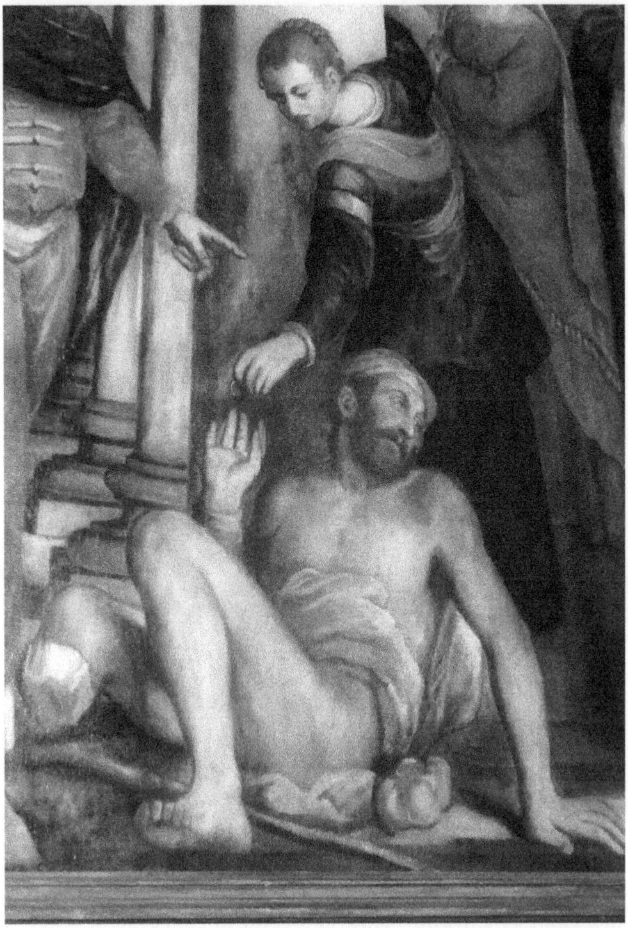

Figure 3.17 Girolamo Dente, *Annunciation*, 1557–1558, Gallerie dell'Accademia, Venice. Photo: author

lavoro alla gente che gente al lavoro" ("if anything, it is rather people who are deprived of work and not positions waiting to be filled by people").[121]

This kind of mentality affords a deeper understanding of one of the most memorable images of the orthopedically impaired from seventeenth-century Italy: Jusepe de Ribera's *Clubfooted Boy* (Plate 17). Although Spanish by birth, Ribera (1591–1652) has been rightly claimed for both the Spanish and Neapolitan schools of painting and hailed as "one of the great masters of Italian seventeenth-century paintings."[122] In fact, Ribera spent all of his professional life in Italy. Already in Rome around 1606, then in Parma by 1611, as attested by one of his early works, and first recorded in Rome in 1612 where he appears in connection with the Accademia di San Luca, after having married the daughter of the Neapolitan painter Giovanni Bernardino Azzolino during the Christmas festivities of 1616 he settled in Naples for the rest of his life.[123] In this town, so renowned for the

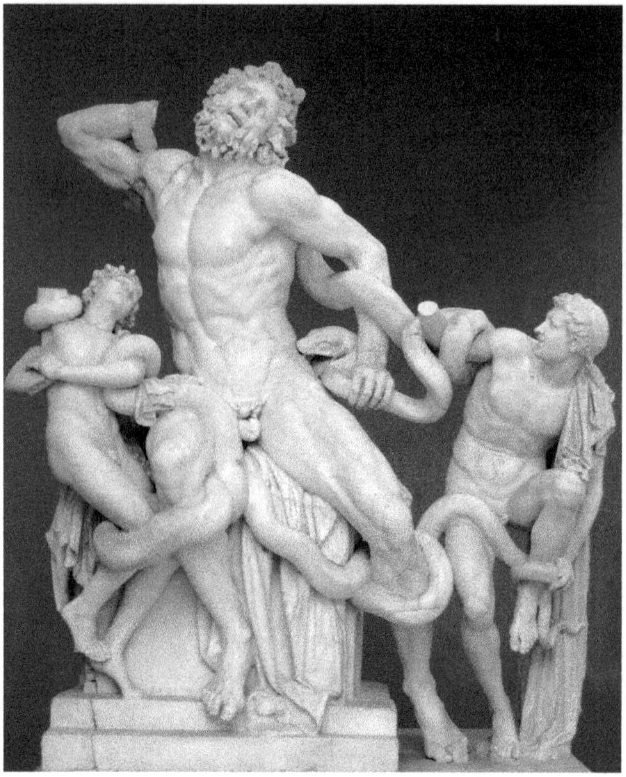

Figure 3.18 Laocoön, first century AD, Rome, Vatican Museums. Photo: author

indolent *lazzaroni*, who were seen as shirking from any type of work even when available, Ribera found the appropriate subject to rebut a common cliché that stigmatized the deprived, especially if lame.

Holding an inscription that declares, "Give me alms for the love of God" ("*Da mihi elemosinam propter amorem Dei*"), this Neapolitan boy is depicted with an endearing smile while holding the ever-present cane and a hat in place of the alms-box. Although on the surface the painting seems an un-idealized depiction of an orthopedically impaired youngster, in fact it not only ennobles him by showing his silhouette from a low viewpoint with his body against a wide expanse of sky – an approach typically reserved for portraits of aristocrats and nobility – but also embodies the idealization of the Counter-Reformation doctrine of salvation through good works.[124] Indeed, the canvas reflects ideas such as those expressed by the Jesuit Daniello Bartoli in his treatise *La Povertà Contenta* (1650) where the poor are considered fortunate, on the one hand, because "they were free from sins afflicting the rich" and, on the other hand, because their "ideal" condition of privation allowed the rich to redeem themselves through charitable works.[125]

Although written with the intention of criticizing and goading the rich to perform charitable deeds, in its message of exaltation of the beggar's state, Bartoli's book – though the

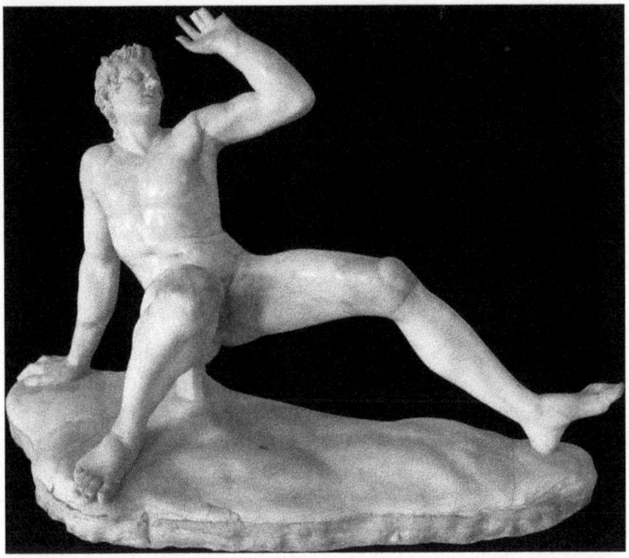

Figure 3.19 *Falling Gaul*, second half of the second century AD, Museo Archeologico, Venice. Photo: author

same could be said of Ribera's painting – was perhaps more pernicious to the poor and the disabled as a social group than those representations that depicted them as roguish vagabonds. If nothing else, representations of the disabled as swindlers were less hypocritical. As Salvator Rosa bitterly quipped in his Satire III, *On Painting*: "The naked and the afflicted beggars receive not a single coin from those who later disburse much money to see them depicted in their paintings. Therefore, from these ragamuffins I learn that the modern princes' inclination is to be prodigal in their luxury, miserly in their piety."[126] With his typical caustic but penetrating observations, Rosa reminded his contemporaries of the schizophrenic attitude they had towards the poor and the disabled members of their communities. While conceptually engaged, and perhaps even interested in the plight of the marginalized, members of mainstream society would avert their eyes and often turn a deaf ear to their condition and fate. In fact, as so many treatises, plays, poems, and manuals on pious and charitable institutions or hospices in the course of the century evince, the attitude that prevailed at the time was a more calloused approach towards those individuals whose fate brought about their "metamorphosis from human to sub-human" creatures.[127]

Given the widespread mistrust of able and pseudo-disabled mendicants in the sixteenth and seventeenth centuries, one might ask how the truly physically impaired fared, caught as they were between the deceitful impostors and a diffident society. As we shall see in the next chapter, in the light of its special position at the heart of Christendom, Papal Rome represents a privileged lens through which one may observe the phenomenon and provides a valuable case study, so to speak, with the creation of the Hospital of San Sisto and its complementary organization, the "Confraternity of the blind, lame and crippled of the Visitation."

Notes

1 Lucian, *The Parasite: Parasitic an Art*, Austin Morris Harmon (ed.), Cambridge and London, 1995, p. 261. Parts of this chapter are adaptations and translations of my articles "Blindness, Lameness and Mendicancy in Italy" and "Simulare disabilità: mendicanti e furfanti a Roma nel Rinascimento," in Philine Helas and Gerhard Wolf (eds.), *Armut und Armenfürsorge in der italienischen Stadtkultur zwischen 13. und 16. Jahrhundert: Bilder, Texte und soziale Praktiken*, Frankfurt am Main, 2006, pp. 371–383.

2 Terence, *The Eunuch*, John Sargeaunt (tr.), Cambridge and London, 1994, p. 259.

3 See note 1.

4 Plato, *Laws*, in *The Collected Dialogues of Plato*, XI, p. 1486. See Ch. 1, p. 24.

5 See Ch. 1, p. 24.

6 2 Thessalonians, 3:6–12.

7 Caner, p. 126, mentions that in 403 Alexander "the Sleepless," "a Greek archimandrite (leader of a flock or fold) who had 'come from the East' and settled in Constantinople with nearly a hundred followers," was among those who believed that one should give indiscriminately to beggars and this comprised perhaps his most radical proclamation. Idem, p. 149.

8 Ibid., p. 168. The problem, of course, as often happens in history, was aggravated when waves of migration due to drought, hail, locusts, famine and invasions forced people to leave their land in search of other means of sustainment. Ibid., pp. 164–165.

9 On the Messalian controversy, see ibid., pp. 83–125. Throughout history, those persons who embraced voluntary poverty were basically following Christ's charge to the apostles, "Cure the sick, raise the dead, cleanse the lepers, cast out devils. You received without charge, give without charge. Provide yourselves with no gold or silver, not even with a few coppers for your purses, with no haversack for the journey or spare tunic or footwear or a staff, for the workman deserves his keep" (Matthew 10:8–10). However, it is clear that for the Messalian vagrants the implications of the final phrase of this quotation from Matthew, "for the workman deserves his keep," was ignored.

10 Caner, p. 178.

11 Quoted in ibid., p. 180.

12 Geremek, *Poverty*, p. 25.

13 Ibid., p. 26.

14 Ibid.

15 Ibid., p. 24.

16 Brian Tierney, "The Decretists and the 'Deserving Poor'," *Comparative Studies in Society and History*, 1 (1959): 365.

17 Ibid., p. 368.

18 Geremek, *Poverty*, p. 22: "As long as voluntary poverty remained an expression of individual aspirations it was tolerated by the Church; but when it began to assume the form of a collective movement and spread to entire communities it became a threat. The creation of mendicant orders was a way of 'taming' and controlling such movements, and at the same time of sanctioning, ethically and religiously, the urban world of money." On the problem that a return to evangelical poverty caused for the papacy and Innocent III's astute reconciliations with those movements that practiced it, see Euan Cameron, *Waldenses: Rejections of Holy Church in Medieval Europe*, Oxford, 2000, esp. pp. 44 and 55. For the Church's response to false beggars see Erik von Kraemer, "Le type du faux mendiant dans les littératures romanes depuis le moyen âge jusqu'au XVIIe siècle," *Societas Scientiarum Fennica: Commentationes Humanarum Litterarum*, Helsingfors, 13:6 (1944): 1–338, esp. pp. 15–20.

19 Vauchez, *Sainthood*, p. 394, and Geremek, *Poverty*, p. 32. Also Pestilli, "Disabled Bodies," p. 90.

20 Goffen, p. 30. Also, Vauchez, *Sainthood*, p. 394.

21 *The Defensor Pacis of Marsilius of Padua*, Charles William Previté-Orton (ed.), Cambridge, 1928, xx, states that Pope John XXII promulgated two bulls in 1322 and 1324 respectively, *Ad conditorem canonum* and *Cum inter nonnullus*, in which he "condemned the spiritual Franciscan belief in absolute poverty of Christ and in the necessity of absolute poverty for the perfect Christian."

22 Vauchez, *Sainthood*, pp. 395–396. Geremek, *Poverty*, p. 31: "The rule was that poverty could reach its apotheosis only as a spiritual value, while real, physical poverty, with its visible degrading effects, was perceived, both doctrinally and by society, as a humiliating state, depriving its victims of dignity and respect, relegating them to the margins of society and to a life devoid of virtue."

23 Lucian's *The Parasite* was translated by Guarino da Verona in 1418. See Leon Battista Alberti, *Momus*, Sarah Knight (tr.), Virginia Brown and Sarah Knight (eds.), Cambridge and London, 2003, p. 387, n. 7. Mollat, p. 255: "With humanism, contempt for the poor took a subtle and perfidious turn, becoming disdainful and philosophical and – height of irony – invoking the dignity of man as justification."

24 Alberti, *Momus*, II, 48, p. 133.

25 *Collected Works of Erasmus: Colloquies*, Craig R. Thompson (tr. and ed.), Toronto, Buffalo and London, 1997, p. 567. Thompson, p. 568, n. 1, elucidates that Irides, "son of Irus," also means "hater of work" in Greek. In a similar vein, Cornelius Agrippa, *De incertitudine et scientiarum et artium*, James Sanford (tr.), London, 1569, chapter 65, p. 105 writes: "[Beggars] will not chaunge theire life with Kinges, so that they maye freely wander where they please and doo what euer they thinke good in warre and peace." Quoted by Thompson, p. 569, n. 17. Cornelius Agrippa, *De incertitudine et vanitate scientiarum declamation invectiva, ex postrema Authoris recognitione*, Cologne, 1584, under Caput LXV, *De mendicitate*: "Sunt alij qui votorum & peregrinationum prætextu provincias obambulant, laborem ex industria fugientes, otiosa paupertate ostiatim mendicantes, atque ij interim, ne cum regibus quidem vitam suam commutate velint, modo illis liberum est, quo libet & velint, vagari, quodcunque collibitum est facere bello & pace."

26 Tom Nichols, *The Art of Poverty: Irony and Ideal in Sixteenth-Century Beggar Imagery*, Manchester, 2007, p. 7, valuably summarizes the differences. The "false beggar" was typically represented in woodcuts, engravings, etchings and drawings depicting genre scenes that were made for the open market and had no fixed location. These images tended to be small in size, were reproduced in mass, were shown in a private, domestic setting, and their monetary and esthetic value was low. The "ideal beggar" was usually depicted in large single-work oil paintings and frescoes of a religious subject that were commissioned by a patron, had a fixed location in a public or institutional location, and had a high monetary and esthetic value.

27 For the sake of clarity, in this chapter, as in the rest of the book, it is obvious that, even though the lame were often mendicants, not all beggars were lame. Nonetheless, it is in the person of the lame mendicant that artists more often than not encapsulated the quintessential image of the beggar. Thus, while the two categories are distinct, in artistic representations it is the lame that subsumes the beggar and not the other way around.

28 Henry G. Bohn, *Polyglot of Foreign Proverbs*, London, 1857, p. 121.

29 See Geremek, *Poverty*, p. 49. See also Camporesi, *Il libro dei vagabondi*, p. 40. The employment of lameness or the lame as negative terms of comparison in proverbs reflects an old tradition that goes back at least as far as the Old Testament. See for example Proverbs 26:7: "Unreliable as a lame man's legs: so is a proverb in the mouth of fools." *The Jerusalem Bible*, Alexander Jones (ed.), Garden City, 1966, p. 968.

30 See the Coda to this book. Geremek, *Poverty*, p. 51: "The beggar's professional technique essentially involved a public display of his external 'weaknesses'; his misery or infirmity justified his appeal for aid. In the general spectacle of ostentatious misery it was often difficult to distinguish the genuine cripple from the impostor: deceit or its suspicion, then as now, invariably accompanies the beggar's profession."

31 Jacobus de Voragine, *The Golden Legend: Readings on the Saints*, 2 vols., William Granger Ryan (tr.), Princeton, 1993, II, p. 300.

32 Ibid.

33 Piero Camporesi, *The Land of Hunger*, Tania Croft-Murray, Caire Foley and Shayne Mitchell (trs.), Cambridge, 1996 (orig. *Il paese della fame*, 1978), p. 167. Furthermore, in various works, such as Fabio Glissenti's *Discorsi morali contro il dispiacer del morire detto athanatophilia* (Moral discourses against the displeasure of dying called *athanatophilia*) published in Venice in 1600, the common treatment of the subject presents lame beggars who exult and thank their "lucky stars" for being

orthopedically impaired: "We greatly rejoice at certain infirmities, indeed it is God's special gift if we have a swollen or cancerous leg, with sores or similar ills. We call it God's leg." For Glissenti's text see Camporesi, *Il libro dei vagabondi*, pp. 457–464, under the chapter heading, "Delle astuzie de' mendicanti, pitocchi e forfanti, e come sono scaltriti nell'esercizio loro, e come simulando vanno ingannando il mondo" ("On the wiles of mendicants, beggars and rogues, on how they slyly practice their trade, and deceive everyone by their simulations").

34 Camporesi, *The Land of Hunger*, p. 187.

35 Biblioteca Apostolica Vaticana V. 682, int. 33, *L'arte della Forfanteria Cantata da Gian Pitocco Fornaro, alla sua amata Signora. Opera Guidonesca dell'Accademico Calcante: Drizzata alla Baronia di Campo di Fiore*, Venice, 1618 (reprinted in Orvieto). My thanks to Pamela Jones for having brought this work to my attention. The text, published by Camporesi in *Il libro dei vagabondi*, pp. 489–495, is dated 1622 and published in Ferrara and Bologna with the name of the author: Giulio Cesare Croce.

36 On the rise of the false beggar imagery especially in northern Europe see Nichols, *The Art of Poverty*, pp. 32–43.

37 The engraving of the lame vendor is taken from the *Arte per via* (1660). See *The Illustrated Bartsch*, 1978, XLII (originally XIX, Part 2), p. 427, n. 152 (304). On the social mindset these prints and others like it reflected and the social implications it had for the dominant and subordinate classes in late sixteenth- and seventeenth-century Italy, see Sheila McTighe, "Perfect Deformity, Ideal Beauty, and the *Imaginaire* of Work: The Reception of Annibale Carracci's *Arti di Bologna* in 1646," *Oxford Art Journal*, 1 (1993): 75–91. Mitelli's *Arti in Bologna* were modeled on Annibale Carracci's well-known figures engraved posthumously in 1646 as *Diverse Figure*. Carracci's original seventy-five drawings have just about all disappeared. There is only one extant drawing in the Ellesmere collection of a *Spazzacamino* or *Chimney Sweeper* that has been attributed to him. See McTighe, p. 89, n. 1.

38 See Erik von Kraemer, "Le type du faux mendiant," p. 19, and Manuel Colmeiro, *Historia de la economia politica en España*, 2 vols., Madrid, 1863, II, p. 35.

39 St. Maximus the Confessor, *The Ascetic Life, The Four Centuries on Charity*, Polycarp Sherwood (tr. and ed.), Westminster, MD, and London, 1955, p. 140, I, 24.

40 Three introductory texts on this topic are Michel Mollat, *The Poor in the Middle Ages: An Essay in Social History*, Arthur Goldhammer (tr.), New Haven and London, 1986 (orig. French edition 1978); Bronislaw Geremek, *Poverty: A History*, Oxford, 1994; Robert Jütte, *Poverty and Deviance in Early Modern Europe*, Cambridge, 1994; Piero Camporesi, *Il libro del vagabondo*, Milan, 2003.

41 Vincenzo Paglia, "La pietà dei carcerati," *Confraternite e società a Roma nei secoli XVI–XVIII*, Rome, 1980, p. 46. Mollat, p. 246: "In general, it has been estimated that a city can sustain a fringe element of up to 10 percent of its population without danger to law and order."

42 Mario Rosa, "Poveri ed emarginati: un problema religioso," *Ricerche per la storia religiosa di Roma*, 3 (1979): 13. All contemporaries agreed on the severity of the situation due to the food shortages of the late 1580s and mid-1590s. See Henderson, "'Mal Francese,'" p. 506. Citing from Sanzio Cicatelli's *Vita di San Camillo de Lellis: fondatore della religione de' chierici regolari, ministri degli infermi*, Rome, 1746, p. 125, Henderson reminds his readers of the dire situation in Rome: "Just in the city of Rome and its region, 60,000 people died, partly through hunger, partly through cold. It is horrible even to read of such a disaster. Imagine then how heartbreaking it must have been for those who saw men in the *contrade* of the city dying under the benches of the butchers and other shops, reduced to feed on grass like sheep in the fields and to eat even cats and dead dogs and any filthy food they could find; so that our [religious] recorded more than once a dead body with his mouth full of grass."

43 Ibid. See also Branislaw Geremek, "Il pauperismo nell'età preindustriale (secoli XIV–XVIII)," *Storia d'Italia, Annali*, Turin, 1978, V, pp. 670–698, esp. pp. 670 and 685. On the percentage of poor people in European cities see Roberto Morozzo della Rocca, "Vecchio e nuovo nell'immagine della povertà agli inizi dell'età moderna," in *La storia dei poveri: pauperismo e assistenza nell'età moderna*, Alberto Monticone (ed.), Rome, 1985, p. 7, who cites from Brian Pullan's "Poveri, mendicanti e vagabondi (secoli XIV–XVII)," *Storia d'Italia, Annali*, R. Romano and C. Vivanti (eds.), Turin, 1973, pp. 981–1047, I. Geremek, *Poverty*, p. 100, claims that beggars and paupers in Late Medieval cities made up 15–20 percent of the population, while in the sixteenth and seventeenth centuries it

was about 25 percent. He also points out (p. 111), that the cities offered possibilites of temporary work that attracted the poor from the countryside: "One could always find work, or at least alms, in the city; there were no dead seasons here, as there were in the country." Richard A. Goldthwaite, "Artisans and the Economy in Sixteenth-Century Florence," in *The Medici, Michelangelo, and the Art of Late Renaissance Florence*, Cristina Acidini Luchinat (ed.), New Haven, 2002, p. 87: "The fall in real wages was evident enough to the Venetian ambassador who in 1588 reported that '[in Florence] the lower classes are poor and go begging' and that there were 'many poor.'"

44 Jacques Le Goff, *Medieval Civilization 400–1500*, Julia Barrow (tr.), Oxford and Cambridge, MA, 2001 (orig. 1964), p. 316.

45 It has been pointed out that the causal relation between diseases such as the plague and the poor in urban environments, where the rich were quick to flee to their country estates when the epidemics broke out – "few but the poor stayed in the city to welcome the plague" – may have been the reverse. Ann G. Carmichael, *Plague and the Poor in Renaissance Florence*, New York, 1986, pp. 98–103 and esp. p. 126. Mollat, p. 247: "People tolerated the beggar but hated the vagabond."

46 Sharon Farmer, "The Beggar's Body: Intersections of Gender and Social Status in High Medieval Paris," in *Monks and Nuns, Saints and Outcasts: Religion in Medieval Society*, Sharon Farmer and Barbara H. Rosewein (eds.), Ithaca, NY, and London, 2000, p. 162.

47 Mollat, p. 70.

48 Geremek, *Poverty*, p. 20.

49 Mollat, p. 106, and Geremek, *Poverty*, p. 20. Philine Helas, "Die Bettler for dem Tempel: Zur Invenzione und Transformation eines Bildmotivs in der Italienischen Malerei der Renaissance (1423–1552)," *Iconographica*, 3 (2004): 69, cites from a sermon delivered in February 1425 by St. Bernardine: "I ricchi e i poveri sono un medesimo corpo, cioè membra d'un corpo. I ricchi sono di necessità alle republiche; e' poveri sono di necessità a' ricchi." ("The rich and the poor are a single body, that is, members of one body. The rich are necessary to the republics; and the poor are necessary to the rich.")

50 Camporesi, *The Land of Hunger*, p. 107, quoting Walter Benjamin.

51 Codice Campori, Biblioteca Estense, y X 2,5, in Camporesi, *Il libro dei vagabondi*, pp. 86–88. "*Rasa*" is derived from the old Venetian dialect word for "fraud," ibid., p. 24.

52 Camporesi, *Il libro dei vagabondi*, pp. 505–514. Geremek, "Il pauperismo nell'età preindustriale," p. 691, n. 1, clarifies that the two documents published by Camporesi had been published previously by Martin Löpelmann in "Il diletteuole Essamine de' Guidoni, Furfanti ò Calchi, altramente detti Guitti nelle Carceri di Ponte Sisto di Roma nel 1598: con la cognitione della lingua furbesca ò zerga commune à tutti loro," *Romanische Forschungen*, 34 (1913): 653–664.

53 See Robert Jütte, *Poverty and Deviance*, pp. 178–185. Pamphlets that explained the outcasts' cant appeared in Florence, Venice, as well as in Germany. For comments on the subject of the beggars' cant and on the imagery of false beggars, such as the one on the frontispiece of the anonymous *Nuovo modo de intendere la lingua zerga, cioe parlare forbescho*, Ferrara, 1545, see Nichols, *The Art of Poverty*, pp. 124–126.

54 Northrop Frye, *Anatomy of Criticism: Four Essays*, Princeton, 1971 (orig. 1957), p. 37: "Tragedy in the central or high mimetic sense, the fiction of the fall of a leader (he has to fall because that is the only way in which a leader can be isolated from his society), mingles the heroic with the ironic." Ibid., p. 43: "In Aristophanes there is usually a central figure who constructs his (or her) own society in the teeth of strong opposition, driving off one after another all the people who come to prevent or exploit him, and eventually achieving a heroic triumph, complete with mistresses, in which he is sometimes assigned the honors of a reborn god. We notice that just as there is a catharsis of pity and fear in tragedy, so there is a catharsis of the corresponding comic emotions, which are sympathy and ridicule, in Old Comedy. The comic hero will get his triumph whether what he has done is sensible or silly, honest or rascally."

55 Pullan, "Poveri, mendicanti e vagabondi," pp. 1012–1013. The document had resurfaced by 1585 – "nella crescente ansia da parte del papa di risolvere il problema della mendicità" – but the earliest edition known is the one from Viterbo of 1621. Idem, p. 1012. Geremek, "Il pauperismo nell'età

preindustriale," p. 697. Also published by Camporesi in *Il libro dei vagabondi*, pp. 247–331. The *biante* (or *beante*) was a vagrant; see Camporesi, *The Land of Hunger*, Cambridge, 1996, p. 96. See note 53.

56 Reprinted in Camporesi, *Il libro dei vagabondi*, pp. 181–246.

57 Ibid., pp. 247–331, esp. p. 264.

58 Ibid., p. 265, the *beanti* were "so called from the verb *beare*, promising each other earthly *beatitude* through their shameful way of finding victuals and enriching themselves." According to Frianoro Rafaele (Nobili Giacinto), *Dell'origine de' bianti, pitocchi, cerretani, o vagabondi*, the Bianti got their name from "Briante prieneo filoso, primo inventore secondo alcuni, dell'arte d'andar vagando e girando per il mondo all'altrui spese." See Camporesi, *Il libro dei vagabondi*, p. 263. A *pitocco* (*pitocchi*, plural) from the Greek ptochos (πτωχός) was an indigent person reduced to beggary. See Mollat, p. 17.

59 Camporesi, *Il libro dei vagabondi*, p. 279: "These individuals are so called because of the *bordone* they use, a round, long staff with some wooden rings, from which hangs a small kerchief with which they falsely claim to be making their pilgrimage to St. James of Galicia [in Santiago de Compostela], to the Madonna of Loreto, to Jerusalem, to Rome and other pilgrimage sites overseas." My translation.

60 Ibid., p. 289.

61 Ibid., p. 293.

62 Ibid., pp. 261 and 331. In Teseo Pini's Latin text the author had comparably ended his work by stating: "Nos ergo oposculum hoc speculum appellemus, ut Medusa suam formam aspiciens vertatur in saxum, hoc est homines ipsis improbis artibus dediti recognoscentes fallacia suas in hoc respiciant et convertantur, vel cogniti minus laedant." Ibid., p. 240.

63 Juan Luis Vives, *On Assistance to the Poor*, Alice Tobriner (tr.), Toronto, Buffalo and London, 1999. Originally published as L. Vivès, *Il modo di sovvenire a' poveri*, Venice, 1545.

64 Quoted by Michele Fatica, *Il problema della mendicità nell'Europa moderna (secoli XVI–XVIII)*, Naples, 1992, p. 74. My translation.

65 Vives, pp. 39–42.

66 Leon Battista Alberti, *De re ædificatoria* (ca. 1450), *Ten Books on Architecture*, Cosimo Bartoli (tr. into Italian) and James Leoni (tr. into English), London, 1965 (from the 1775 edition), V, p. 91: "For there is hardly any so maimed but what may do some Work or other; even the blind Man may turn a Rope-maker's Wheel, if he can do nothing else." Giovanni Botero, *Della Ragion di Stato Libri Dieci, con tre libri delle cause della Grandezza e Magnificenza delle Città*, Venice, 1589, IV, p. 131: "e non sono comportati in modo alcuno i scioperati, e gli otiosi: i ciechi, e gli stroppiati s'impiegano, per quanto le loro forze comportano; e non s'ammettano à gli hospedali, se non quei che sono affatto impotenti."

67 See Chapter 1 and note 4 above.

68 For the *Landscape with Five Beggars* see Walter L. Strauss, John T. Spike and Isabelle de Ramaix (eds.), *The Illustrated Bartsch*, XL (Commentary, Part 1), New York, 1987, p. 265), *The Illustrated Bartsch*, XL, formerly XVIII (Part 2), New York, 1982, p. 14, for the Italian. For the *Birbante*, see John T. Spike (ed.), *The Illustrated Bartsch*, XLII, formerly XIX (Part 2), New York, 1981, p. 449. The authorship of the *Five Beggars* engraving is disputed. Listed as the work of Francesco Brizio, it may have been executed by Pietro Stephanoni or Vaccini. See *The Illustrated Bartsch*, XL (Commentary, Part 1), p. 265.

69 "Vivemus ex rapto; nam quas fortuna negavit,/furto quaerit opes ingegnosa manus./Qui simulat caecum, si quid sors obtulit olli,/lynceis oculis surripienda videt./Qui claudo titubat gressu si rapta reportet,/currentem aligeros credis habere pedes./Arte sibi victum stulti quesisse laborent/non ulla ars melior, quam piceata manus." My thanks to Inge Weustink for translating this passage.

70 The couplets in Italian read as follows: "Questi di varie rase sei monelli/Raminghi vanno in quella parte, e'n questa./L'Orbo quante città, ville e castelli/Hà veduto a compagni manifesta./La Grimma i scorsi chiassi e i borselli/Leccati il Guerzo: il Muto tienli in festa/Con novelle: il Calcante ultimo è raro,/Che di tutte le fiere hà il calendaro." ("These six roaming rogues go swindling here and there. The blind one reveals to the others the many cities, villas and castles he has seen. The old woman the alleys frequented [in the past – "chiasso," a narrow street but also

a brothel] and the cross-eyed the many purses he has 'licked': the mute one keeps them amused with his tales: the last beggar is unique, as he carries the calendar of all the fairs." The sixth rogue mentioned in these couplets refers to the infant carried in a barrel-like container on the back of the vagabond in the middle of the group.

71 On this common European phenomenon, see Jütte, pp. 146–150. See also, Geremek, *Poverty*, p. 146: "The laws against vagrancy issued by the French government were harsh: vagrancy became a crime, to be combated by repression: those caught were sent to the galleys or sentenced to forced labour in the city."

72 *The Illustrated Bartsch*, XLII, p. 449, app. 11. My translation.

73 Niccolò Tommaseo, *Dizionario della lingua italiana*, Turin, 1916, VII, p. 1602: "Trionfare: 5. Godersela a tavola manginado e bevendo." Salvatore Battaglia, *Grande dizionario della lingua italiana*, Turin, 2002, XXI, p. 360: "Trionfare: 16. Godersela, spassarsela, far bisboccia, festeggiare in allegra compagnia; mangiare e bere di gusto e in abbondanza." Giovanni Della Casa, *Galateo*, Ruggiero Romano (ed.), Turin, 1975, p. 28: "sì come il bere e il godere si nominano per beffa trionfare."

74 Tommaso Garzoni, *La Piazza Universale di tutte le Professioni del Mondo*, Venice, 1617, under Discorso LXXII, "De' Guidoni, O Furfanti, O Calchi," pp. 251r–251v: "Si trovano alcuni, che non tanto da inopia, e da miseria tratti, quanto da una pigritia mera, abbonda[n]te l'arti, e le scienze si danno à una vita talmente otiosa, e negligente, che la maggior quiete, ò felicità non istimano, che con una pazza furfanteria mendicar del continuo il cibo, ed il vitto; reputando questa vita per la più, e più beata al mondo, che' esser possa . . . . Hora la furfantesca professione di costoro non consiste in altro salvo, che in ingannare il mondo, e con occulto intendimento alle spalle d'altrui sguazzare, e trionfare." My translation.

75 In this context it is worth citing Camporesi, *Il libro dei vagabondi*, p. 171: "Il 'mestiere di vagabondo' fu quasi sempre frutto di un duro bisogno, non di libera scelta: perfidia, simulazione e satanismo conseguenze necessarie e dirette del crudele 'stato di necessità' che costringeva poveri, diseredati, disoccupati e mendicanti a una continua mimetizzazione, a una dolorosa girandola d'invenzioni nuove per sopravvivere e per tirare, in qualche modo, avanti." ("The 'vagabond's craft' was almost always the outcome of a harsh reality, not of free choice: perfidy, simulation and satanism [were] the direct and necessary consequence of the cruel 'state of necessity' that forced the poor, the disinherited, the unemployed and beggars to [rely on] a constant masquerade, a painful slew of new ploys in order to survive and, somehow, make ends meet.")

76 Giovan Battista Scanarolo, *De visitatione carceratorum*, Rome, 1655. Quoted by Roberto Morozzo Della Rocca, "Il potere, la sicurezza, l'ordine," in Monticone (ed.), *La storia dei poveri*, p. 162.

77 A comparable depiction of disabled mendicants north of the Alps is provided, of course, by Hieronymous Bosch's phenomenal series of drawings at the Albertina, Vienna. For these images see Nichols, *The Art of Poverty*, pp. 62–63.

78 This print is reproduced in Helen Langdon's "Bari, zingare e venditori ambulanti," in *Il genio di Roma, 1592–1623*, Beverly L. Brown (ed.), Milan, 2001, p. 46, fig. 12. Although it is recorded as being in the Bibliothèque nationale de France, Paris, the librarians have failed to find it in this collection. No less condemning of the whole category of beggars, although in this case it is a representation of a (fake?) blind man with dog and cane, is an engraving by Pietro Faccini executed in the 1590s below which the inscription reads, "Andei vù à lavorà fiévi de porche, Mà non havè besogn' de lavorà, Perche à disnà v'aspettano le forche." ("Go to work, you sons of bitches. However, you have no need to work, since the gallows await you for dinner.") See *The Illustrated Bartsch*, XL, p. 145, no. 2 (272).

79 Civiche Raccolte Grafiche e Fotografiche, Civica Raccolta delle Stampe Achille Bertarelli, Castello Sforzesco, Popolari Profane m 13–5.

80 See Paolo Preto, "Gli emarginati," in *Mentalità comportamenti e istituzioni tra Rinascimento e decadenza 1550–1700*, Giuseppe Galasso (ed.), Milan, 1988, p. 171. A third variant is reproduced in Giorgio Lise and Claudio Salsi, "Emilia e Romagna, ovvero Mitelli e Soliani," in *Pittura votiva e stampe popolari*, Milan, 1987, p. 200, by the title, "Abito e vita di forfanti."

81 These didactic prints were collected not just by the bourgeoisie as a form of art more accessible to the "average" person but also by people of the "better" kind. See Camporesi, *The Land of Hunger*, p. 12.

82 Pier Luigi Fantelli, "I pitocchi nell'arte veneta del XVII secolo," in *La pittura nel Veneto: il Seicento*, 2 vols., Mauro Lucco (ed.), Milan, 2001, II, p. 712.

83 Helen Diane Russell, *Jacques Callot: Prints and Related Drawings*, Washington, 1975, p. 4.

84 Ferdinand Braudel, *The Structures of Everyday Life: The Limits of the Possible (Civilization and Capitalism: 15th–18th Century)*, Berkeley and Los Angeles, 1992, also quoted by Luciano Nasto, *La questione della mendicità nello stato pontificio (sec. XVIII–XIX)*, Rome and Pisa, 2001, p. 170.

85 Barry Wind, *"A Foul and Pestilent Congregation": Images of "Freaks" in Baroque Art*, Cambridge, 1998, p. 60.

86 See Russell, *Jacques Callot*, especially Wenzel Hollar's prints after Callot, nos. 42–44.

87 See Francesco Porzio, "Aspetti e problemi della scena di genere in Italia," in *Da Caravaggio a Ceruti: la scena di genere e l'immagine dei pitocchi nella pittura italiana*, Francesco Porzio (ed.), Milan, 1998, p. 35, especially Giovanni Battista Corlone's *Group of Rogues* (*La compagnia dei baroni*), cat. no. 72, fig. p. 199.

88 For the impact these prints had, see Porzio, as in note 87, cat. no. 72, p. 199, and Russell, as in note 86, plate nos. 42–44.

89 Anna Orlando, entry no. 72, p. 391, in F. Porzio.

90 Ibid.

91 Cesare Ripa, *Iconologia*, Piero Buscaroli (ed.), Milan, 1992, pp. xiv–xv.

92 The proverb is quoted from Quintilian's *De Institutione Oratoria*, in *The Institutio Oratoria of Quintilian*, H.E. Butler (tr.), 4 vols., Cambridge, MA, and London, 1989, book IV, ii, 91.

93 Ibid., pp. 45–46. My translation.

94 McTighe, p. 83, rightly points out how these images of distorted or deformed bodies "had the function of strengthening the hegemony of a ruling élite, by deeply embedding the stigma of labour and its distortion of the physical body into the mentality of those who could not escape the necessity of work."

95 Mark J. Zucker (ed.), *The Illustrated Bartsch*, XIV, Commentary Part 1, *Early Italian Masters*, New York, 1999, p. 103.

96 For Enea Vico's *Senectus*, after a drawing probably by Francesco Salviati, see *The Illustrated Bartsch*, XXX, formerly XV (Part 3), *Italian Masters of the Sixteenth Century*, New York, 1985, p. 79, fig. 88.

97 *The Illustrated Bartsch*, XIV (Part 1), pp. 103–105, fig. 001.

98 Seneca, *Ad Lucilium Epistulae Morales*, 3 vols., Richard M. Gummere (tr.), Cambridge and London, 1989, I, 12.5, pp. 66–68.

99 Cicero, *De senectute*, William Armistead Falconer (tr.), Cambridge and London, 2001, xix, 71, p. 83.

100 For Marcellus II, see Ludwig von Pastor, *The History of the Popes from the Close of the Middle Ages*, Ralph Francis Kerr (tr.), 40 vols., London, 1891–1941, VI, pp. 303–340.

101 Spike (ed.), *The Illustrated Bartsch*, XLII, formerly XIX (Part 2), *Italian Masters of the Seventeenth Century*, New York, 1981, p. 39.

102 Paolo Bellini and Mark Carter Leach (eds.), *The Illustrated Bartsch*, XLIV, formerly XX (Part 1), *Italian Masters of the Seventeenth Century*, New York, 1983, p. 89.

103 Tom Nichols, "Secular Piety, Sacred Poverty: Picturing the Poor in Renaissance Venice," *Art History*, 30 (2007): 139–169, explains how in sixteenth-century Venetian art commissioned by the state, and in keeping with poor legislation, the poor were removed from representations of the public space. Instead, the poor and an emphasis on charitable deeds became prominent in paintings commissioned by the non-ruling class, especially by the *scuole* (lay confraternities) in large-scale narrative paintings.

104 Roland H. Bainton, *Here I Stand*, London, 1950, p. 261, relates how, when Luther was taken to task for having translated into German St. Paul's "justification by faith" as "justification by faith alone," he responded that he was translating the concept and not the words. "Through all the revisions of his lifetime he would never relinquish that word 'alone'." John Dillenberger, *Martin Luther: Selections from his Writings*, Garden City, 1961, p. xxvi, n. 7: "The phrase 'justification by grace through faith' (cf. Ephesians 2:8) or 'justification by faith' (Romans 5:1) is a slogan which points

the way in which Luther broke through the medieval development at a central point through the medieval Pauline understanding. In our day, it is better to speak of 'grace' and 'freedom,' defining them, than to continue to use the term 'justification.' In that way, Luther's classical insight can more readily become our own."

105 Dillenberger, pp. xxvi–xxvii.

106 The same concept is repeated in Romans 5:1: "So far then we have seen that, through our Lord Jesus Christ, by faith we are judged righteous and at peace with God, since it is by faith and through Jesus that we have entered this state of grace in which we can boast about looking forward to God's glory."

107 Dillenberger, p. 69.

108 Brian Pullan, "Catholics, Protestants, and the Poor in Early Modern Europe," *The Journal of Interdisciplinary History*, 35:3 (2005): 447.

109 Philip Hughes, *A Popular History of the Reformation*, Garden City, 1960, p. 141.

110 Philip Hughes, *A Popular History of the Catholic Church*, Garden City, 1962, p. 164.

111 "When I say by faith alone, I do not mean, as those inventors of novelties do, a mere credulity and confidence in God, by which, to the seclusion of charity and the other duties of a Christian mind, I am persuaded that in the cross and blood of Christ all my faults are unknown; this, indeed, is necessary, and forms the first access which we have to God, but it is not enough. For we must also bring a mind full of piety towards Almighty God, and desirous of performing whatever is agreeable to him; in this, especially, the power of the Holy Spirit resides." For Sadolet's letter and Calvin's reply see http://www.monergism.com/thethreshold/sdg/calvin_sadolet.html (last accessed March 21, 2016). For John Calvin's reply and general support of "justification by faith alone," see Dillenberger, pp. 81–118.

112 *Decrees of the Ecumenical Councils*, II, pp. 671 and 673.

113 Anthony Blunt, *Artistic Theory in Italy*, London, Oxford and New York, 1973, p. 116.

114 Nichols, "Secular Charity, Sacred Poverty," p. 144, mentions that in works produced in Protestant countries, pictures portraying almsgiving tend to be "anti-clerical, suppressing all reference to religious charity."

115 See Tom Nichols's discussion of the appropriateness of such Classical models for Christian art as dictated, for example, by Giovanni Andrea Gilio in 1564. Nichols, *The Art of Poverty*, pp. 160–161.

116 Ibid., p. 161. Nichols attributes the popularity of this statue in Venetian art to the transfer of this statue in 1523 from the Grimanis' Palazzo San Marco in Rome to Palazzo Grimani in Venice.

117 Blunt, p. 126.

118 Nichols, "Secular Charity, Sacred Poverty," p. 152, makes a comparable observation indicating how, "in the imagery of official charity, the poor are depicted in the same naturalistic manner used for the donor portraits."

119 Brian Pullan, "Poveri, mendicanti e vagabondi," p. 1046. My translation. Also Porzio, p. 39.

120 Pullan, "Poveri, mendicanti e vagabondi," p. 1046.

121 Giuseppe Palmeri, *Riflessioni critiche sull'arte della Guerra*, Naples, 1761, cited by Fatica, p. 276.

122 Ellis Waterhouse, in the catalogue to the exhibition *Ribera* held at Fort Worth in 1982. Quoted by Pierre Rosenberg, "Da Ribera a Ribot, dal naturalismo all'accademismo: la fortuna di un pittore alla ricerca della sua nazionalità e della sua definizione stilistica," in *Jusepe de Ribera 1591–1652*, Alfonso E. Pérez Sánchez and Nicola Spinosa (eds.), New York, 1992, p. 96. Rosenberg traces Ribera's perceived nationality by the European connoisseurs through the centuries and points out that after his death his work was preserved from oblivion because the painter "veniva collocato tra i pittori di Napoli." The painting was probably executed for Don Ramiro Felipe de Guzmàn, duke of Medina de las Torres and viceroy of Naples from 1637 to 1644. He married as his second wife Anna Carafa Aldobrandini, princess of Stigliano. The picture remained in the collection of the princess of Stigliano, then passed to the La Caze collection at an unknown date, and eventually entered the Louvre in 1869. See the catalogue to the exhibition *Civiltà del Seicento a Napoli*, 2 vols., Naples, 1984, I, pp. 171–172 and 418–419 as well as Denise Maria Pagano's entry for the painting in *Jusepe de Ribera 1591–1652*, p. 254.

123 José Milicua, "Da Jàtiva a Napoli," in *Jusepe de Ribera 1591–1652*, p. 17. See also Guillaume Kazerouni and Guillaume Kientz (eds.), *Ribera à Rome, autour de l'Apostolado*, Rennes, November 7 to February 8, 2015, Strasbourg, February 28 to May 31, 2015, and more recently Giuseppe Porzio and Domenico Antonio D'Alessandro, "Ribera between Rome and Naples: New Documentary Evidence," *The Burlington Magazine*, CLVII, October 2015, pp. 682–683.

124 See Pagano's entry as in note 121 and E.J. Sullivan, "Ribera's *Clubfooted Boy*: Image and Symbol," *Marsyas*, 19 (1977–1978): 17–21, and Wind, pp. 49–65.

125 Wind, p. 60. Also, Luigi Fiorani, "Religione e povertà: il dibattito sul pauperismo a Roma tra Cinque e Seicento," *Ricerche per la storia religiosa di Roma*, 3 (1979): 123.

126 Salvator Rosa, *Satire e vita di Salvator Rosa*, Florence, 1833, p. 170: "Così i vivi mendichi afflitti, e nudi,/Non trovan da coloro un sol danaro,/Che ne' dipinti poi spendon gli scudi./Così ancor io da quegli straccioni imparo,/Che dei moderni principi l'istinto/prodigo è ai lussi, alla pietade avaro."

127 Camporesi, *The Land of Hunger*, p. 121.

4 Papal Rome

> If you are questioning us today about an act of kindness to a cripple, and asking us how he was healed, then I am glad to tell you all, and would indeed be glad to tell the whole people of Israel, that it was by the name of Jesus Christ the Nazarene ....
>
> (The Acts of the Apostles, 4:9–10)

Of the three theological virtues – Faith, Hope and Charity – the last has always been the most important. As St. Paul remarked: "And now abideth faith, hope, charity, these three; but the greatest of these is charity" (1 Co 13:13).[1] And since "the supreme charity is God's love for us," by loving others with the desire to unselfishly satisfy them, the Christian carries out "the essential commandment of the Law, which is love of God and neighbour."[2] Indeed, this concept was so entrenched in Christian ideology that in Gratian's *Decrees* of about 1140 it was deemed the fundamental premise to the faithful's hope for salvation: "Lay people may have a wife, till the earth, judge and bring lawsuits, lay the offerings on the altar, pay tithes. If they have done this, they can be saved, provided they avoid vice through the practice of charity."[3]

This emphasis on charitable deeds has always held true for Christian communities at large but particularly so for the popes, who, as heads of Christendom, made it one of their foremost preoccupations, if not the very first of their concerns. That this has been so at least since the Edict of Milan in AD 313, when Constantine and Licinius granted religious freedom throughout the Roman Empire, is proven by the fact that, starting from its foundation, St. Peter's also functioned as a center of assistance for the poor.[4] Indeed, as indicated by the *Liber Pontificalis* – the biographical accounts of the vicars of Christ starting from St. Peter in the first century through the ninth-century popes – charitable acts towards the indigent and the marginalized were most important to their pastoral mission. Among the many popes whose charitable nature is emphasized by the biographers of these *Lives*, one finds Symmachus (498–514), who "constructed accommodation for the poor" in the basilicas of St. Peter, St. Paul and St. Lawrence,[5] and Pope Pelagius (579–590), who a century later "made his own house into an almshouse for the aged poor."[6] In the biography of Zacharias (741–752) one learns of the earliest *domuscultae* – the papal estates that were established in the *campagna* around Rome to procure provisions for the poor – and that "this blessed pope laid down that on frequent days the victuals and provisions which are even now called *eleemosyna* [alms] should be taken from the venerable patriarchate by the cellarers and dispensed to the poor and the pilgrims who doss at St Peter's; and he decreed that this *eleemosyna* of provisions should likewise be distributed to all the destitute and the sick living in all this city of Rome's regions."[7] Like Zacharias, his successor Stephen II (752–757) was "quick to provide help for Christ's poor"[8] and, by the end of the century, Hadrian I (772–795) seems to have espoused the beggars' cause with the greatest solicitude:

> His thrice-beatitude [Hadrian I] decreed and promulgated under mighty ties and interdicts that every day a hundred of our brethren Christ's poor, and even more, should be gathered at the Lateran patriarchate and be stood in the portico close to the stairs going up into the patriarchate, where the painting of the poor is; and 50 loaves, each loaf weighing 2 lb, and 2 *decimatae* of wine, each *decimata* weighing 60 lb, and also cauldrons full of broth should be disbursed every day to these poor by the hands of a trusty cellarer, each of them receiving a portion of bread, a drink of wine, that is 1 beaker containing 2 cupfuls, and a ladle of broth. So his bountiful thrice-beatitude, with the sacerdotal college, laid down and promulgated that the revenues of the produce and the various properties of this domusculta should be disbursed or expended on no other needs, but all the profit should be for, and should be disbursed for ever on, the assistance and daily sustenance of these our brethren Christ's poor.[9]

Of course, among the destitute, invalids and pilgrims who "doss[ed] at St. Peter's" one would have found sufficient numbers of crippled or lame individuals who precariously survived from day to day by relying on the papal donations. While all of the indigent, who must have intensely populated the square portico and the stairs leading up to the Early Christian basilica, could be taken as symbols of Christian *caritas*, the lame were particularly important to the vicars of Christ for the way they had been metaphorically employed in the Bible.

It is not coincidental that St. Peter's first miracle should be the healing of a lame man by the Temple entrance called the Beautiful Gate (Plate 18).[10] After all, St. Luke, the most likely author of *The Acts of the Apostles*,[11] could have employed any other disabled individual to make the point in his narrative. Surely, one would think that an equally effective way of showing how Peter, the rock on which Christ founded his church,[12] was able to cure individuals as his Master did would have been the healing of a blind person. In truth, since miraculous cures were metaphorically meant to represent the spiritual healing of a person, a blind individual regaining his or her sight would have been a powerful way of alluding to that person's ability to finally see the "true" faith. Still, this choice was not made and it is significant that the *Healing of the Lame Man* (Acts 3:1–11) should have been preferred over other miracles.

The fundamental text that regulated the rapport between humanity and divinity in the Old Testament, that enumerated the impediments of the Jews to the priesthood, is Leviticus 21:17–21, where Yahweh clearly proclaims to Moses:

> None of your descendants, in any generation, must come forward to offer the food of his God if he has any infirmity – no man must come near if he has an infirmity such as blindness or lameness, if he is disfigured or deformed, if he has an injured foot or arm, if he is a hunchback or a dwarf, if he has a disease of the eyes or of the skin, if he has a running sore, or if he is a eunuch. No descendant of Aaron the priest must come forward to offer the burnt offerings of Yahweh if he has any infirmity; if he has an infirmity, he must

> not come forward to offer the food of his God. He may eat the food of his God, things most holy and things holy; but he must not go near the veil or approach the altar, because he has an infirmity, and must not profane my holy things; for it is I, Yahweh, who have sanctified them.

From this text it is clear that the rapport of the Old Testament God with his people through the intercessory role of the priestly caste is one that does not admit of physical ailments because, if the disabled priest is to approach God and share in his sanctity, these would be an affront to the One who created the universe without blemishes.[13] In this perspective, the blind and the lame were unfit creatures for the sacerdotal task, as were blind, lame and diseased animals for celebrating the divine service, as they polluted the altar and were evidence of the priest's disrespect for Yahweh.[14] In fact, during the capture of Jerusalem from the Jebusites, one reads not only that "as for the blind and the lame, David hated them in his soul" but also that this gave rise to the saying, "the blind and the lame shall not come into the house" (2 Sa 5:8–9).[15]

The evangelists, however, took the Old Testament tradition and, so to speak, turned it upside down. That is, in all of the neo-evangelical stories that deal with the blind and the lame – but also with other infirmities – they show how in their community those individuals, who until then had been marginalized, were given pride of place. Thus Luke reports Jesus' admonition on choosing which guests to invite to one's home: "When you give a lunch or a dinner, do not ask your friends, brothers, relations or rich neighbours, for fear they repay your courtesy by inviting you in return. No; when you have a party, invite the poor, the crippled, the lame, the blind; that they cannot pay you back means that you are fortunate, because repayment will be made to you when the virtuous rise again" (Lk 14:12–14).

Of course, in the New Testament the infirm appear primarily as the co-protagonists of miraculous events that serve as examples of Christ's thaumaturgic powers and, as such, their ailments are characteristically redressed prior to their admittance into able-bodied society.[16] Nonetheless, the treatment and acceptance of the disabled by the Christian community is in sharp contrast with the way they had been considered previously.

As heirs of St. Peter, the popes had a particular interest in emphasizing the special healing powers the first vicar of Christ had inherited from Him, for, in their millennial contention on ecclesiastical hierarchy with those who believed that "the congregation of apostles was of greater authority than was Peter or any other apostle alone," it was to the popes' benefit that the bishop of Rome be seen as "first among equals."[17] This is one of the reasons why, when Paolo Romano sculpted the relief for Sixtus IV (1471–1478) that graced the baldachin over the tomb of Peter in the old basilica (Figure 4.1) or Raphael designed the cartoons for the tapestries that would hang in the Sistine Chapel beneath the fifteenth-century frescoes by Perugino, Botticelli, Ghirlandaio and others, they were asked to represent the *Healing of the Lame Man* (Plate 18).[18] To any viewer approaching the site near the tomb of the saint or any privileged dignitary who was allowed to go beyond the *cancellata* – the grate that separated the laymen from the more privileged clergymen area in the Sistine Chapel – the meaning would have been clear as they would have been aware of a tradition that from Arator to Bede as well as the *Glossa ordinaria*[19] interpreted the lame man as representing Israel being introduced by Peter into Christ's Church[20] and lameness as a symbol of the need for faith.[21] The biblical passage merits a full citation:

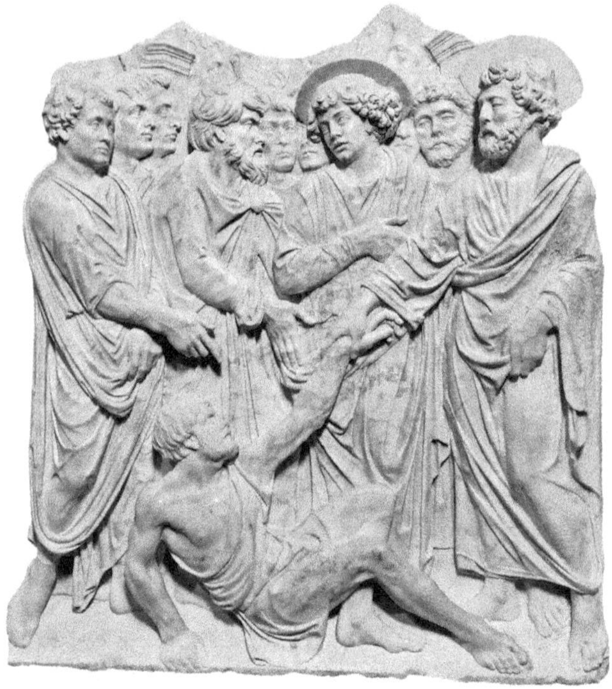

Figure 4.1 Paolo Romano, *Healing of the Lame Man*, St. Peter's Basilica, Ottagono di Simon Mago – Archivio Storico Generale

Once, when Peter and John were going up to the Temple for the prayers at the ninth hour, it happened that there was a man being carried past. He was a cripple from birth; and they used to put him down every day near the Temple entrance called the Beautiful Gate so that he could beg from the people going in. When this man saw Peter and John on their way into the Temple he begged from them. Both Peter and John looked straight at him and said, "Look at us." He turned to them expectantly, hoping to get something from them, but Peter said, "I have neither silver nor gold, but I will give you what I have: in the name of Jesus Christ the Nazarene, walk!" Peter then took him by the hand and helped him to stand up. Instantly his feet and ankles became firm, he jumped up, stood, and began to walk, and he went with them into the Temple, walking and jumping and praising God. Everyone could see him walking and praising God, and they recognized him as the man who used to sit begging at the Beautiful Gate of the Temple. They were all astonished and unable to explain what had happened to him.

Everyone came running towards them in great excitement, to the Portico of Solomon, as it is called, where the man was still clinging to Peter and John. When Peter saw the people he addressed them,

> Why are you so surprised at this? Why are you staring at us as though we had made this man walk by our own power or holiness? *You are Israelites, and it is the God of Abraham, Isaac and Jacob, the God of our ancestors, who has glorified his servant* Jesus, the same Jesus

> you handed over and then disowned in the presence of Pilate after Pilate had decided to release him. It was you who accused the Holy One, the Just One, you who demanded the reprieve of a murderer while you killed the prince of life. God, however, raised him from the dead and to that fact we are the witnesses; and it is the name of Jesus which, through our faith in it, has brought back the strength of this man whom you see here and who is well known to you. It is faith in that name that has restored this man to health, as you can all see.
>
> (Ac 3:1–16)

It is clear that in this neo-evangelical context the lame was symbolically exploited by the Christians to disparage the Jewish nation for having failed to recognize the Messiah (Ac 3:11–16). As Bede glossed, "the beautiful gate of the temple is the Lord. Whoever enters through him will be saved. Enfeebled Israel, being unable to walk to this gate, was brought there by the words of the law and the prophets, so that they might request help from those who were entering into the interior places of the wisdom of the faith which they were to hear"[22] and Peter was the guide into the temple.

Perhaps the decision to employ the healing of the lame by the Beautiful Gate to underscore this anti-Judaic concept, instead of a miracle relating the healing of a blind person, was dictated by the fact that the appearance of "a cripple from birth," at least in the eyes of some, might be more indicative of a physical and spiritual disability than the image of a blind man could provide. Nevertheless, there may be an additional reason that might justify the choice of this particular physical impairment.

The first-century *Apocryphon of Ezekiel* – a text that has survived in five fragments, the longest of which was found in rabbinic literature and in the writings of Epiphanius – relates the story of two disabled men, one blind and the other lame, who, being the only ones not invited to the king's feast, decide to retaliate by destroying trees in the king's garden or, according to the Hebrew version, by eating the choice fruit. Given their respective disabilities the two agree to collaborate. After having braided a rope, the lame threw it to the blind, stating: "Come to me, be [my] feet and carry me, and I will be your eyes, guiding you from above to the right and left." Although they succeed in their intentions, their plan is unmasked by the king, who "made the lame man ride upon the blind and . . . judged them as one." The author of the text clarifies: "So the Holy One, blessed be He, brings the spirit and placing it in the body, He also judges them as one."[23] Cited well into the Middle Ages and taken as the prototype of a sixteenth-century image for *Mutual Aid* by Andrea Alciati in his *Book of Emblems* (*Emblematum libellus*) (Figure 4.2)[24] and included in Hertel's 1758–1760 edition of Cesare Ripa's *Iconologia* as emblematic of *Friendship*,[25] this apocryphal story was interpreted on a spiritual level as the doctrine of the resurrection of *both* body and soul. Accordingly, like the blind and the lame, the body and the soul while indissolubly united on Earth were believed to be reunited on Judgment Day in a resurrection where they would both receive their just rewards. Still, what is significant for the present discussion, is that while the blind 'stood' for the body, it is the *lame* who represented the *soul*.[26] Thus, the inclusion of the *Healing of the Lame Man* by the Beautiful Gate in the *Acts of the Apostles*, besides having come to symbolize Israel in the Christian tradition, probably responded more poignantly than any other miracle to St. Luke's intentions of providing an obvious and powerful metaphor for humanity's spiritual healing and ultimate rebirth of the soul.

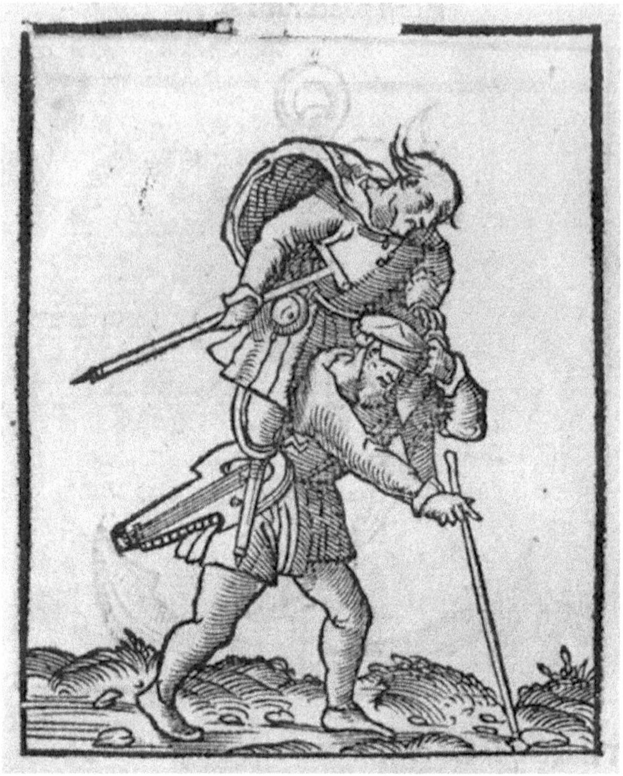

Figure 4.2 Andrea Alciati, *Mutual Aid*, *Emblematum libellus*, 1536. Photo: in the public domain

As mentioned earlier, the particular attention the popes devoted to the destitute and the disabled was a fundamental feature of their pastoral mission. Therefore, images that reflect this concern logically appear in contexts that relate to the papacy. This occurred not only because it was objectively true but also because such images of papal charity could be used propagandistically to extol the popes' role in the secular and the spiritual realms. Inevitably, this very image also appeared where one would expect it most: in St. Peter's basilica. Understandably, Ludovico Cigoli's (1559–1613) *Healing of the Lame* (Figure 4.3) was one of the six very large paintings that were executed for Clement VIII (1592–1605) and meant to "prove irrefutably the historical, doctrinal and moral rightness of the Petrine order."[27] Placed on the south side of the south-west giant pier that sustains the vast dome above, and facing squarely the pope when saying mass on the main altar in the apse of the basilica, the painting would have reminded the popes of what was expected of them as successors of Peter, and it offered the reassuring "message to the faithful . . . that of all St Peter's virtues as first pope, the administration of charity to the poor demanded his special attention."[28] Thus, it comes as no surprise that one of the most beautiful frescoes in the Vatican should feature the lame and the indigent (Plate 19).

The chapel of Nicholas V, painted by Fra Angelico ca. 1448–1450, was decorated with major scenes from the lives of two proto-martyrs: St. Stephen and St. Lawrence.

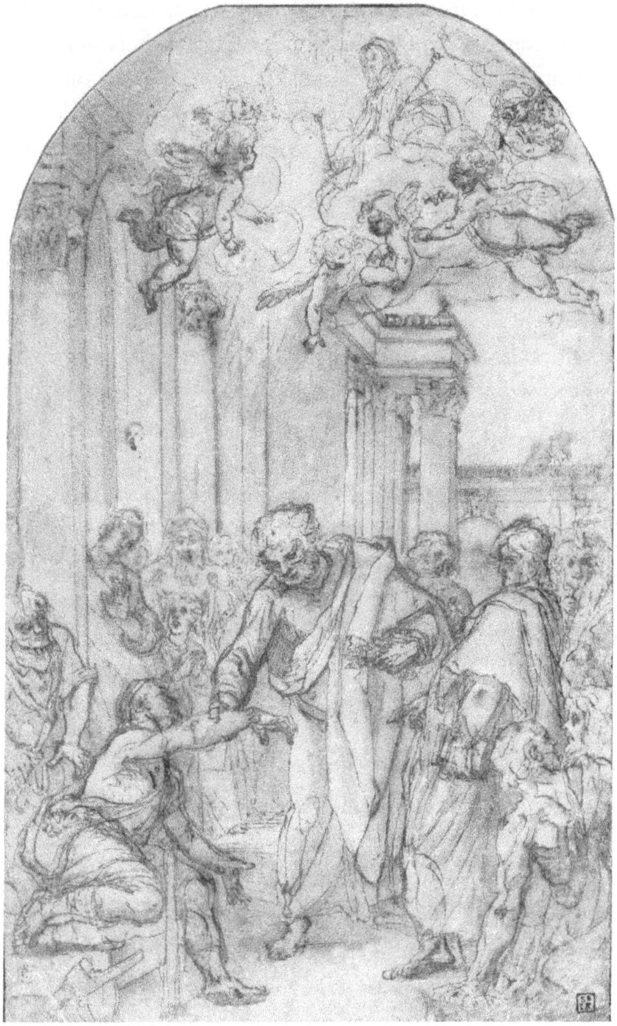

Figure 4.3 Lodovico Cigoli, *St. Peter Heals the Lame Man*, 1603–1606. Museo del Prado, Madrid. Photo: © Madrid, Museo Nacional del Prado

The former, one of the first seven deacons elected by the Christian community, was stoned to death for having upheld the superiority of the Christian over the Jewish faith in the Sanhedrin, the Jewish legislative body.[29] The latter was ordained deacon by Sixtus II, and before the pope's death in 258 was instructed to give the Church treasures to the poor. When he refused to surrender the treasures to the imperial authorities he was martyred by burning on a gridiron.[30]

It has been noted that the iconography of the chapel of Nicholas V reaffirmed the authority of the papacy.[31] In fact, the attempt to reassert the papacy's religious leadership had been the most salient aspect of the pontificates of Eugene IV (1431–1447) and

Nicholas V (1447–1455). The latter, especially, would see the Church of Rome through the last phase of the power struggle known as the "Age of the Councils."[32] After the Great Schism of the fourteenth century, which had divided Europe between allegiance to the Avignonese or the Roman line of popes, the ensuing Age of the Councils saw a rigid monarchic government upheld by the Church of Rome.[33] Through the political maneuvers of Nicholas V, the papacy prevailed and by 1449 the "separatist" cardinals had recognized Nicholas V's authority and the seat of Peter once again became the sole center of Catholic authority.[34]

By commissioning Fra Angelico to depict scenes from the lives of the two proto-martyrs, Nicholas and his advisers chose to reassert graphically the legitimacy of papal supremacy by showing that, contrary to the conciliarists' allegations, papal authority was founded on the continuity between the Early Church in Jerusalem led by Peter (upper register) and the Early Christian Church of Rome led by the popes (lower register).[35] The iconographic program for the chapel specifically avoided any reference to the principal biblical allusions employed to support claims of papal supremacy.[36]

Given the political and religious tensions of the first half of the fifteenth century, three frescoes from the life of St. Lawrence play a significant role in the papal chapel: *Saint Lawrence is Ordained Deacon by Sixtus II*, *Sixtus II Confides to Saint Lawrence the Treasures of the Church* and *The Charity of Saint Lawrence* (Plate 19). These scenes address the problematic issue mentioned earlier of ecclesiastical governance raised by the conciliarists, who would have agreed with Marsilius of Padua's claim that "it is … clear that neither Saint Peter nor any other apostles had pre-eminence or power over the others in the distribution of the temporal offerings."[37] Contrary to their view, the frescoes make clear that continuity existed between present-day papacy and Early Christian papal governance of the ministries and its treasure. Any educated individual entering the chapel would have understood the parallel narratives in the upper and lower register: just as Saint Peter had ordained St. Stephen in Jerusalem, so Sixtus II ordained St. Lawrence in Rome. Both Peter and Sixtus are shown offering the chalice and paten to Stephen and Lawrence respectively, who, as deacons of the church, were responsible for the daily masses and the church administration. In both instances, the act of proffering the treasures of the church to the two proto-martyrs signaled that only the "Vicar of Christ" had the authority to ordain priests and that only these could officiate the Eucharist.[38] Lest one miss the point that the pope was the legitimate heir of Peter, the painter twice replaced the portraits of Sixtus II in the lower register with those of the reigning pope, Nicholas V. What is more important in the context of this chapter, however, is that the lame are featured as co-protagonists in the scene *The Charity of Saint Lawrence*. When asked by the prefect of Rome for the Church treasure, St. Lawrence indicated "the decrepit, the blind, the lame, the maimed, the lepers, orphans, widows and maidens," and responded: "Here are the treasures of the Church."[39]

It is obvious that, despite the primary role played by the mutilated and the lame in Fra Angelico's fresco of *The Charity of Saint Lawrence* – it is not coincidental that iconographically the first to receive the alms is the mutilated man in the foreground – they remained subsidiary to the papal ideological agenda. In fact, their presence was dictated by the need to depict scenes that exalted the pope as the ultimate religious authority and the legitimate heir to the

Petrine tradition. Far from constituting the subject of a work of art in their own right, the lame in Nicholas V's fresco would have reminded the viewer of the pope's charity towards the Romans since he had created a large almshouse in the Vatican.[40] What is remarkable in the fresco, however, is that a consistent part of humanity, which traditionally had been kept on the margins of society, should now be exalted ideologically and pictorially as the Church's most valuable "capital." In keeping with the enhanced papal appreciation of the disabled, in this Roman fresco the orthopedically impaired body asserted its presence at the center of the viewer's visual field.

While the papacy was certainly not the only institution to monopolize care of the poor and the disabled, the hope, if not the assurance, that alms and a more tolerant government were to be found in Rome made this city a definite pole of attraction not just for pilgrims.[41] Indeed, contrary to other Italian cities Rome was not afflicted by transient vagrancy. Since the evangelical tradition made Christian charity one of its most important reasons for being, when vagabonds reached Rome they normally became part of the permanent poor population.[42] In fact, if a 1670 census of three Roman neighborhoods has any validity for the city as a whole, in comparison with other Italian cities Rome had two to three times as many poor people.[43] With an overall population of 27,092, the poor in the three *rioni* of Ponte, Regola and Trevi amounted to 11,160 – that is, 41 percent of the population. Assuming that this percentage is somewhat representative of the entire city, it makes the 15 percent registered in Cremona in the year 1610 and the 11 percent in Modena in 1621 seem insignificant.[44]

Consideration of this serious problem in Rome through the creation of a public structure with an official organization that would care for the indigent goes back to St. Philip Neri's creation of the Confraternita della Santissima Trinità, also called Confraternity of the Pilgrims and Convalescents ("Confraternita dei pellegrini e convalescenti") in 1548.[45] In fact, through a series of edicts, *avvisi* and papal bulls, starting with Paul III, also in 1548, the popes tried to contain the rising problem of widespread poverty, roaming mendicants and related issues, by creating what has been described as "a sort of charitable segregation."[46] These attempts culminated with an "Edict in Favor of the Poor Mendicants" issued by Gregory XIII in February 1581, in which, besides intimating that the poor report and be registered within six days at the hospital of the Santissima Trinità, "every faithful Christian" was encouraged to subsidize as much as one could this "most holy enterprise," with the assurance that "the alms would be given only to the truly poor."[47] This edict was followed by a more serious *avviso* on February 27, when, under pain of incarceration, begging was forbidden throughout the city and it was decided that all disabled mendicants be confined under one roof.[48]

On that very date, after having congregated by the oratory of the Santissima Trinità and having heard Mass, those mendicants who had opted to sacrifice their personal freedom for the sake of a secure shelter and food solemnly began a procession (somewhat akin to the one evoked by Ludovico Carracci's drawing of a group of lame mendicants marching through the Roman forum[49]) (Plate 20) that would lead the disabled indigent to what a contemporary eyewitness, Camillo Fanucci, described as the "longed for haven of San Sisto" ("desiato porto di San Sisto"). Following the members of the Confraternita dei Pellegrini e Convalescenti, came the mendicants grouped according to their ailments:

> One could see the partially lame [marching] in double file, the blind guided, and the cripple in carts pulled by the same mendicants. These individuals were followed by fourteen carriages loaded with many persons so disabled and infirm that it would have been impossible to escort them any other way. A truly pitiful but marvelous spectacle, the likes of which perhaps will never be seen again. Finally came the chief officer [*Primicerio*], the guardians and other officials of the confraternity, along with a multitude of people who had come not only to witness this unique event but also to obtain the indulgences that were granted by the pope to all those who accompanied the procession. There were 850 mendicants, between men and women, young and old, climbing and descending as they did the Capitoline Hill more triumphantly than the ancient Romans: finally, they reached the longed-for haven of San Sisto, where they were piously and charitably welcomed.[50]

That it should have been a Bolognese pope to initiate such repression of the mendicants in Rome is hardly surprising since the first Italian city to adopt such measures and to compel the truly poor into imposed seclusion was Bologna in 1563.[51] Nonetheless, there were a couple of problems with the original site chosen for these mendicants, since this former convent of the Dominican Nuns at San Sisto (Figure 4.4), besides being considerably distant from the city proper – the convent was situated near the Baths of Caracalla in the uninhabited south side of town near the Aurelian walls – was located in an area believed to be malarial.[52] Therefore, under the next pope, Sixtus V (1585–1590), with the promulgation of the papal bull *Quamvis infirma* of 1587 the pontiff announced his intention to create a hospice (*domum hospitalem instituire*) in which all the poor disseminated throughout the city streets and squares (*per via et plateas tota Urbe dispersi*) would find food, clothing and shelter. Soon after, in 1588, the hospice of San Sisto was inaugurated next to Ponte Sisto, named after an earlier pope, Sixtus IV, who had built the bridge, as well as the more renowned Sistine Chapel (Figure 4.5).[53]

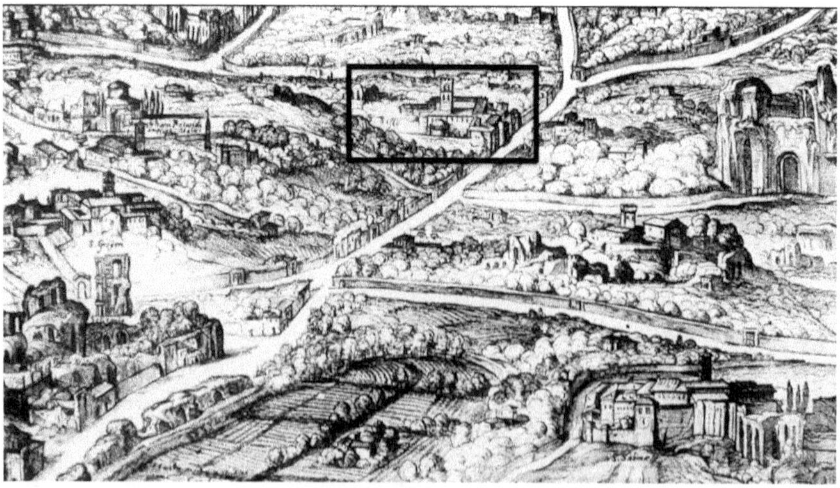

Figure 4.4 Antonio Tempesta, *Convent of San Sisto by Baths of Caracalla*, 1693, from Pietro Frutaz Amato (ed.), *Le piante di Roma*, Rome, 1962, III, pl. 369

Despite this more conveniently located hospice, what did not change was the spectacle that confronted anyone visiting this "grand Theater of human misery" ("gran Teatro dell'umane miserie"), where, according to an eyewitness, "everywhere one sees blind people, paralytics, lame and crippled individuals, old, decrepit men and women whose bodies have been altered through the years, maimed of their feet, or arms, disfigured, deaf, their physical appearance blemished either by bad luck or Nature, and incapable of earning a living."[54] Also unchanged was the situation in the city itself, since the Ospedale di San Sisto was unable to take care of all the beggars in Rome who, regardless of the papal edicts and *avvisi*, continued begging in every corner of the city because of personal choice or the inability of the Ospedale to accommodate them. Indeed, it soon became evident to the authorities that they had to be very selective not to succumb to the great numbers of those who requested shelter. Being poor, old, blind, crippled and unable to work was not sufficient to be taken into the Ospedale if the individual was still able to earn a living by begging.[55]

Thus, comparably to what occurred in other Italian and European cities, neither notices nor injunctions succeeded in controlling the tide of mendicants who, like the gypsies and the vagabonds, came to the city and contributed to the swelling crowds of beggars.[56] So much so that, especially in the late sixteenth century, when the Roman *campagna* yielded meager harvests, Rome was known as "the international capital of the poor."[57]

The great significance this institution had for the reigning Sixtus V is testified by one of the two large, high reliefs that flank the kneeling pontiff on his tomb in Santa Maria Maggiore (Figure 4.6). Foremost among the important accomplishments of his brief but incredibly productive papacy for which the pope wished to be remembered, was his charity to the destitute. Echoing the Latin inscription beneath, "for the people who were begging for food all over the city he built the building in which they are being fed" ("Victum per urbem ostiatim quaerentibus/domum in qua alerentur aedificavit"), the surmounting relief commemorates the pope's charitable deeds by displaying the near life-size personification of Christian Charity

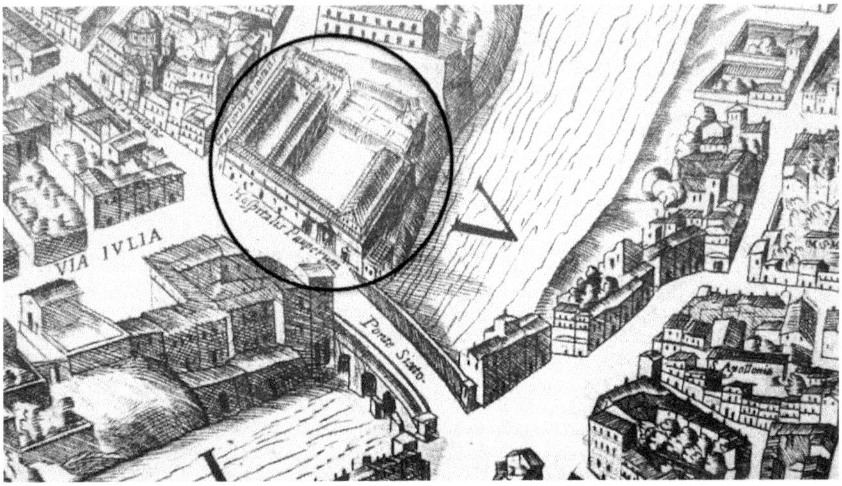

Figure 4.5 Antonio Tempesta, *Hospice of S. Sisto*, 1693, from Pietro Frutaz Amato (ed.), *Le piante di Roma*, Rome, 1962, III, pl. 374

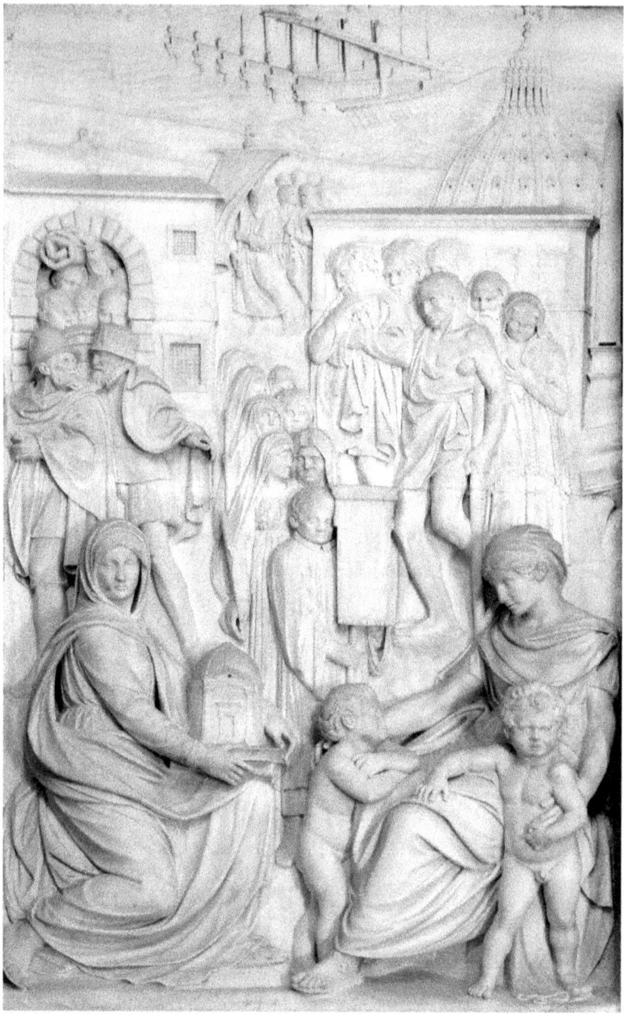

Figure 4.6 Govanni Antonio Paracca (Valsoldo), *Creation of the Hospice of S. Sisto*, Sistine Chapel, Santa Maria Maggiore, Rome. Photo: author

(the woman with two children by her side at bottom right) over which, first among a crowd representing Rome's poor, is the figure of a lame man supporting himself on crutches as the group approaches, ideally, the newly founded hospice.[58]

Despite these considerable efforts, improvement for beggars and society at large was not really in sight. The same Fanucci who informs us of the "triumphal march" of the beggars to the top of the Capitoline Hill, gives us an indication of the situation in the streets in 1601, when there were about 110,000 people living in the city:

> in Rome one sees nothing but poor beggars, and they are so numerous that it is impossible to stand or walk in the streets without being continually surrounded by them, which

> results in bad feelings both towards the people and the beggars themselves. In said hospital [of San Sisto] there are very few of them [beggars] and, as far as I know, between the poor, the overseers and the staff, there are usually no more than one hundred and fifty persons, and frequently fewer.[59]

Thus, even with the creation of the San Sisto hospice there were still many mendicants who continued to beg all over town, either because the structures were unable to accept all of the needy or because some of the beggars were unwilling to submit to confinement. This, in turn, led to the papal sanction of the founding of a confraternity that would allow the poor blind and lame to look after their own interests: the *Compagnia dei ciechi, zoppi e stroppiati della visitazione*.[60]

Legally founded on 27 September 1613,[61] and far from being an innovation on the European scene,[62] this confraternity of blind and lame people was originally placed under the protection of the Visitation of the Blessed Virgin, also called "*Salute degli infermi*."[63] Oddly, when a second invocation and dedication was added to St. Elizabeth as the other protagonist of the evangelical story of the Visitation, the confraternity of the lame and blind became more commonly known as the *Compagnia di Sant'Elisabetta*.[64] However, at the root of this seemingly incongruous dedication to the biblical St. Elizabeth undoubtedly was the confusion between St. Elisabeth, cousin of the Virgin Mary, and her homonym, St. Elisabeth of Hungary.[65] In fact, it was the daughter of King Andrew II of Hungary who, having converted to the ideals of St. Francis of Assisi, devoted her life to the destitute and thus had been the patron saint of beggars ever since 1235, when she was canonized.[66] Thus, in a woodcut from Jacobus de Voragine's *Golden Legend* dated 1483 (Figure 4.7),[67] she is depicted in a visual synecdoche, while giving alms to a single lame mendicant as a representative of the "profession" at large.[68] Again, in keeping with her role as patron saint of mendicants and charities, this is how she appears in a print by an anonymous master after Guglielmo Caccia (also known as Moncalvo) and in another by Nicolas Beatrizet, after Girolamo Muziano, dispensing solace and riches to the destitute and the infirm.[69]

While one reason for the creation of the Confraternity of St. Elizabeth was probably that of providing the blind with guidance by the lame,[70] it has also been suggested that the primary motive for founding this congregation was the desire on the part of the truly disabled mendicants to unite against a notice by the local government.[71] In fact, in an attempt to repress idleness and vagrancy, an *avviso* dated September 15, 1612 announced that "seeing the daily influx and multiplication of vagabonds and lazy people in this city, Monsignor the Governor [of Rome] has ordered the ministers of justice to carry out inflexibly the proclamations published against them by imprisoning, as they have been doing, those vagabonds who have been previously banished under threat of incarceration."[72]

Whatever reasons are adduced to a better understanding of the causes that gave rise to the congregation, from the statutes of the Compagnia di Sant'Elisabetta it is evident that, like all respectable Roman confraternities after which it was modeled,[73] this one looked after the interests of its members very assiduously, as did, for an analogy in a non-Roman context, the Scuola degli Zotti (Confraternity of the Lame) in Venice since 1392.[74] Although only local mendicants could be part of the *compagnia*, in special cases a temporary permit was given to foreigners as well, perhaps worn on their persons as does a "lame" beggar with cap in hand in a drawing attributed to Annibale Carracci (Plate 21).[75] The normal

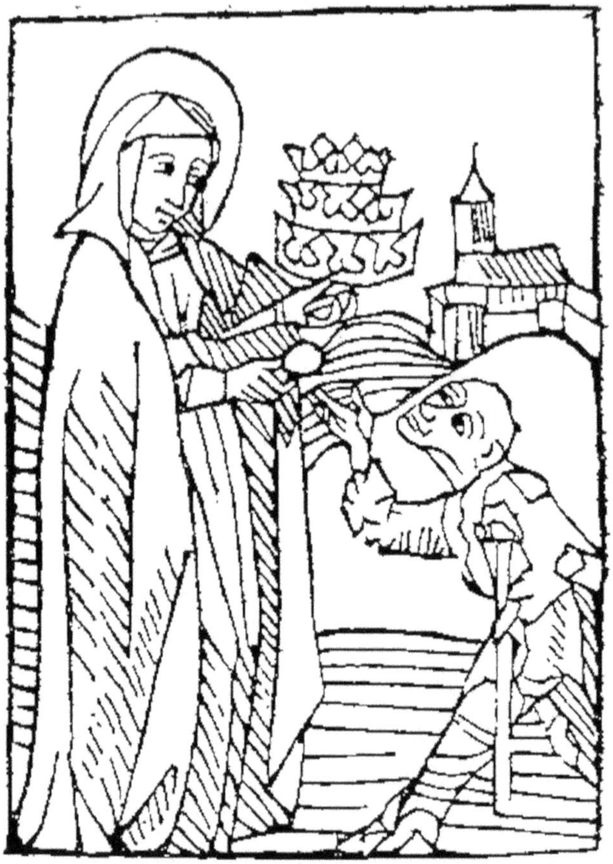

Figure 4.7 *St. Elizabeth*, from William Caxton's edition of Jacobus de Voragine's *Golden Legend*, 1483. Photo: in the public domain

modicum fee the "brethren" had to contribute was the monthly payment of *mezzo grosso*.[76] Of course, the visiting paupers were asked to pay a higher tax to the confraternity than the homegrown mendicants for the privilege of begging in town.[77] Nevertheless, when members failed to pay their dues for more than four months, they were deprived of the "tool of their trade": the alms-box with the image of St. Elizabeth, the Madonna and a mendicant; an image that must not have been very different from the print of the *Visitation* engraved by Oliviero Gatti (Figure 4.8).[78]

Wearing the confraternity's distinguishing garment of a deep blue color, the disabled mendicants paraded themselves through town by visiting four churches four times per year: in November, April, June and on July 2, Feast of the Visitation. Moreover, during the month of May of each year the brethren had to visit the seven major basilicas of Rome after having gathered and received Holy Communion at the church of St. Francis of the Mendicants, adjacent to the hospice of San Sisto (Figure 4.5).[79] On these occasions those members who were not able to walk were exempt from participating in the procession

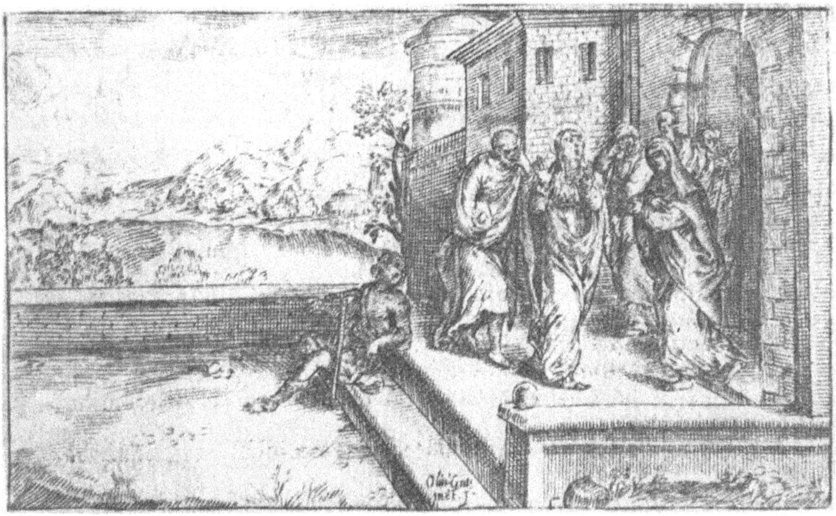

Figure 4.8 Oliviero Gatti, *Visitation of St. Elizabeth*. Photo: from *The Illustrated Bartsch*, XLI, p. 18

but were obliged to recite the rosary. Instead, those able-bodied mendicants who failed to show up had to pay a small fine.[80] On Sundays the *camerlengo* (chamberlain), always a lame person, along with the *signore* (supervisor) and the *guardiano* (custodian), always two blind people, accompanied by "two violins, a viola and a poet," would make the rounds collecting alms for their patron's feast day while giving their benefactors a pinch of tobacco from a snuff-box.[81] Furthermore, those brethren who were so ill as not to be able to beg were given a subsidy of two *giulii* and, if necessary, were hospitalized at the expense of the confraternity.[82]

Ultimately, what really emerges from these statutes is that the confraternity wished to have a complete monopoly on mendicancy.[83] The confraternity's real concern regarded those mendicants who not only refused to join their ranks and comply with official decrees but also disobediently pestered devout citizens with their lamentations. In fact, as proven by the written complaints of parish priests and sacristans of forty Roman churches during the Holy Year of 1625, these unruly mendicants disturbed the faithful by lying on the floor inside the churches or in the atria, moaning, asking for alms during Mass, and causing such attrition that the priests or sacristans were forced to call the police to keep them from pestering the parishioners[84] – a disturbance beautifully captured at bottom right of Raphael's fresco of *The Donation of Constantine* (ca. 1521), which portrays an orthopedically impaired older man importuning a faithful bystander inside old St. Peter's, who, annoyed by the beggar's timing, gestures towards the emperor, who is making his historically momentous donation to Pope Sylvester (Plate 22).[85] It is for this reason that the statutes of the Compagnia di Sant'Elisabetta exhorted the members to "never go begging for alms inside the church but humbly remain outside the door as not to impede the way of those [faithful] who wish to enter."[86] What the confraternity really objected to was that these "freelancers" might ruin their reputation as law-abiding mendicants and deprive the authorized beggars of their donations.

However, and perhaps most importantly in this context, the document never attacks or mentions those impostors who were the primary target of so much visual and literary censure.

Despite the noble intensions of the papacy, as well as those of the hospice of San Sisto and the Compagnia di Sant'Elisabetta, the subsequent history of the blind and the lame in Rome is marked by a progressive decline in the efficacy of the measures taken to solve the problems raised by their mendicancy. Thus, if the "carrot" of coerced enrollment in a papal or lay establishment did not work, then the Papal State reverted to the "stick." In an "Edict for Vagabonds, Beggars and the like, who loiter around the portico and stairs of the Churches" of 1628 one senses all of the inefficacy and inadequacy of an incomplete social-aid or poor-relief system: "We hereby alert and command that all and every one of the aforementioned Vagabonds, Cheats, Beggars, fake or real, who do not have a license ... leave those places where they take shelter ... under pain of incarceration, and of the whip/to be carried out immediately, for those who have come of age, and for the minors twenty-five lashes to be executed in public, and banishment from Rome and its region in perpetuity."[87] Indeed, during the seventeenth and eighteenth centuries governments all over Europe distinguished themselves because of the greater restrictions they imposed on the marginalized, thus justifying Foucault's designation of the whole period as the age of "the Great Confinement."[88] Notwithstanding the popes' good intentions and the recurring propagandistic imagery that affirmed their prodigality towards the poor – as in a 1658 Bernini drawing of a silver *scudo* for Alexander VII (Figure 4.9) where a lame individual represents the poor *par excellence* – the papal government followed the general trend and adopted comparable restraining laws.

On October 2, 1692, in a final attempt to eliminate mendicancy and vagrancy, Innocent XII promulgated a bull ordering Roman beggars to appear in the portico of Santa Maria in Trastevere to be registered by the papal authorities.[89] The mendicants were initially to be *rinchiusi* ("confined") and *sostentati* ("cared for") in the Lateran Palace that now took the name of *Hospitium Apostolicorum Pauperum Invalidorum* (*Apostolic Hospice of the Poor and the Invalid*) (Figure 4.10).[90] This building – the official seat of the bishop of Rome that had been left vacant by the popes – was thus renovated and modified to serve the new purpose[91] and, ultimately, became one of three hospices that was eventually absorbed by the vast eighteenth-century complex of San Michele a Ripa (Figure 4.11).[92] Individuals who were considered truly needy and unable to work, received a special symbol to be placed on their person that would identify them as legitimate mendicants. Those who proved to be healthy and able to work were forbidden to beg under pain of imprisonment and physical punishment.[93] This remedy concerned *all* mendicants, real and false. Therefore, the brethren of the Compagnia di Sant'Elisabetta organized a demonstration and went to the Quirinal Palace asking for an audience with the pope.[94] Two among them, who had been chosen as representatives to Innocent XII, offered the pope 4,000 *scudi* a year if he would only allow the members of the confraternity to continue begging in the city.[95] They also showed him a copy of the bull issued by Sixtus V, which had stated that the members of the *compagnia* could not be confined. To their disappointment the pope answered that "he wanted them either out of Rome or confined in the serraglio."[96] Given that the word *serraglio* was typically used to describe the Roman Jewish Ghetto created in 1555 by Paul IV to segregate the Jewish members of the Roman community, it might seem that by the end of the seventeenth century the popes could not have distanced themselves more from their Early Christian predecessors and had

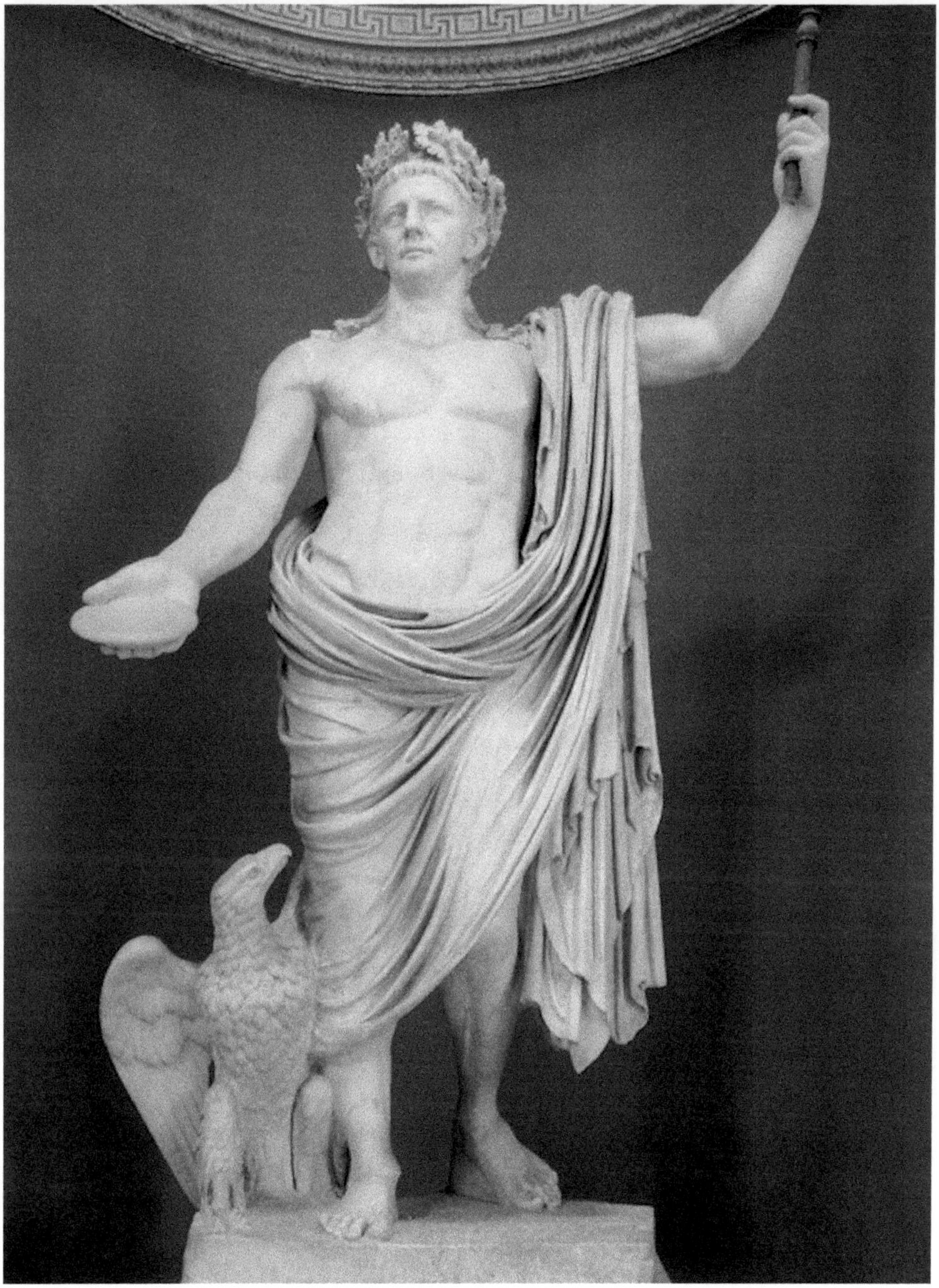

Plate 1 The Deified Claudius, Vatican Museums. Photo: author

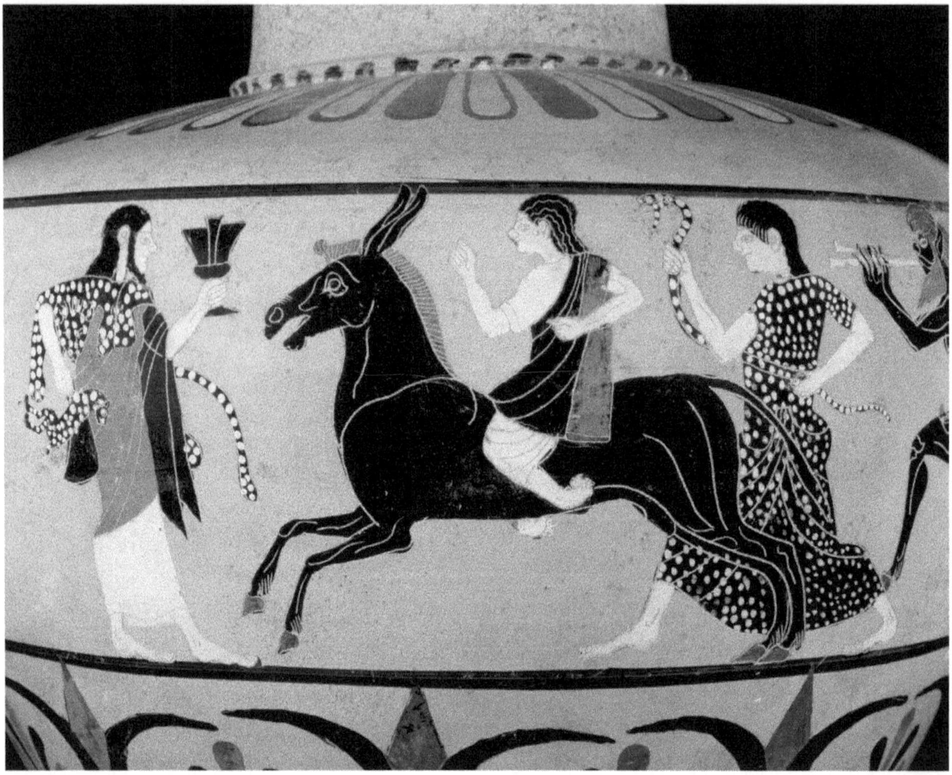

Plate 2 The Return of Hephaistos to Olympus, Vienna, Kunsthistorisches Museum. Photo: Kunsthistorisches Museum, Wien

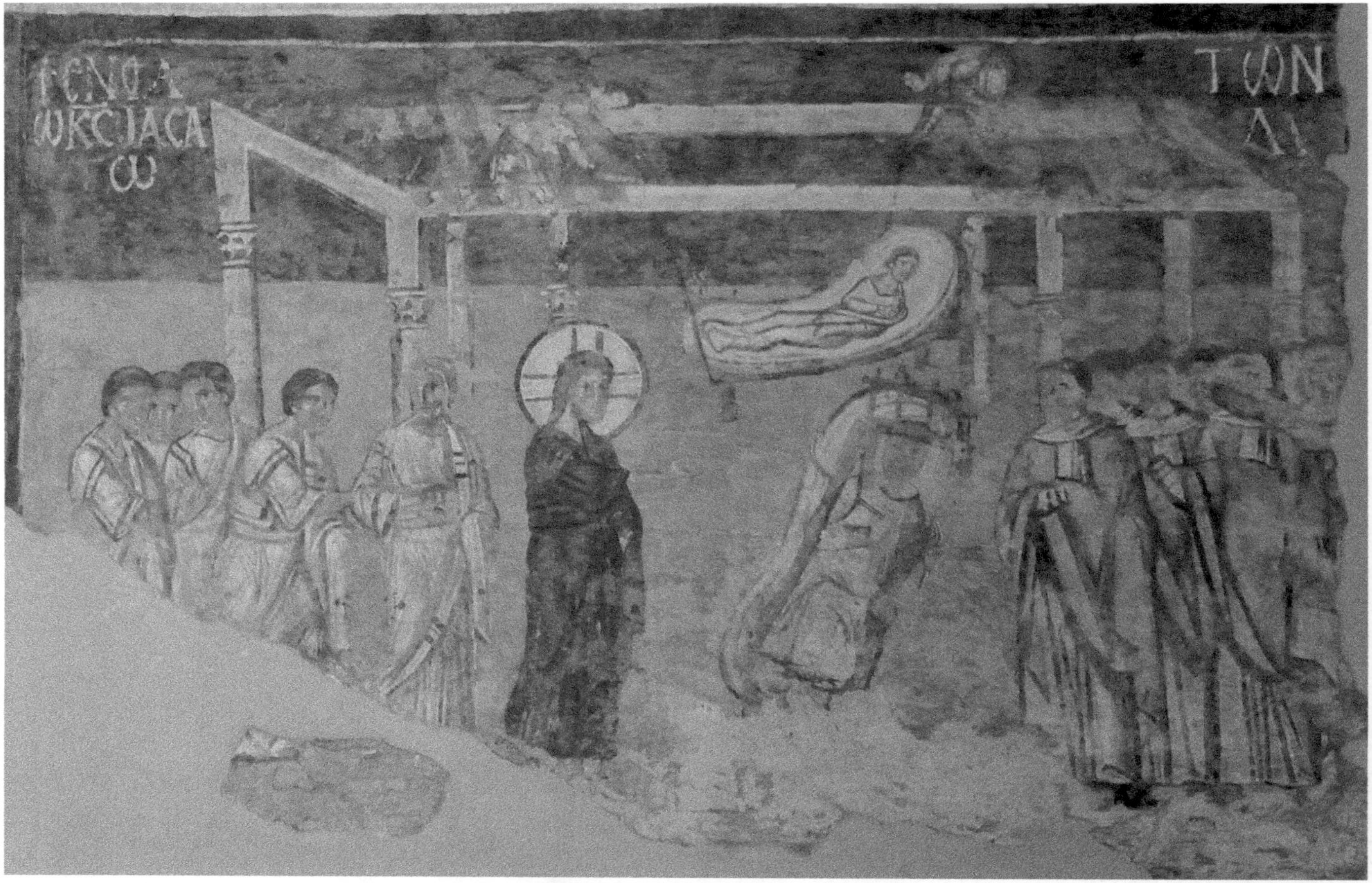

Plate 3 Healing of the Paralytic, San Saba, Rome. Photo: author

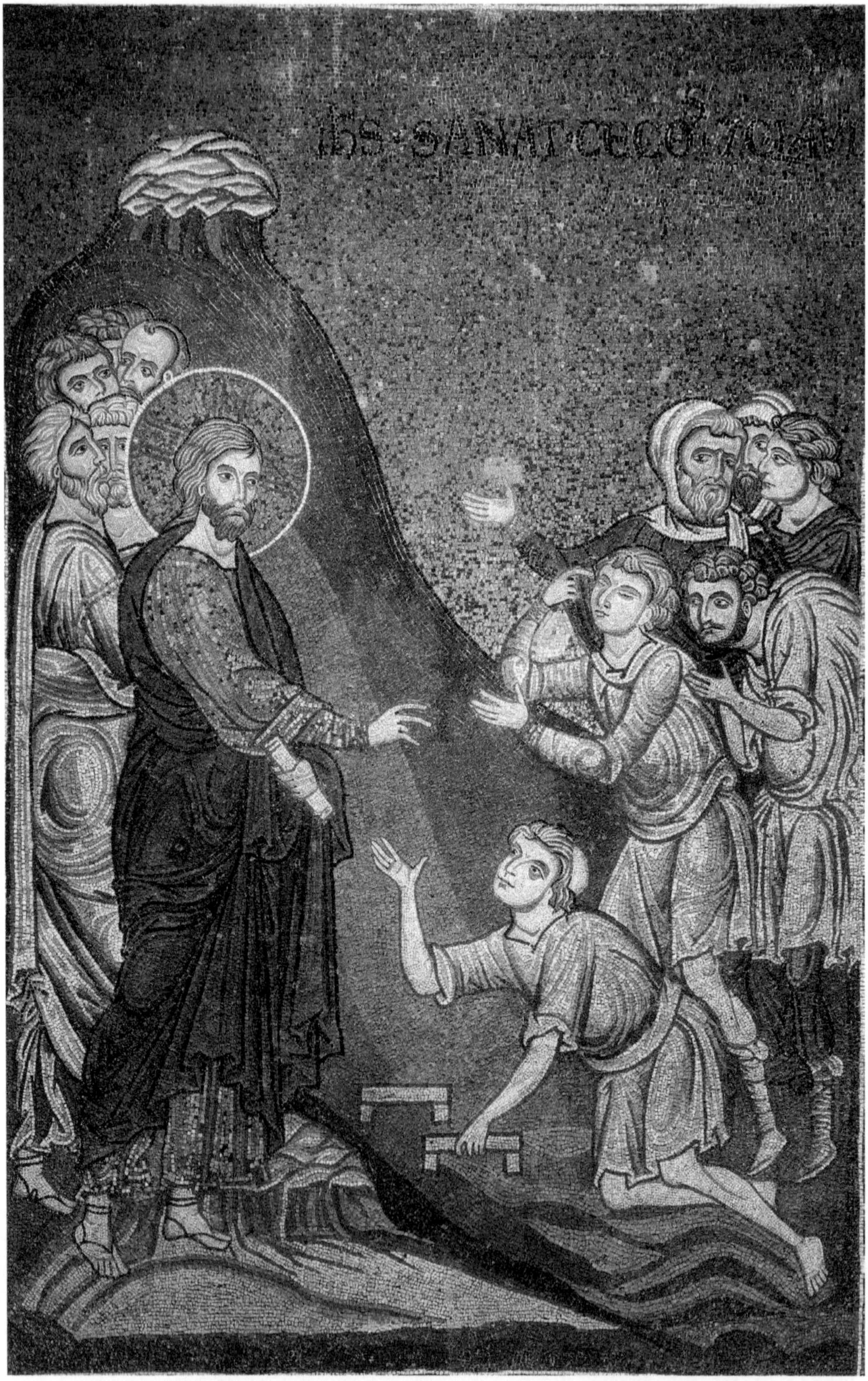

Plate 4 Christ Healing the Infirm, Cathedral, Monreale. Photo: © 2015. A. Dagli Orti/Scala, Firenze

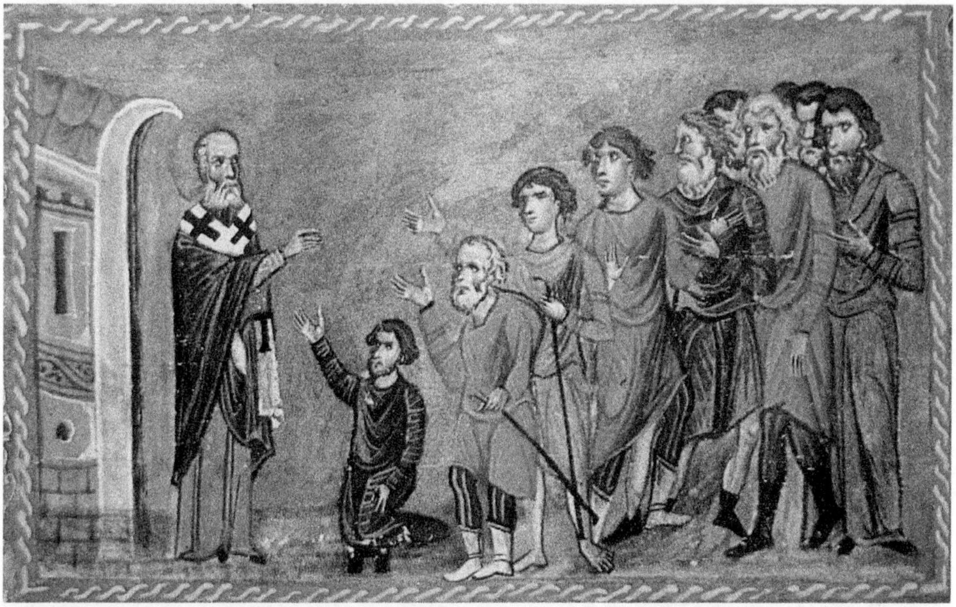

Plate 5 *St. Nazianzus and the Poor*, Cod. 339, Monastery of St. Catherine, Mt. Sinai. Photo: from Kurt Weitzmann and George Galavaris, *The Monastery of Saint Catherine of Mount Sinai: The Illuminated Greek Manuscripts*, Princeton, 1990, I, pl. XXIII

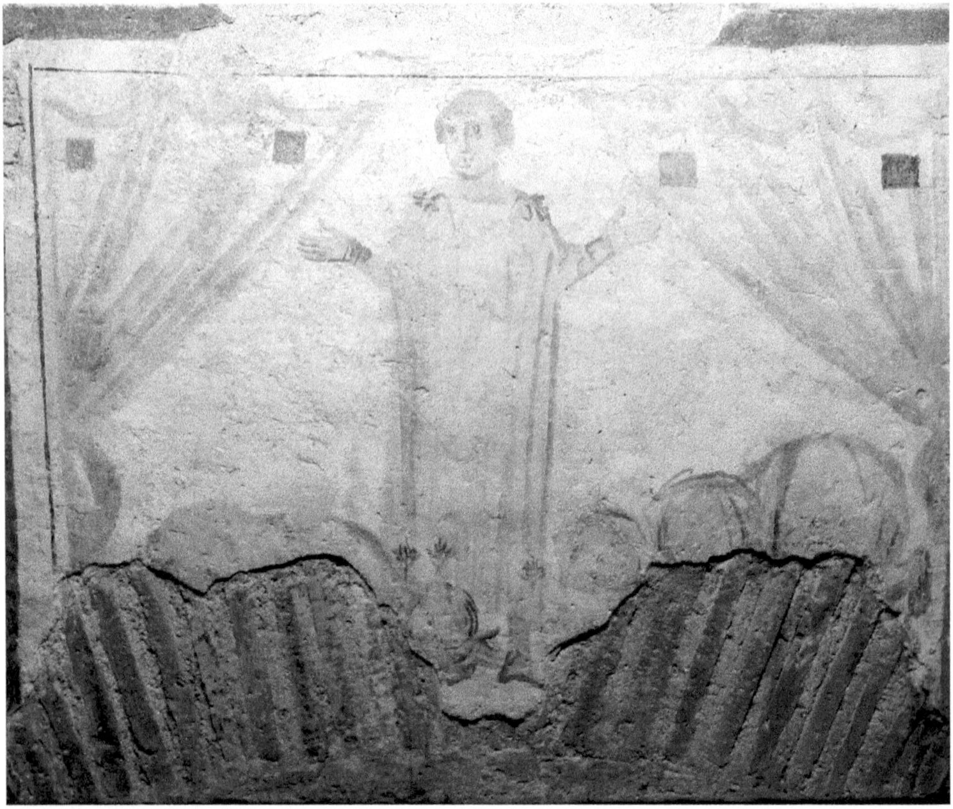

Plate 6 Praying Saint with Two Prostrated Devotees, ca. 400, Santi Giovanni e Paolo, Rome. Photo: author

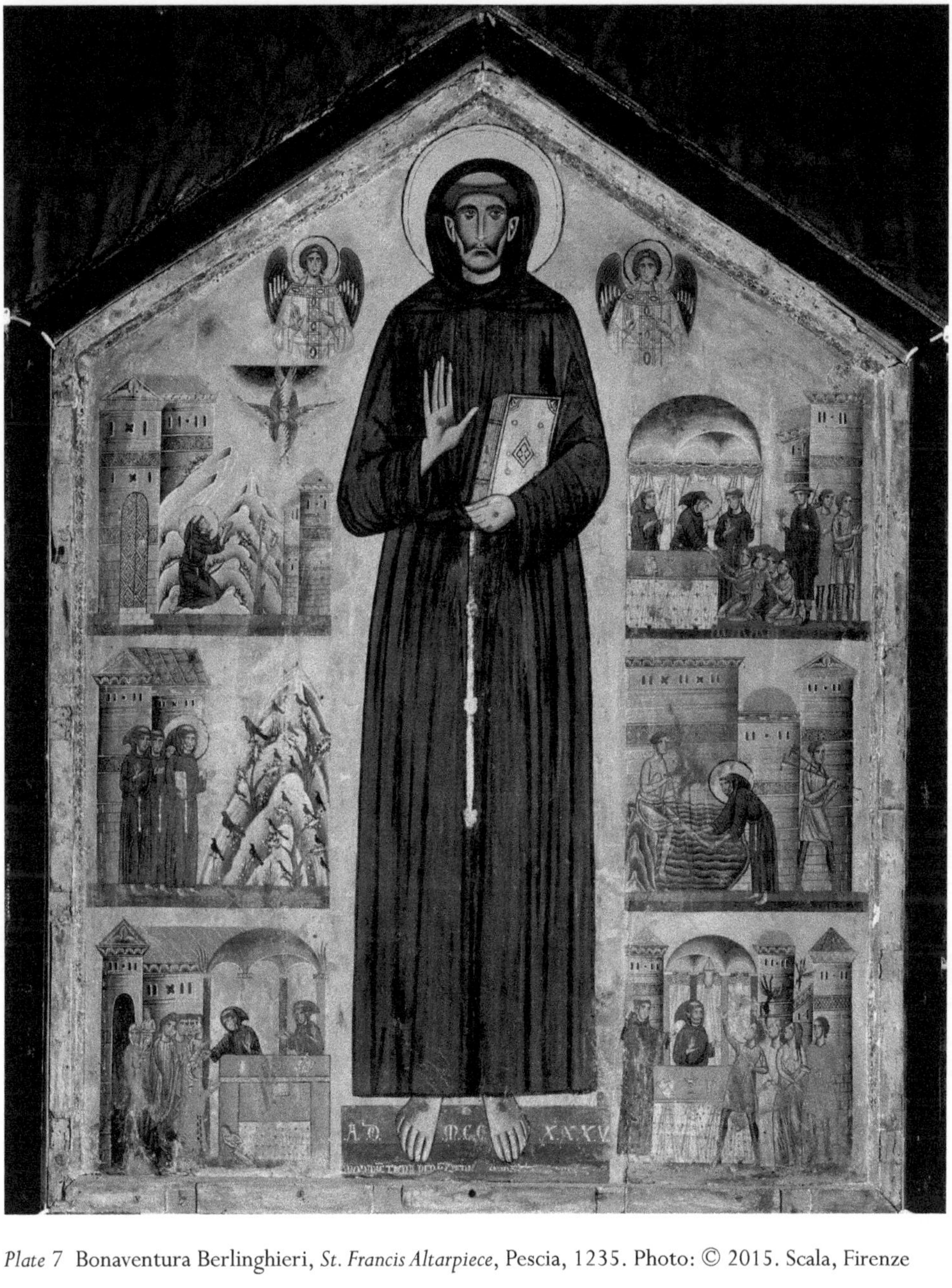

Plate 7 Bonaventura Berlinghieri, *St. Francis Altarpiece*, Pescia, 1235. Photo: © 2015. Scala, Firenze

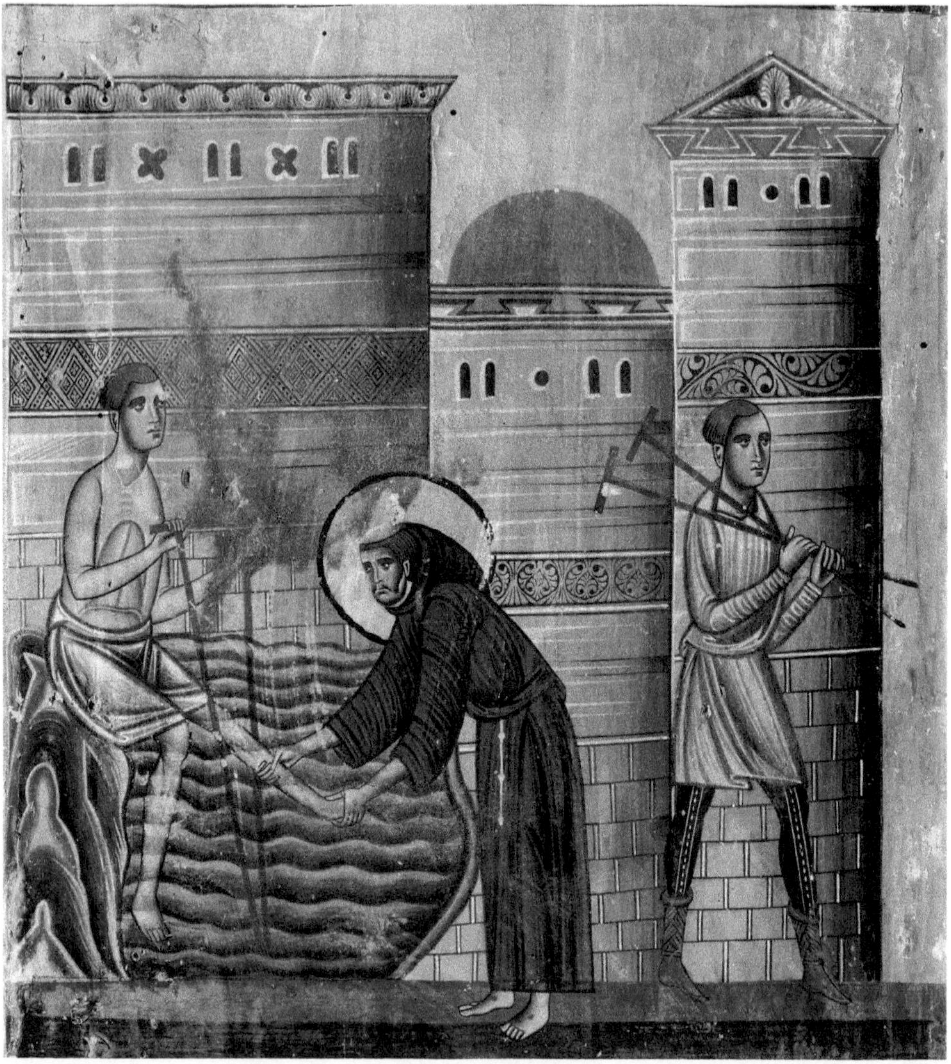

Plate 8 Bonaventura Berlinghieri, *Healing of Bartolomeo da Narni*, detail of Plate 7. Photo: © 2015. Scala, Firenze

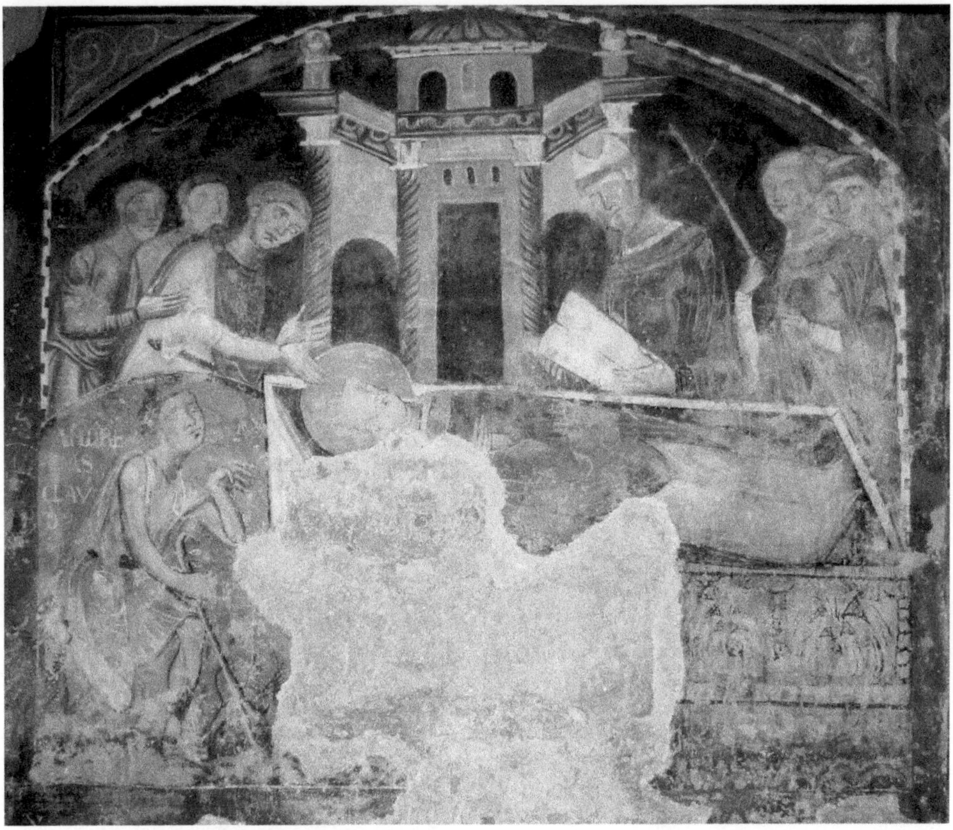

Plate 9 *Healing of the Crippled Doorman Andrew by the Sarcophagus of St. Magnus*, crypt of the cathedral of Anagni. Photo: author

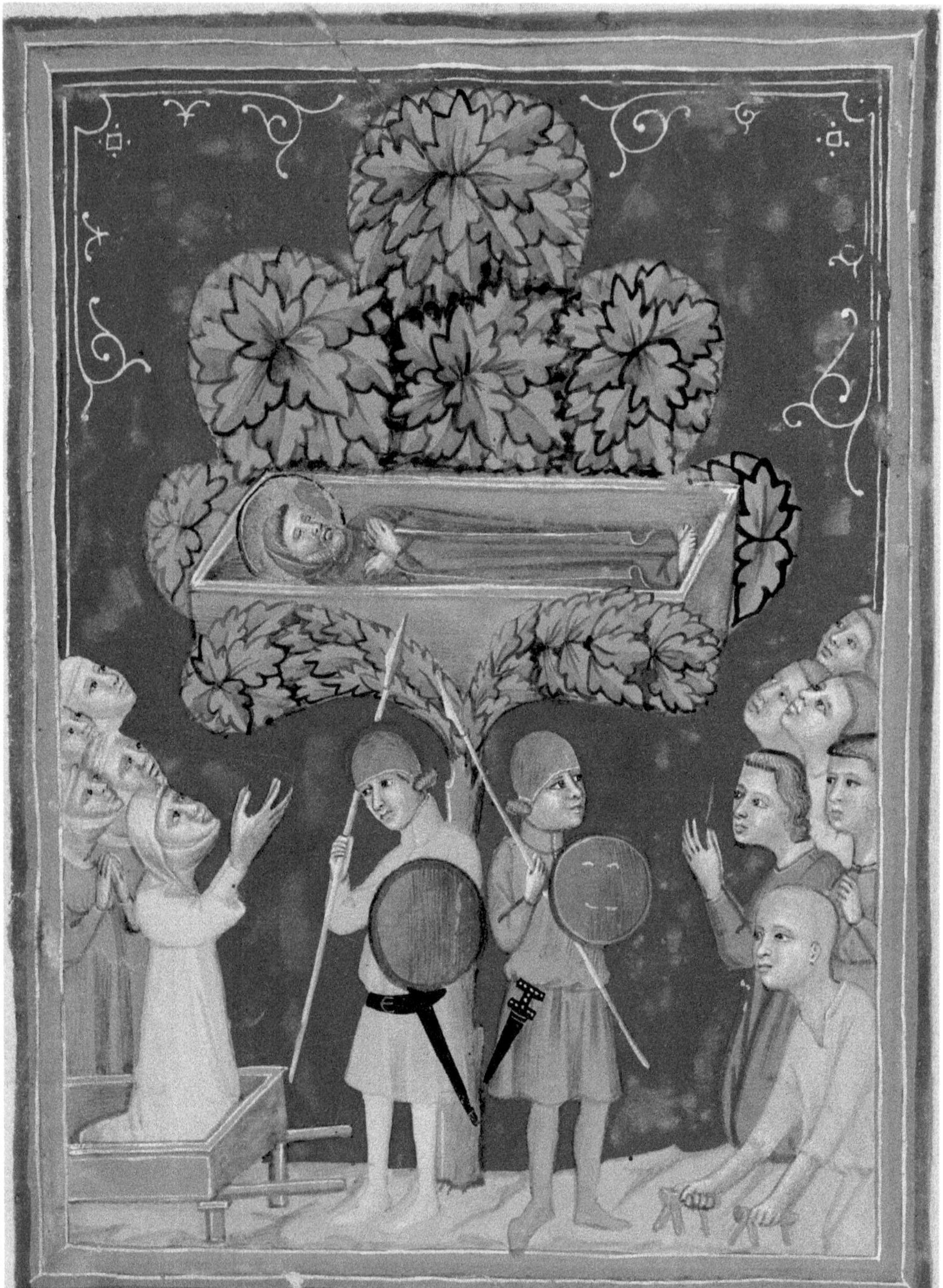

Plate 10 The Body of the Blessed Gerard of Villamagna Guarded by Two Guards from Disabled Supplicants, The Pierpont Morgan Library, New York. MS M.643. Purchased by J.P. Morgan (1867–1943) in 1919

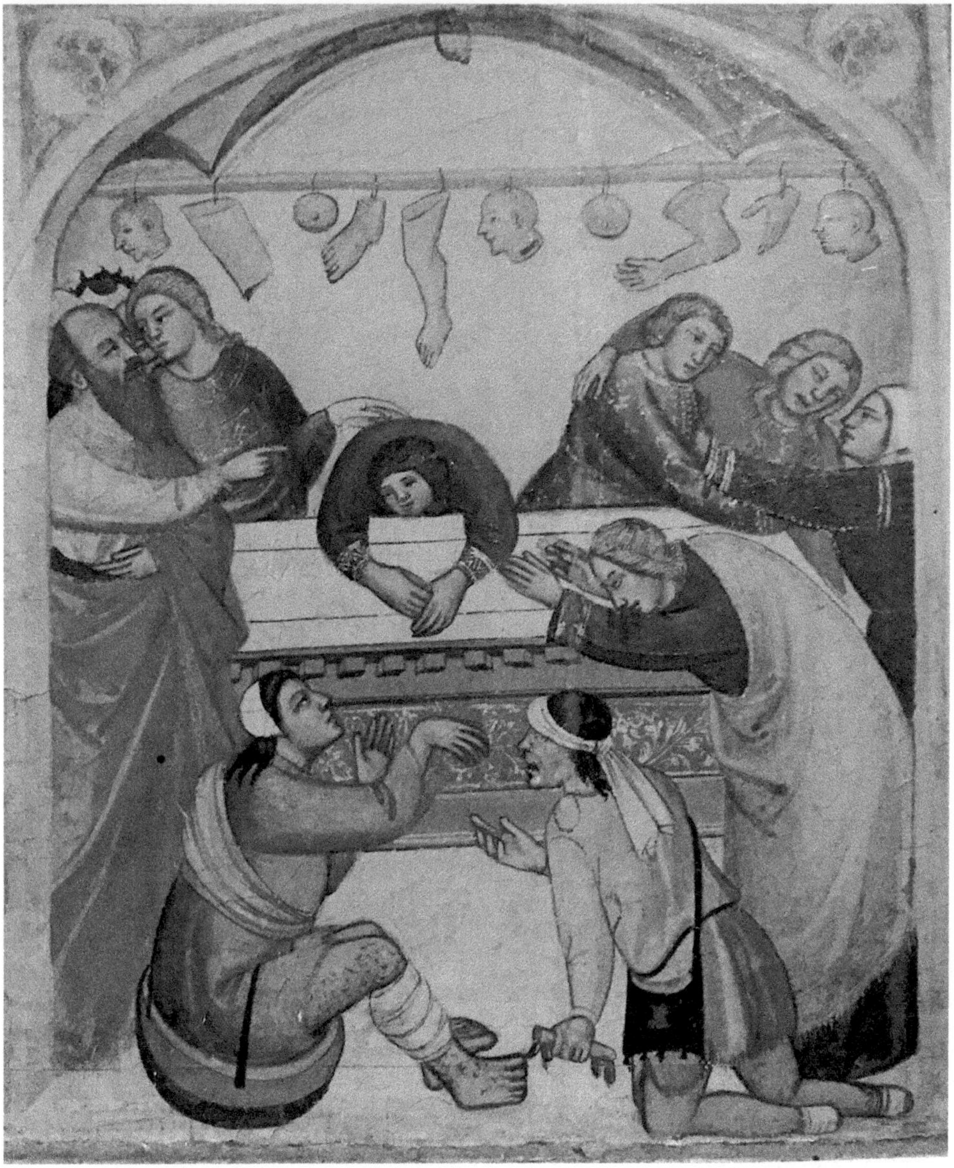

Plate 11 School of Turino Vanni, *Supplicants at the Tomb of St. Margaret*, ca. 1400, Vanni Altarpiece, Pinacoteca Vaticana. Photo: author

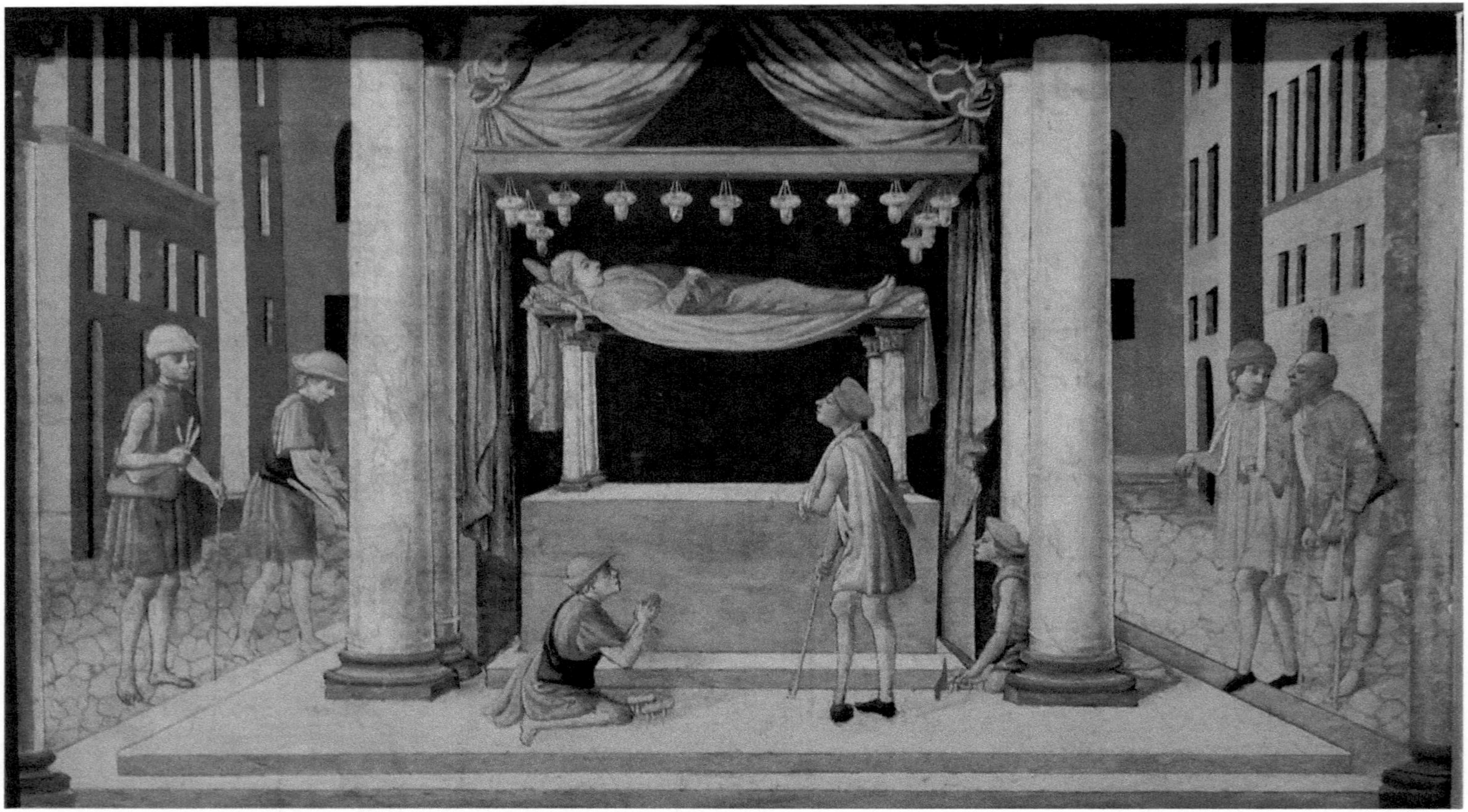

Plate 12 Disabled Supplicants by St. Barbara's Sepulcher, Pinacoteca Vaticana. Photo: author

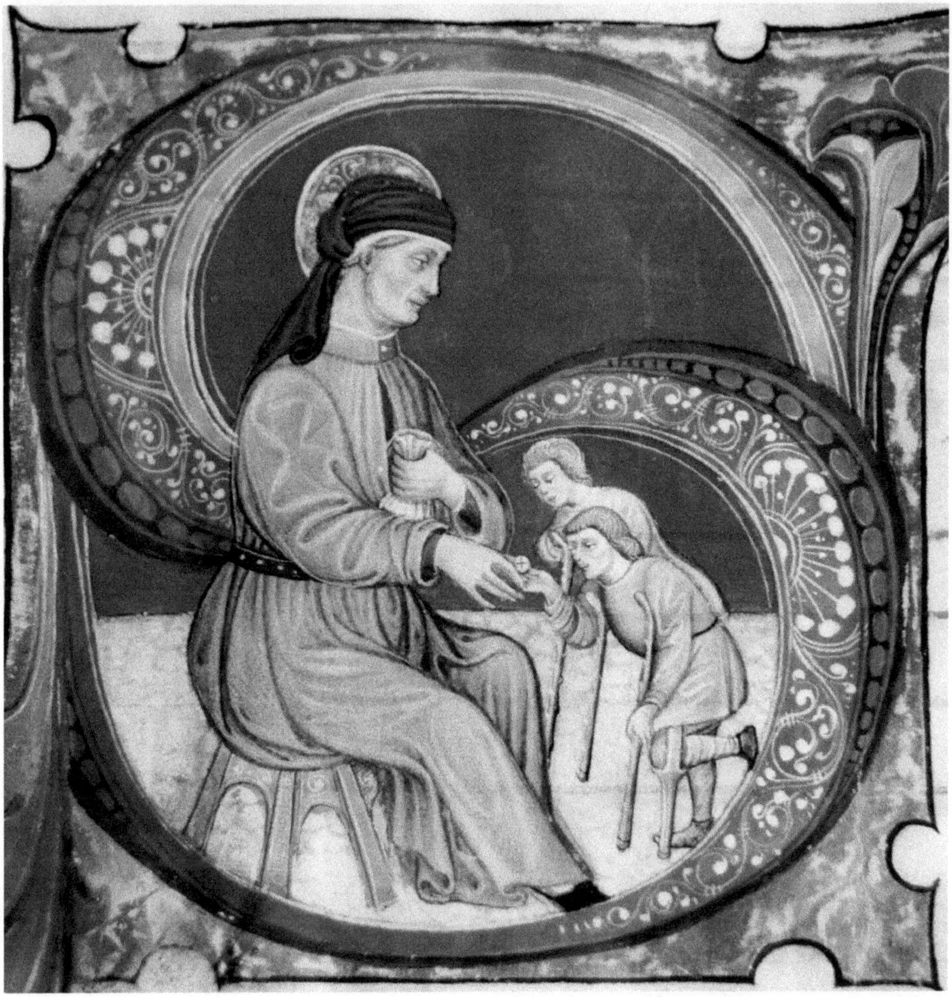

Plate 13 St. Homobonus Donating Alms to the Poor, Cod. IX, no. 224, Ufficio Beni Culturali Ecclesiastici della Diocesi di Cremona

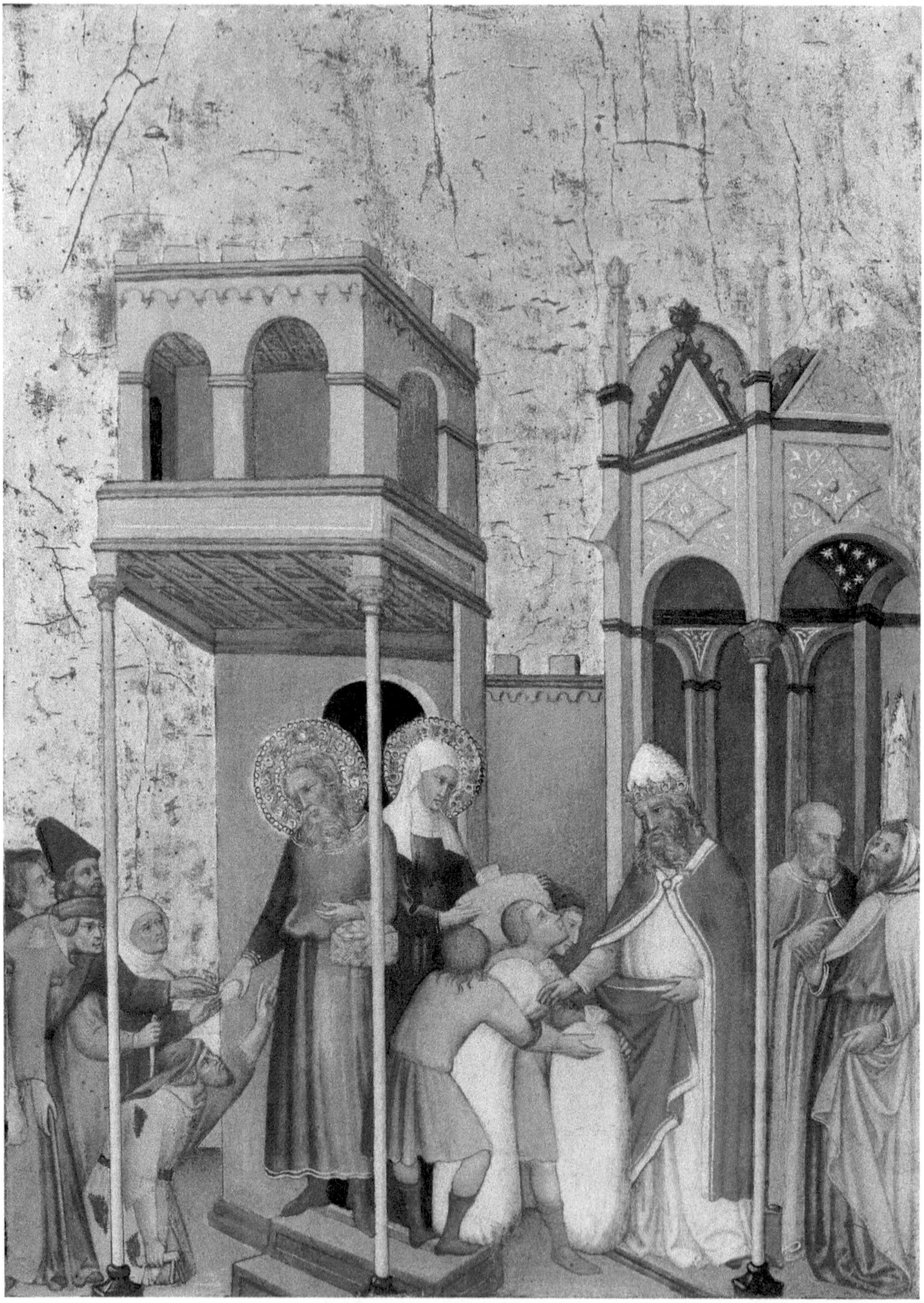

Plate 14 Andrea di Bartolo, *Joachim and the Beggars*, ca. 1400, Washington National Gallery. Photo: Washington National Gallery

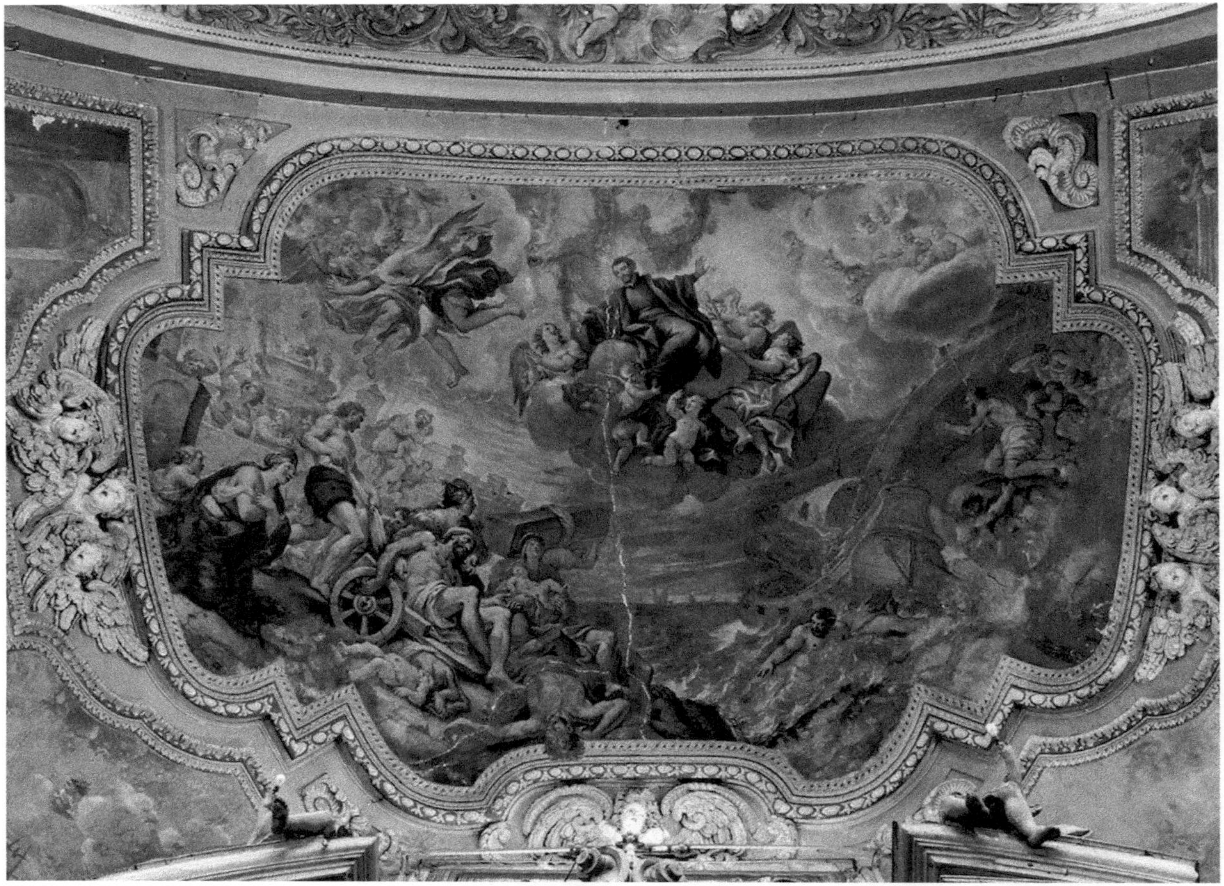

Plate 15 Paolo de Matteis, *St. Francis Xavier in Glory Protecting the City from Hunger, Plague, and Fire, and the Shipwrecked from Drowning*, 1693, San Ferdinando, Naples. Photo: Claudio Garofalo, Naples

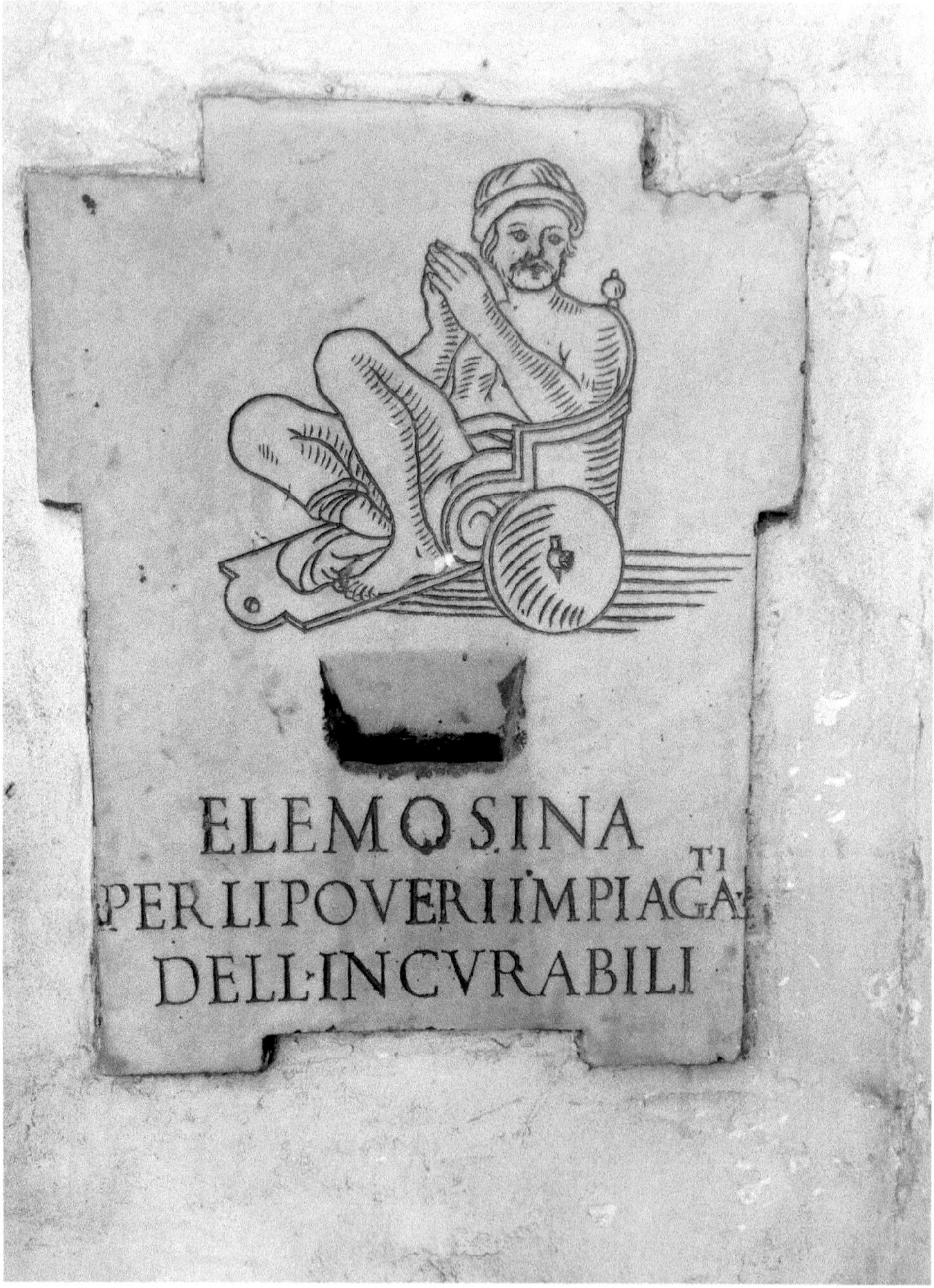

Plate 16 Victim of Syphilis, first half of the sixteenth century, plaque in Santa Maria in Porta Paradisi (Hospital of San Giacomo degli Incurabili, Rome). Photo: author

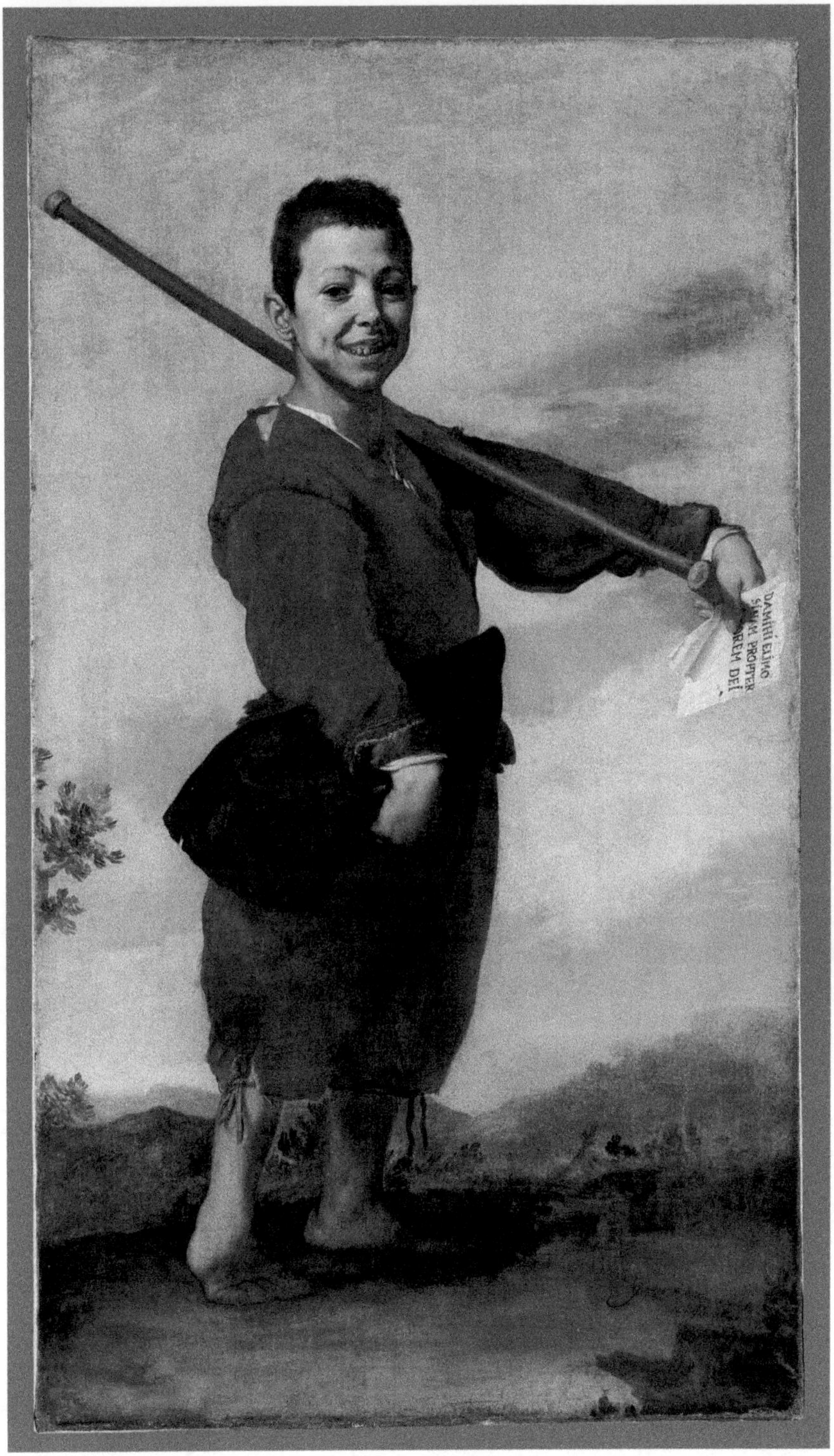

Plate 17 Jusepe de Ribera, *Clubfooted Boy*, 1642, Musée du Louvre, Paris. Photo: © RMN-Grand Palais (musée du Louvre)/Stéphane Maréchalle

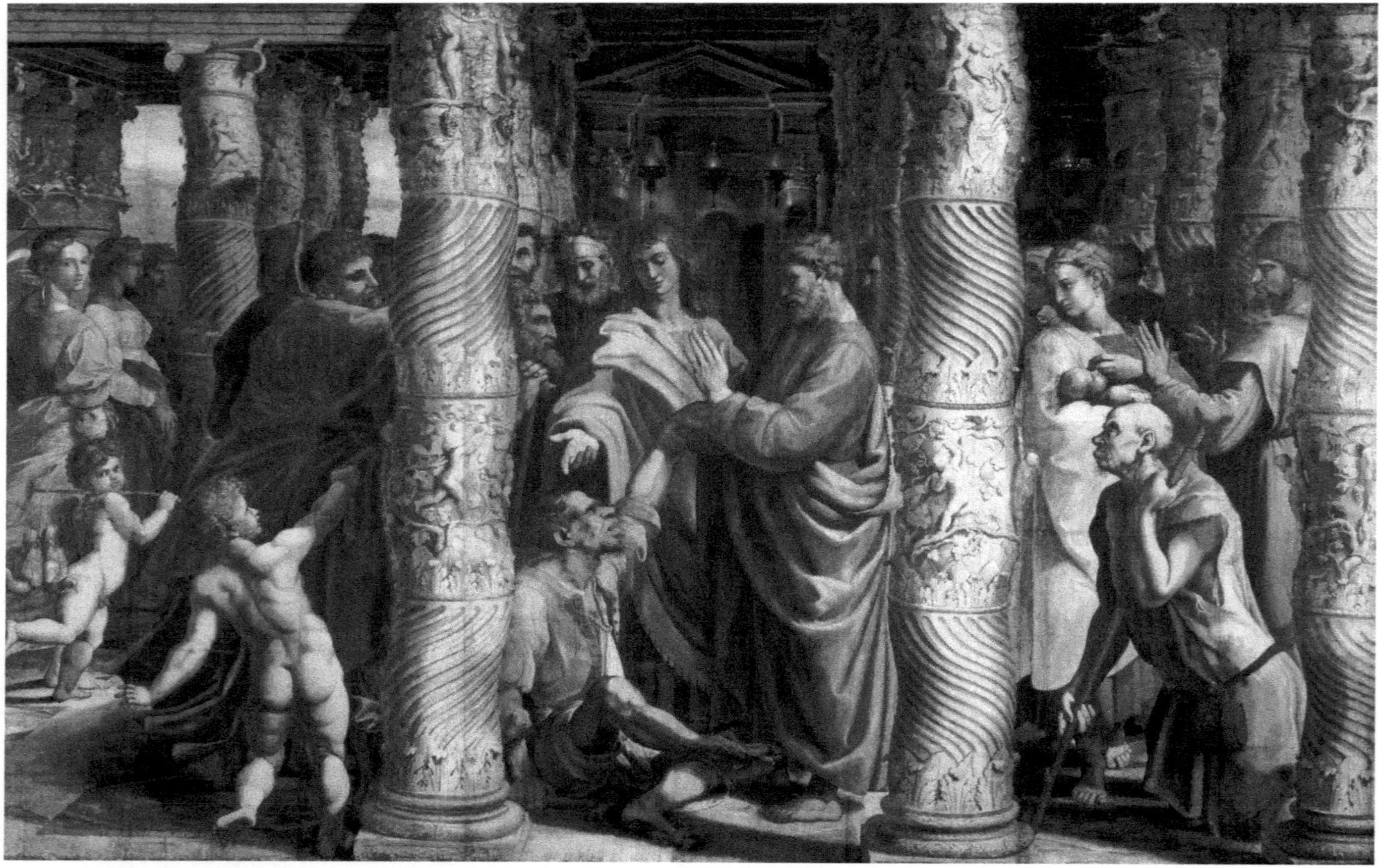

Plate 18 Raphael, *Healing of the Lame Man*, 1515, Victoria and Albert Museum, London. Photo: © 2015. Foto Scala Firenze/V&A Images/The Royal Collection, on loan from HM the Queen

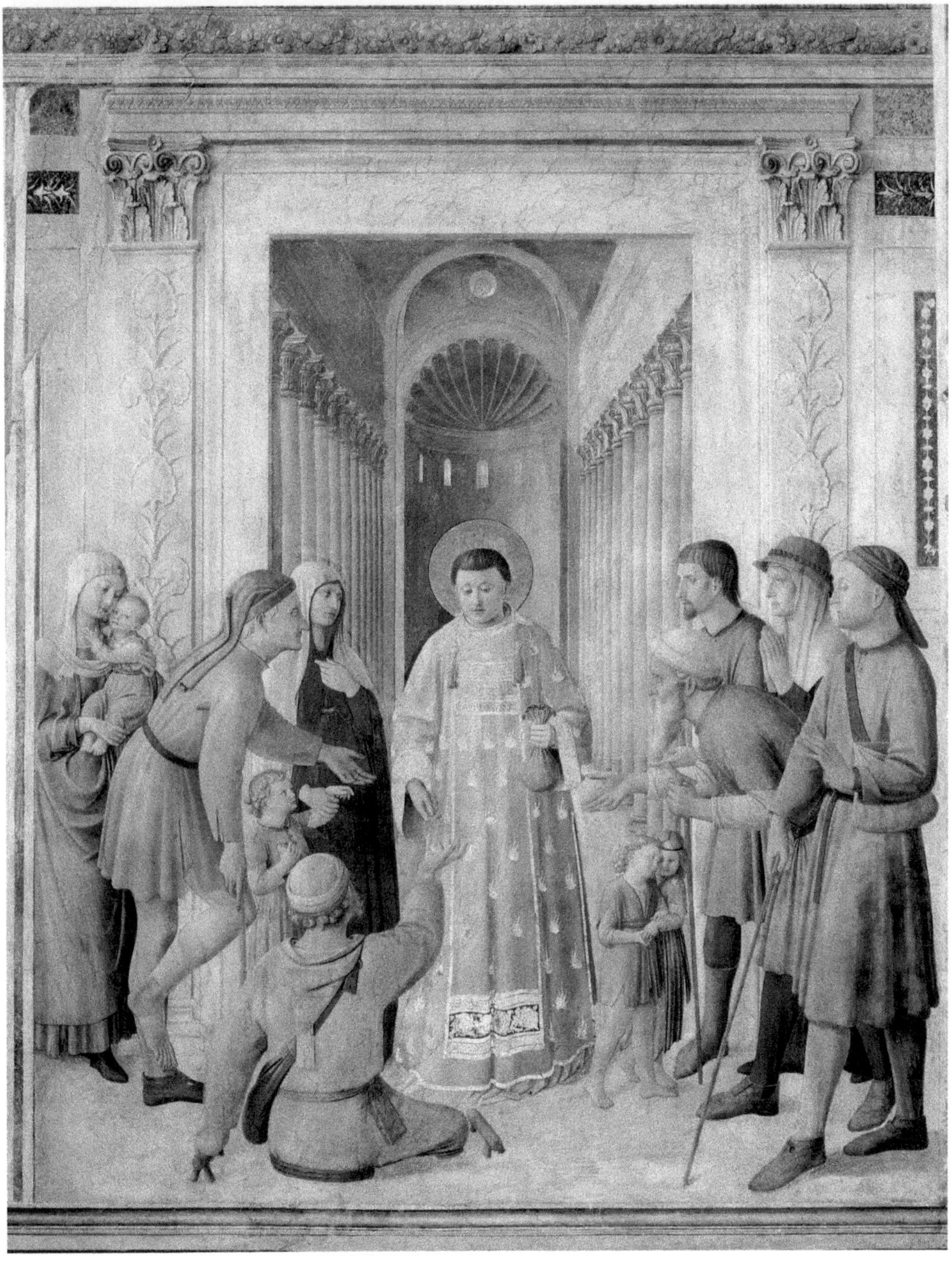

Plate 19 Beato Angelico, *The Charity of St. Lawrence*, Cappella Nicolina, Apostolic Palace, Vatican City. Photo: © 2015. Scala, Firenze

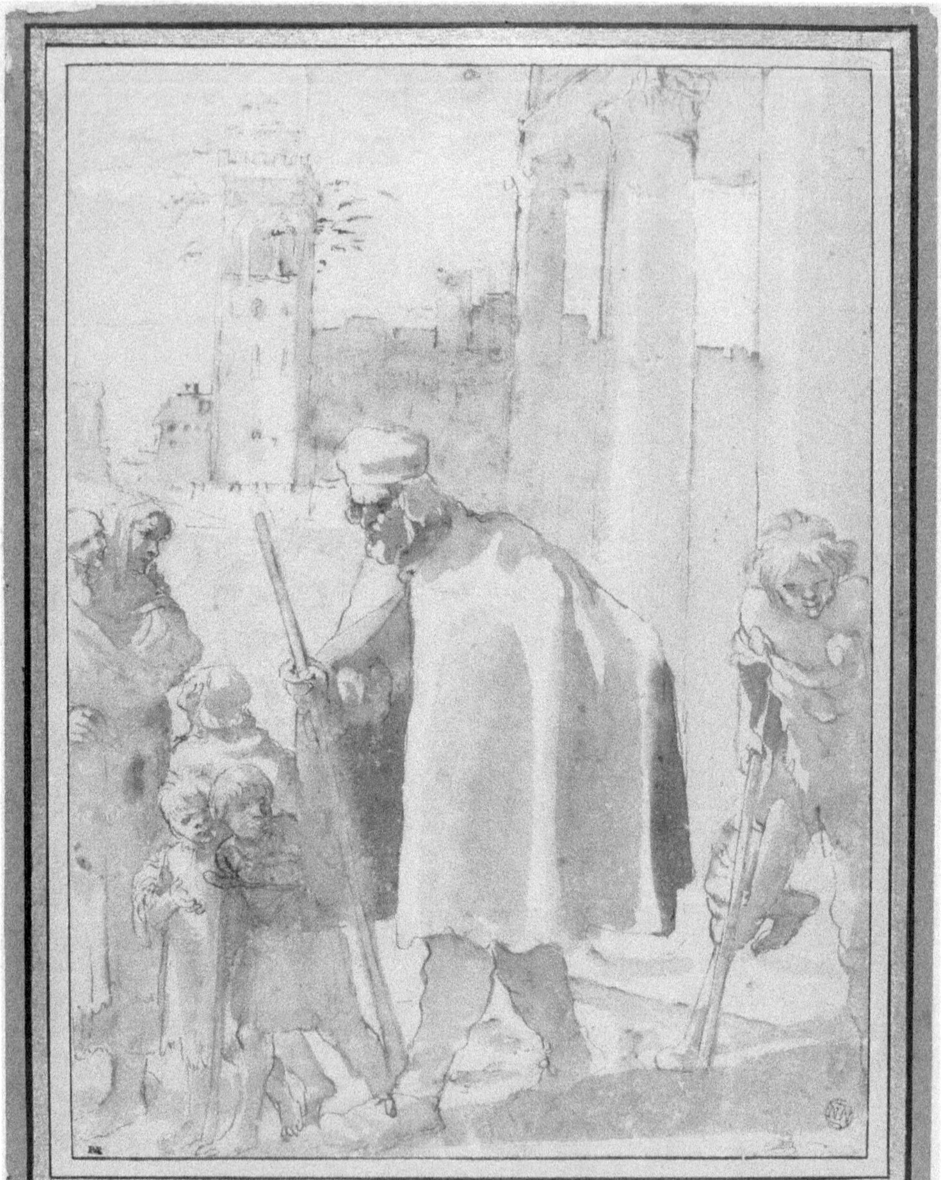

Plate 20 Ludovico Carracci, *Group of Mendicants*, Cabinet des dessins, Musée du Louvre, Paris, © RMN-Grand Palais (musée du Louvre)/Richard Lambert

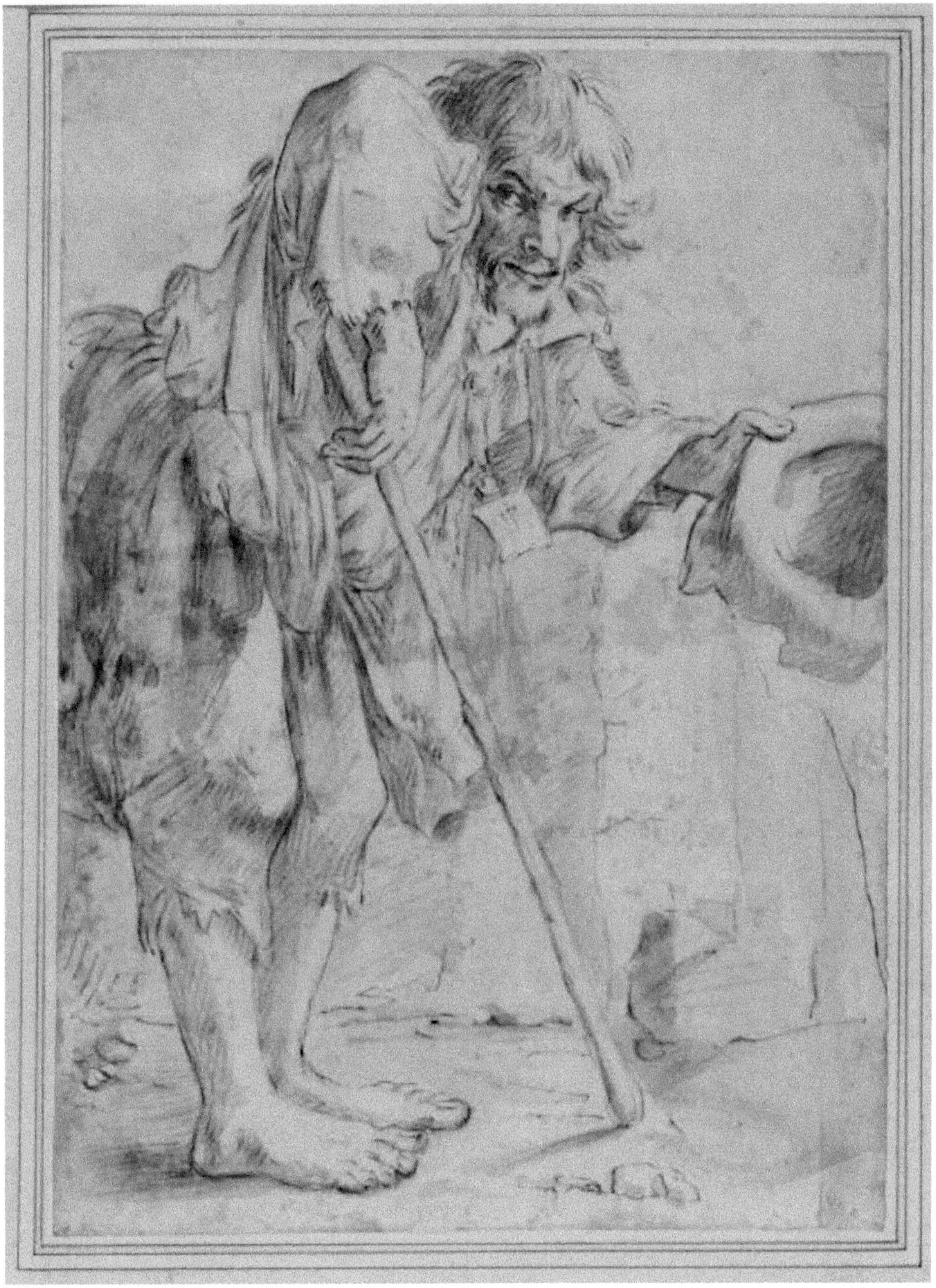

Plate 21 Attributed to Annibale Carracci, *Lame Beggar*, http://en.wahooart.com/Art.nsf/O/8DNVXU/$File/Annibale-Carracci-Crippled-beggar.JPG

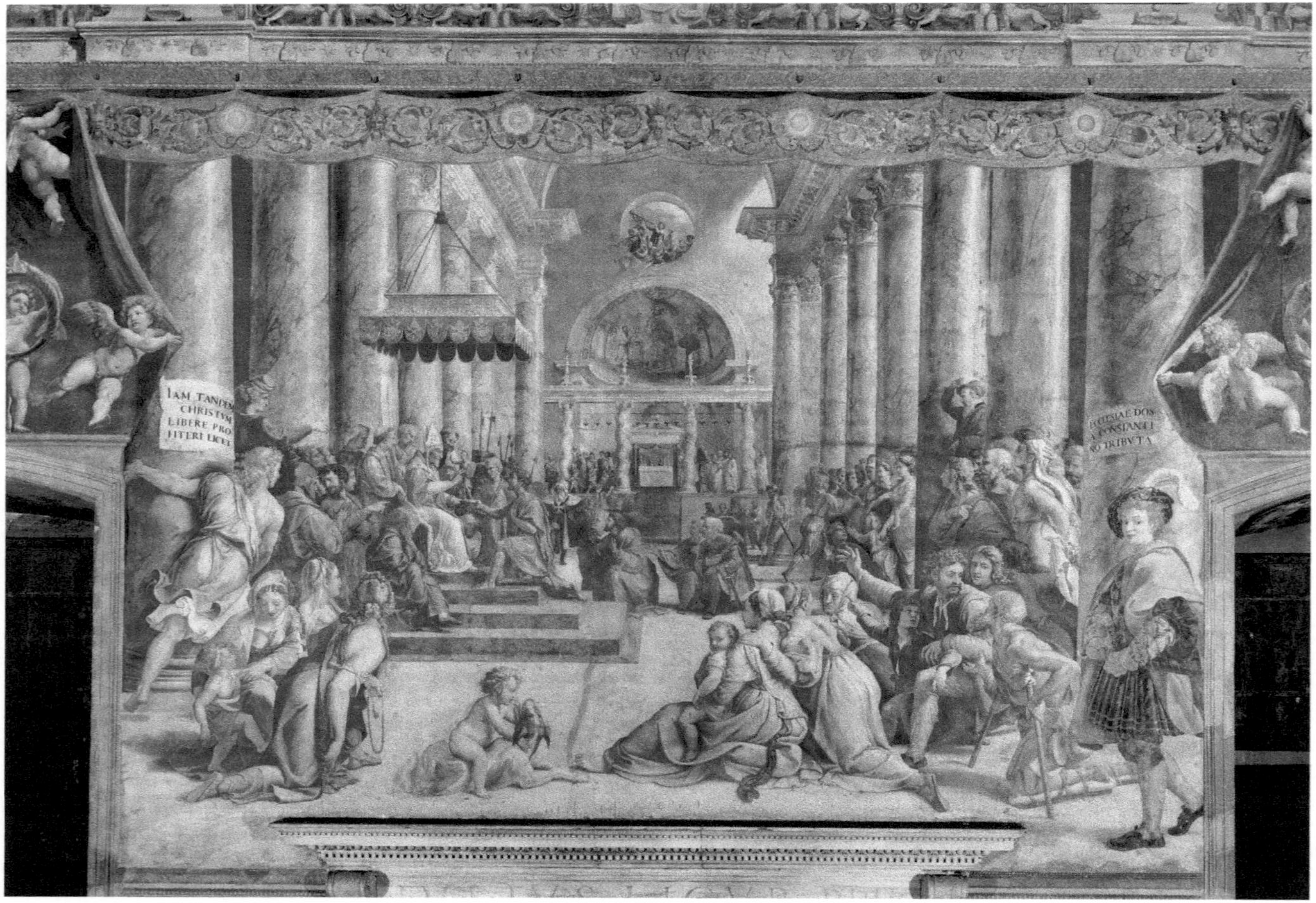

Plate 22 Raphael, *Donation of Constantine*, Sala di Costantino, Apostolic Palace, Vatican City. Photo: © 2015. Scala, Firenze

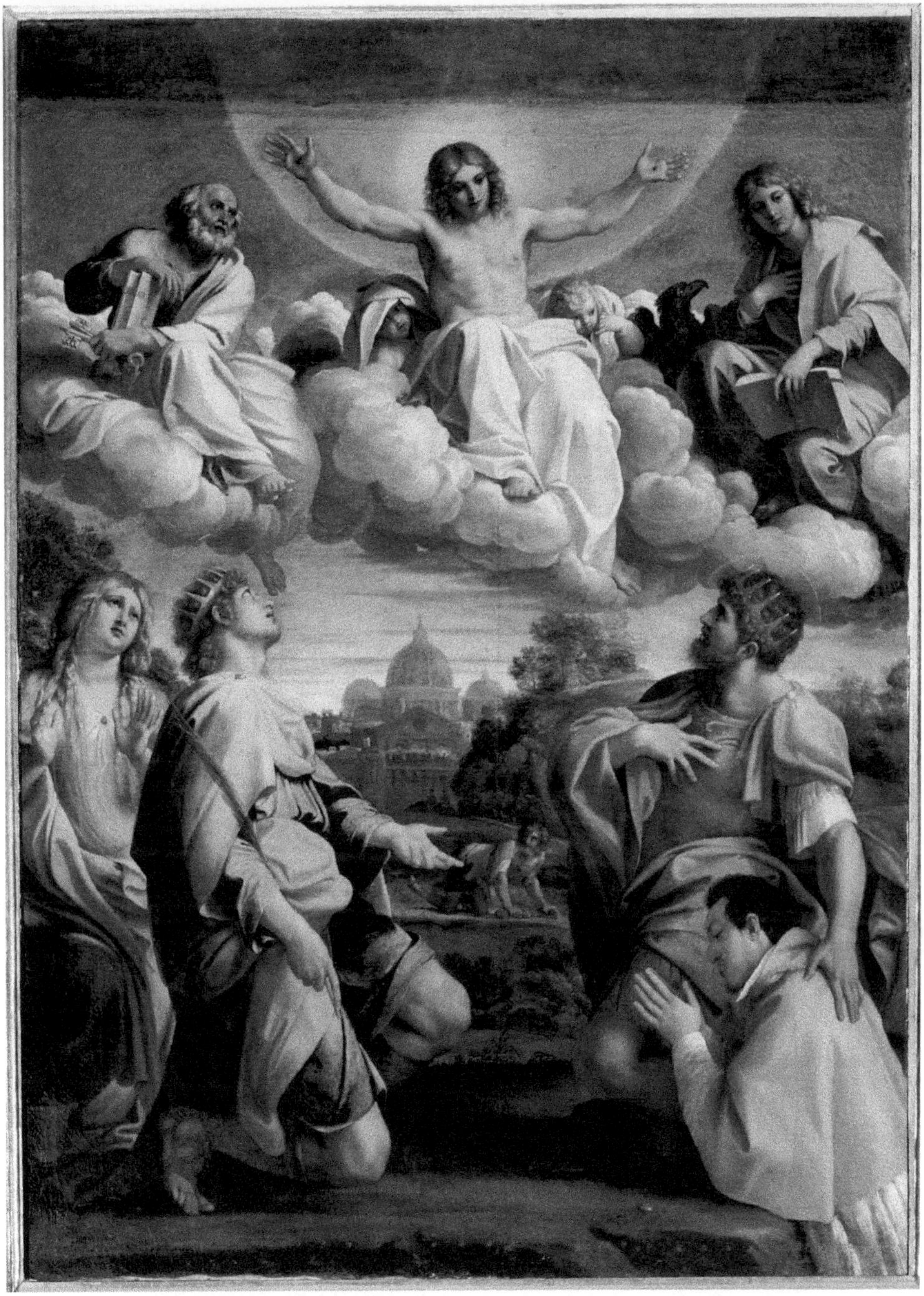

Plate 23 Annibale Carracci, *Christ in Glory with Sts. Peter, John the Evangelist, Mary Magdalen, Ermenegildo and St. Edward of England with Odoardo Farnese*, Pitti Palace, Florence, ca. 1600. Photo: Scala/Art Resource, NY

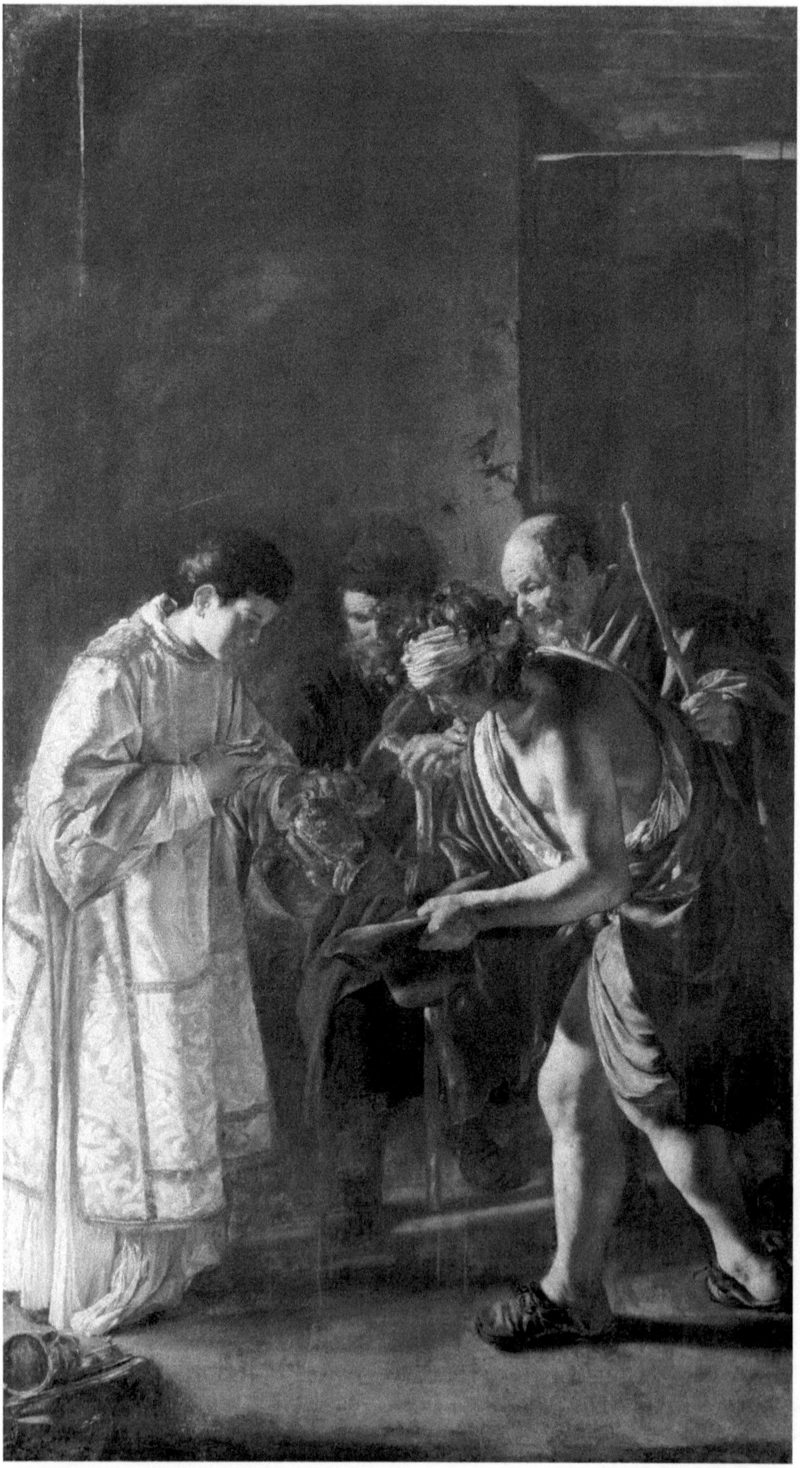

Plate 24 Giovanni Serodine, *St. Lawrence Distributing Alms*, Museo Archeologico di Casamari, ca. 1615. Photo: Abbazia di Casamari

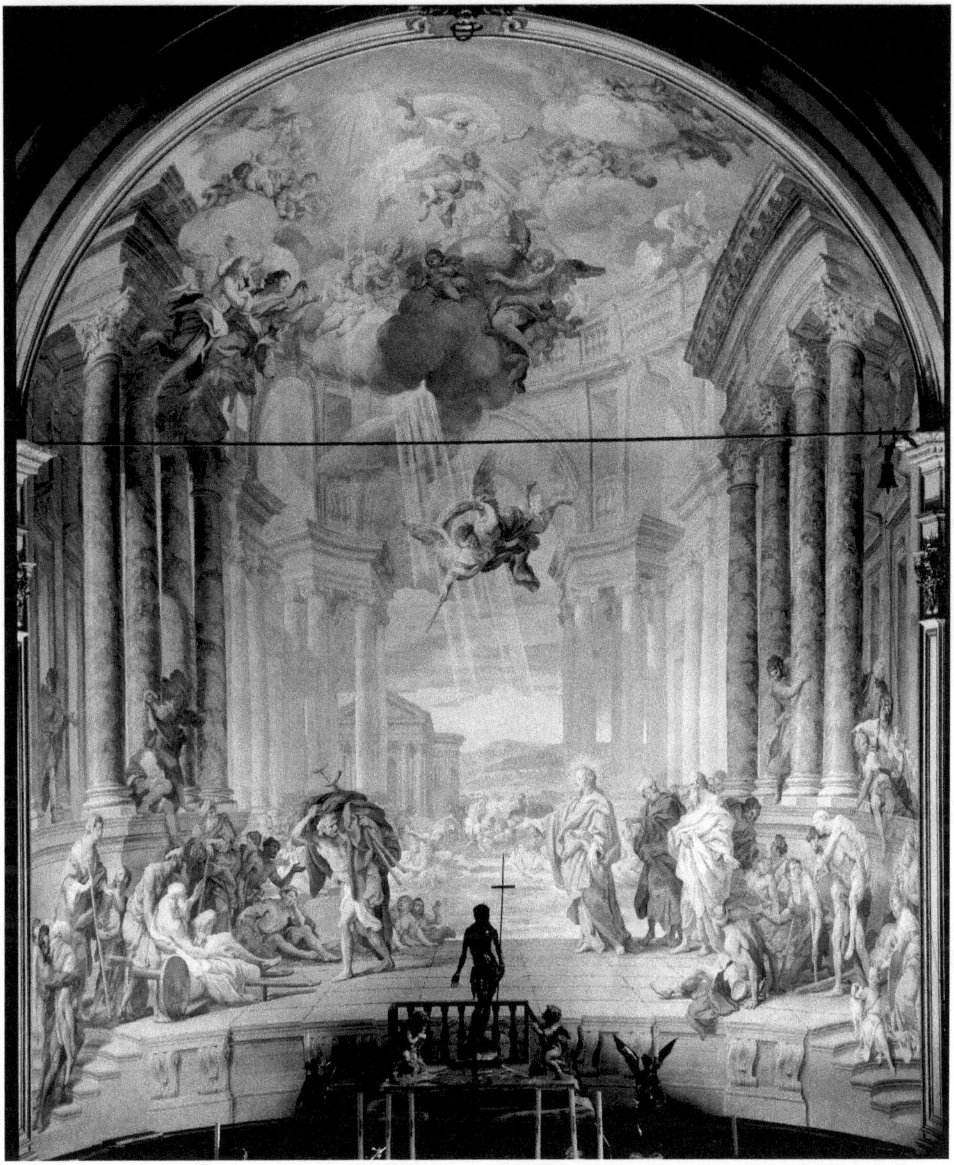

Plate 25 Sebastiano Conca, *Healing of the Cripple at the Pool of Bethesda*, 1731, chapel of the Spedale di Santa Maria della Scala. Photo: © *Foto LENSINI Siena*

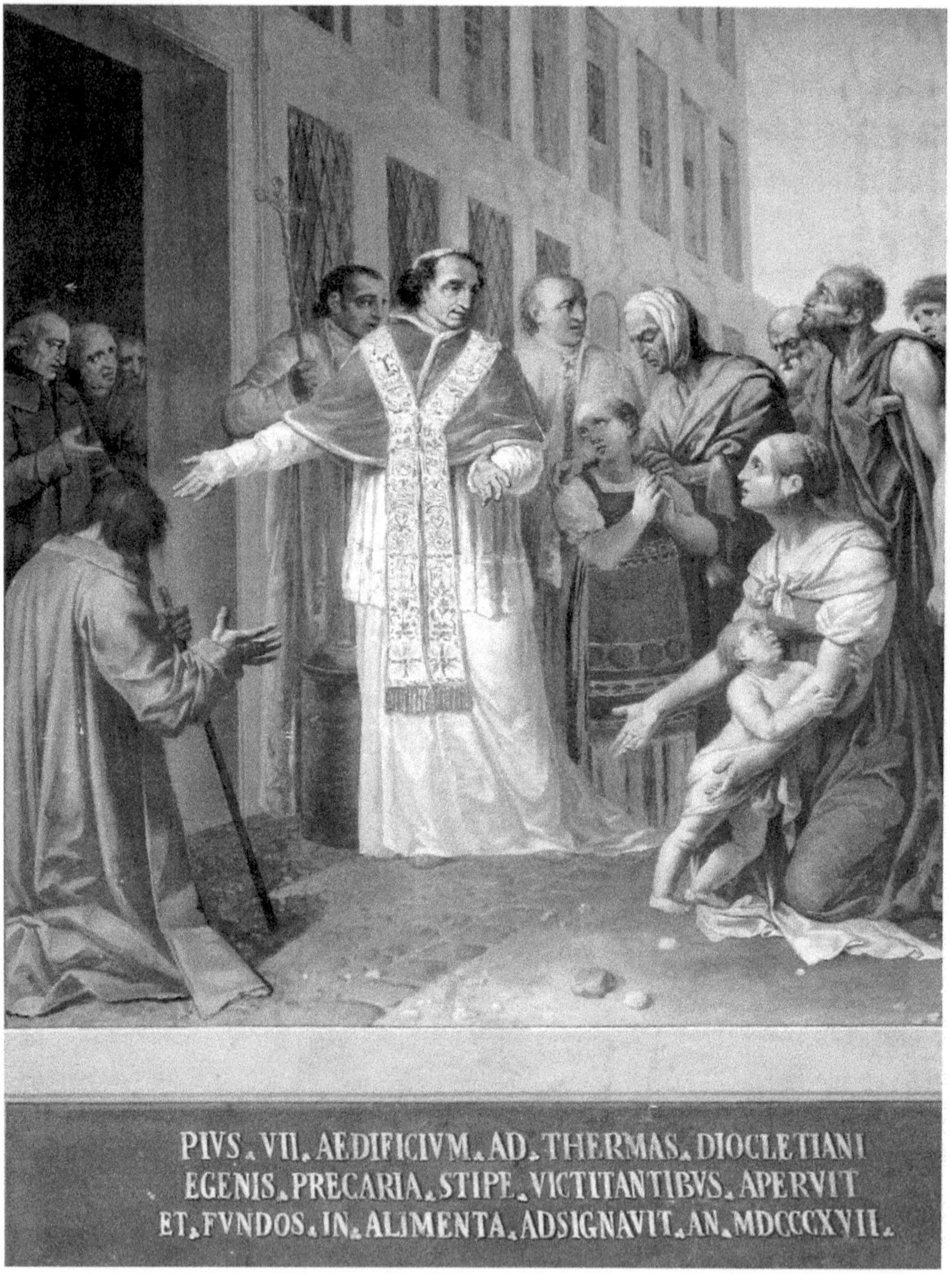

Plate 26 Domenico del Frate, *Pius VII Founding a Hospice for the Poor*, Galleria Clementina, Vatican Museums, 1817. Photo: author

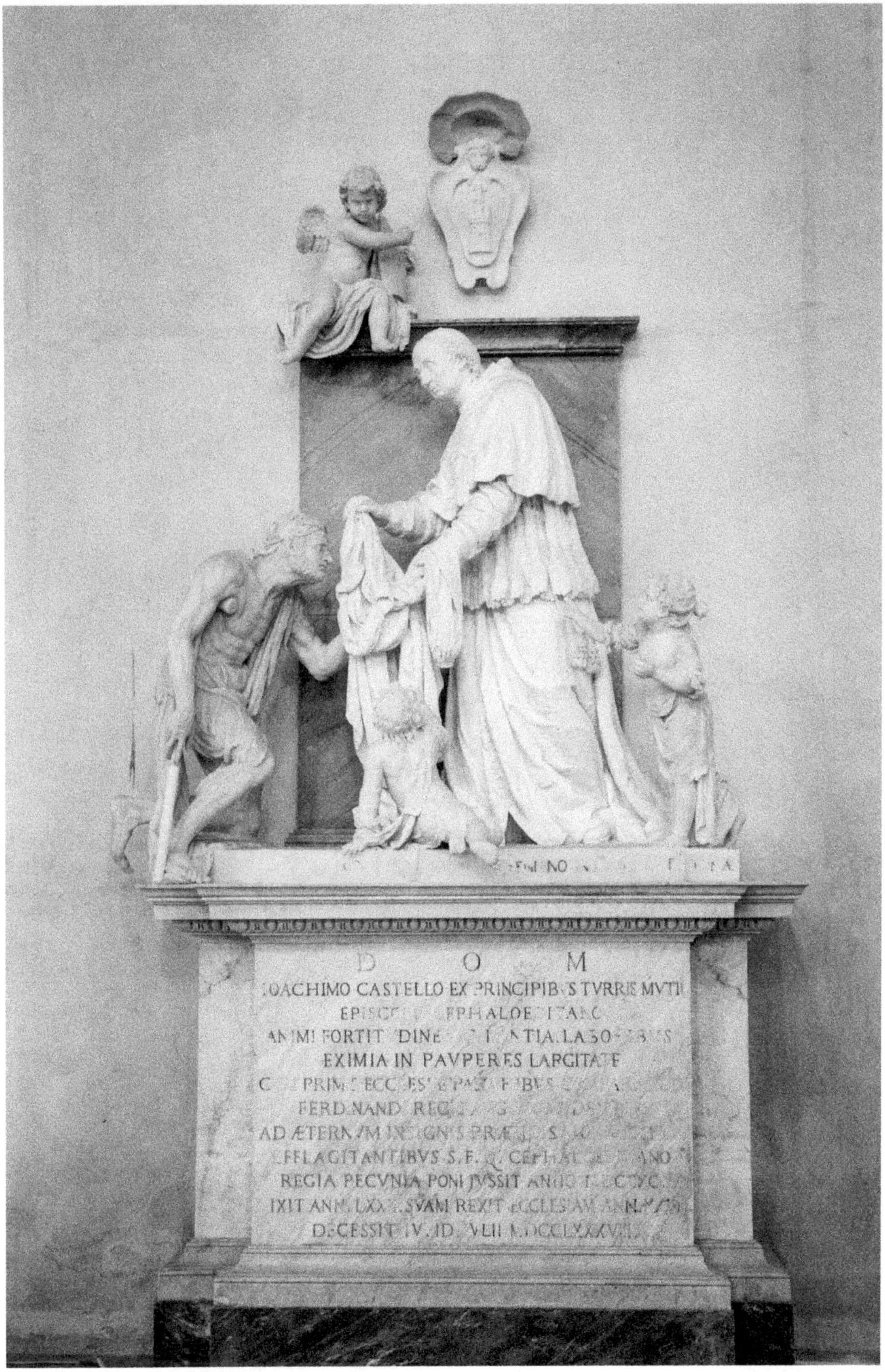

Plate 27 Leonardo Pennino, *The Charity of Bishop Gioacchino Castelli*, ca. 1788, Cefalù, Cathedral. Photo: author

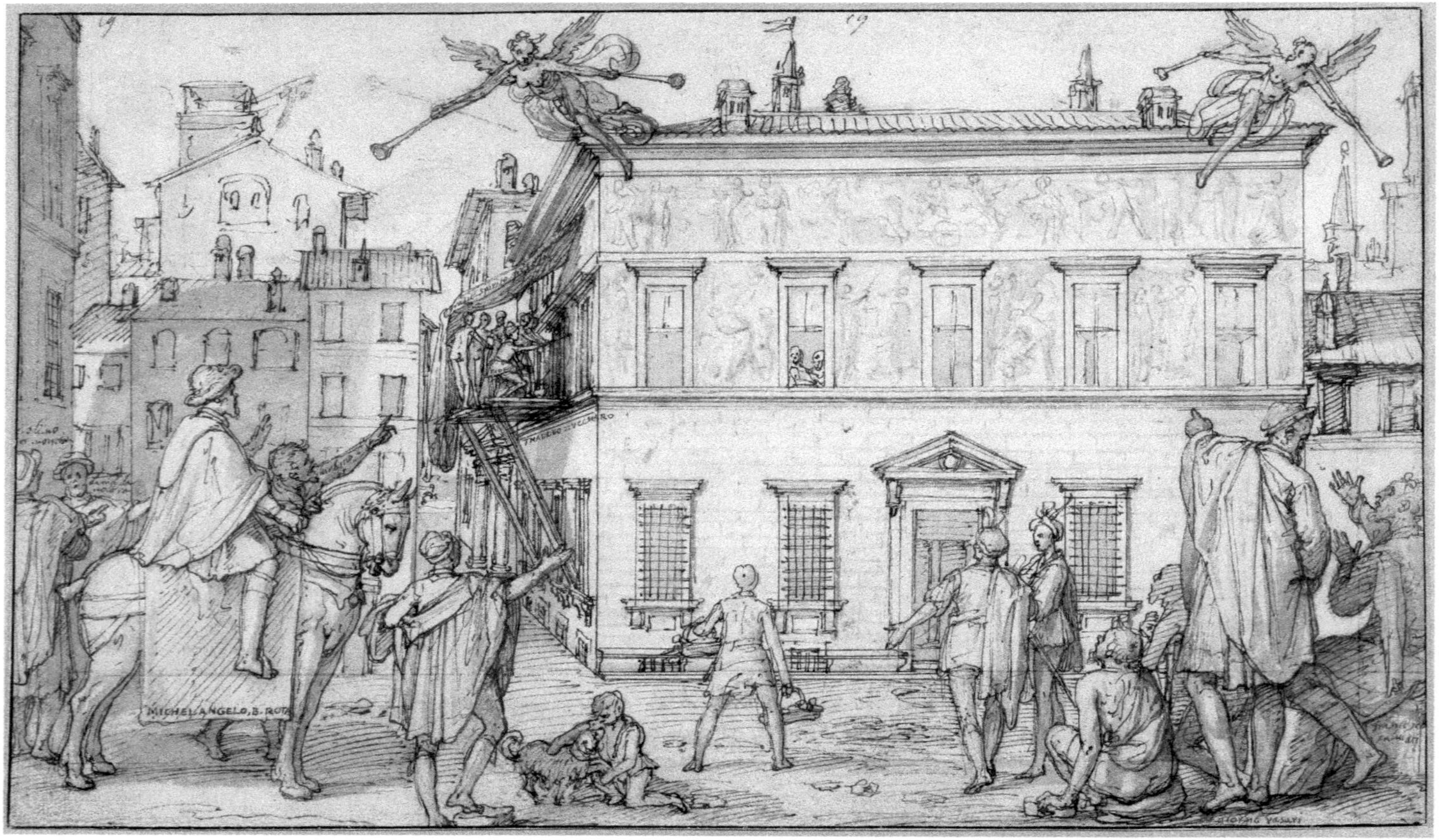

Plate 28 Federico Zuccari, *Taddeo Zuccari Frescoeing Palazzo Mattei*, ca. 1595, Los Angeles, The Getty Museum. Photo: The Getty Museum

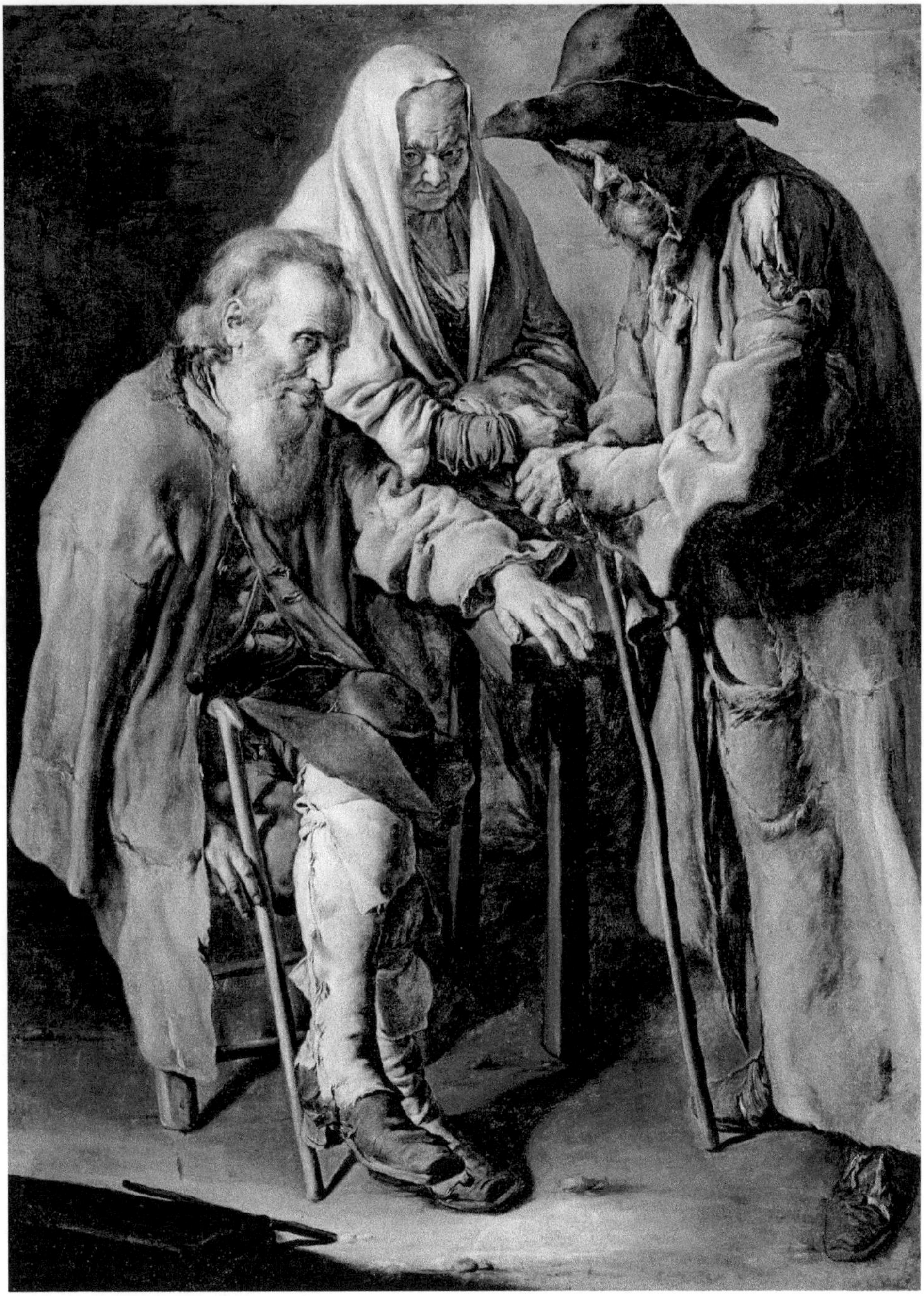

Plate 29 Giacomo Ceruti, *Three Beggars*, ca. 1736, Fundación Colleción Thyssen-Bornemisza, Madrid. Photo: © Museo Thyssen-Bornemisza, Madrid

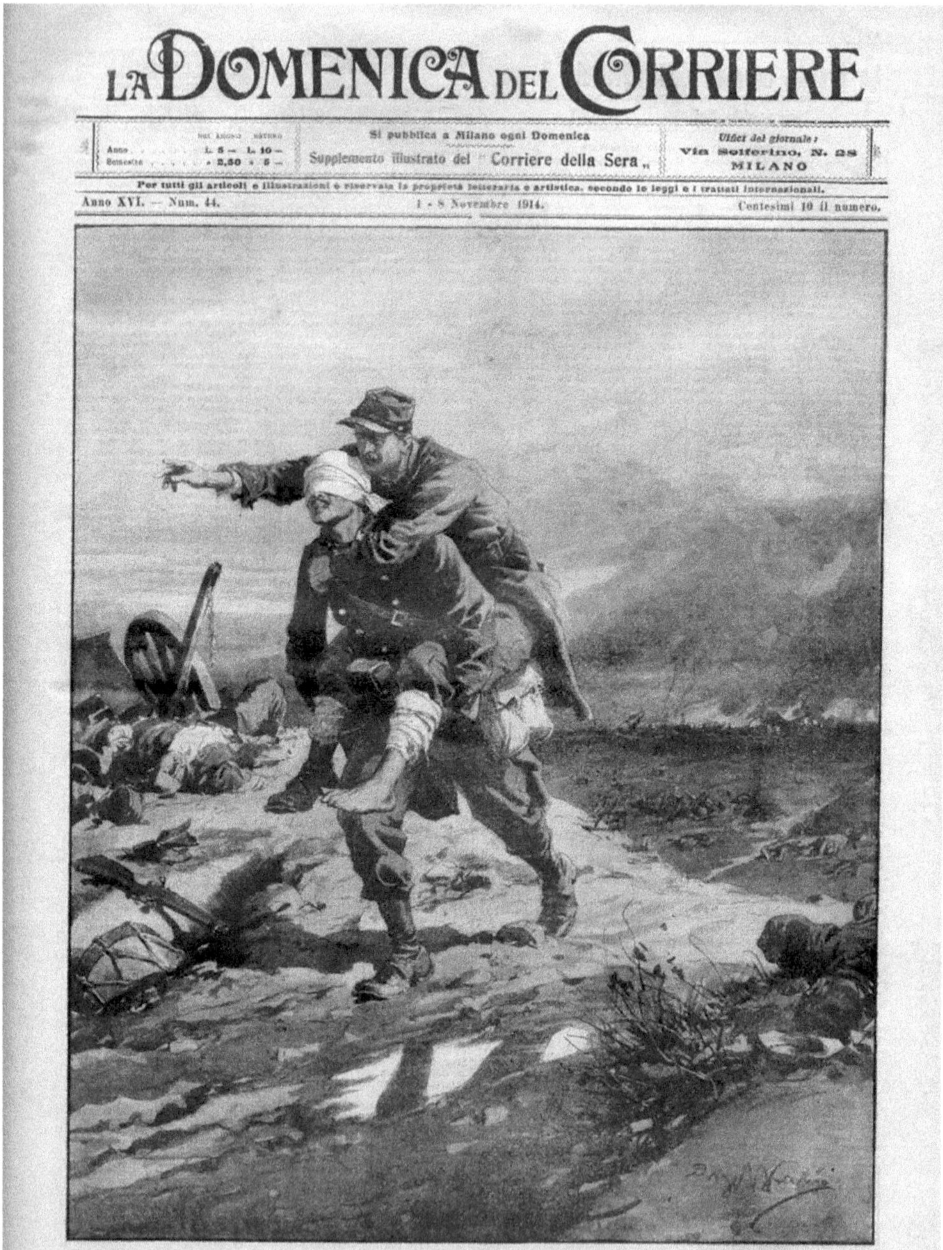
LA DOMENICA DEL CORRIERE

Anno . . . . . L. 5 — L. 10 —
Semestre . . . . . » 2,50 » 5 —

Si pubblica a Milano ogni Domenica
Supplemento illustrato del "Corriere della Sera"

Uffici del giornale:
Via Solferino, N. 28
MILANO

Per tutti gli articoli e illustrazioni è riservata la proprietà letteraria e artistica, secondo le leggi e i trattati internazionali.

Anno XVI. — Num. 44. 1 - 8 Novembre 1914. Centesimi 10 il numero.

Episodi di guerra: due soldati francesi, uno accecato ed uno ferito ad una gamba si aiutano a vicenda per raggiungere l'ambulanza.

(Disegno di A. Beltrame)

Plate 30 Achille Beltrame, *Mutual Aid*, La Domenica del Corriere, November 1–8, 1914.
Photo: Corriere della Sera

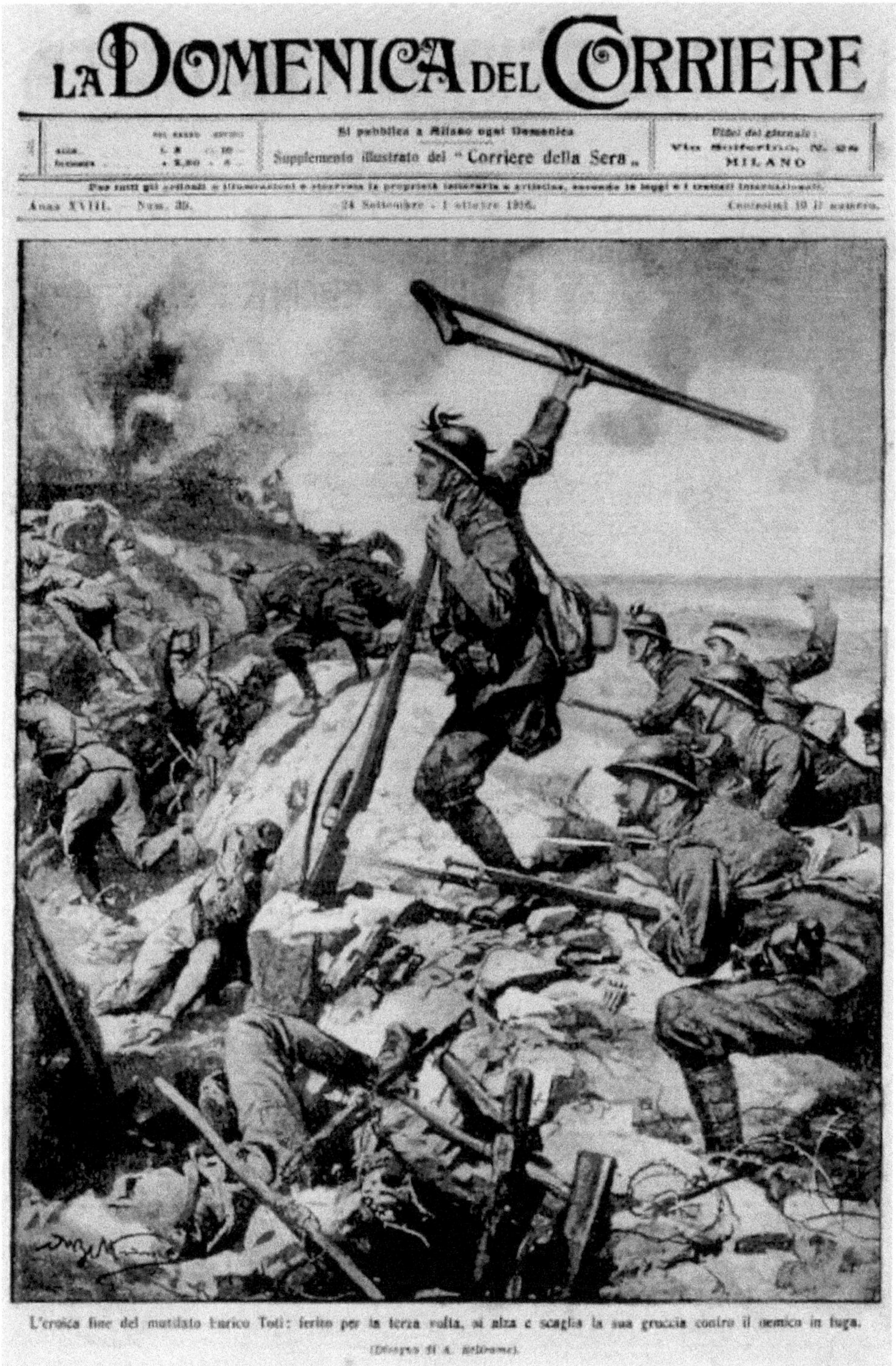

Plate 31 Achille Beltrame, *Enrico Toti Throwing his Crutch Towards the Austro-Hungarian Soldiers*, La Domenica del Corriere, September 24–October 1, 1916. Photo: Corriere della Sera

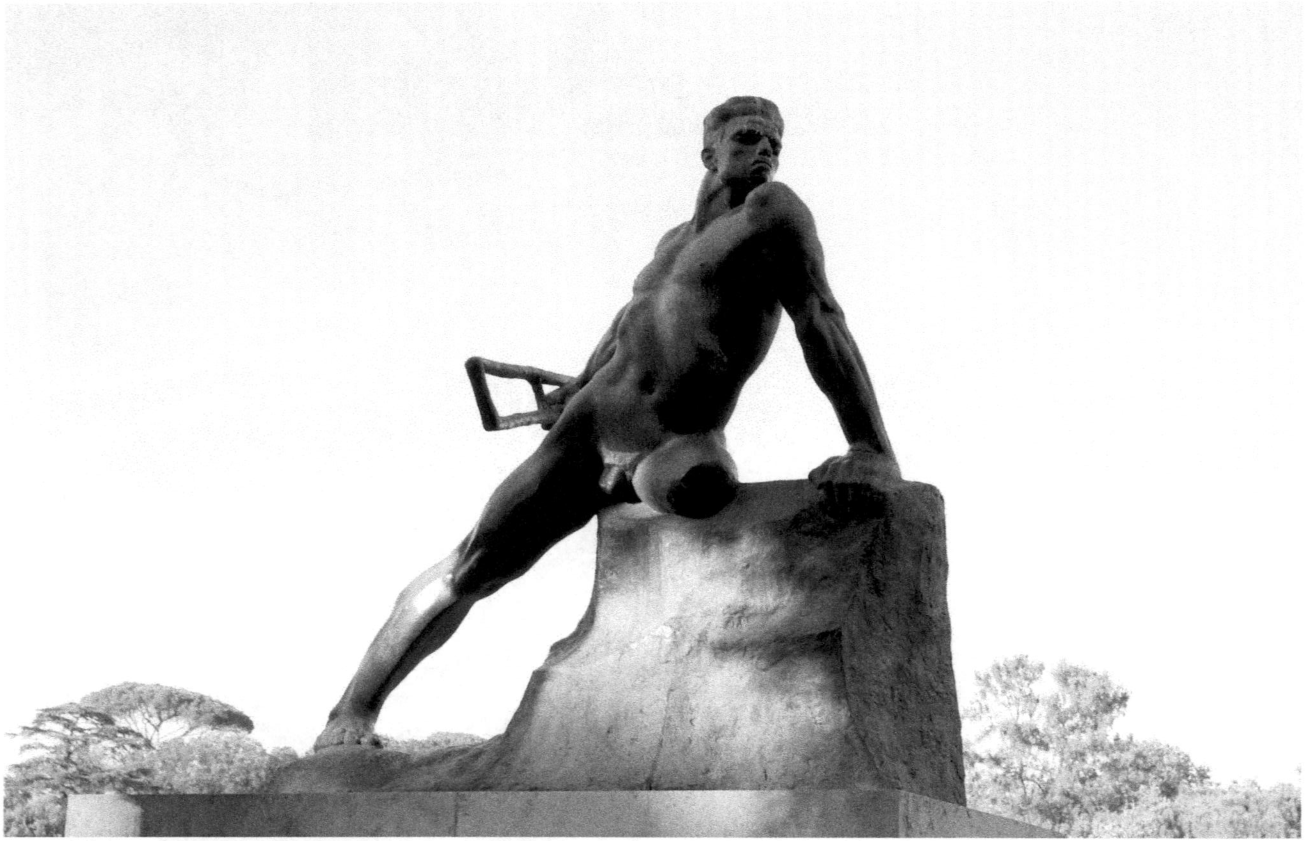

Plate 32 Arturo Dazzi, *Enrico Toti*, 1922, Villa Borghese, Rome. Photo: author

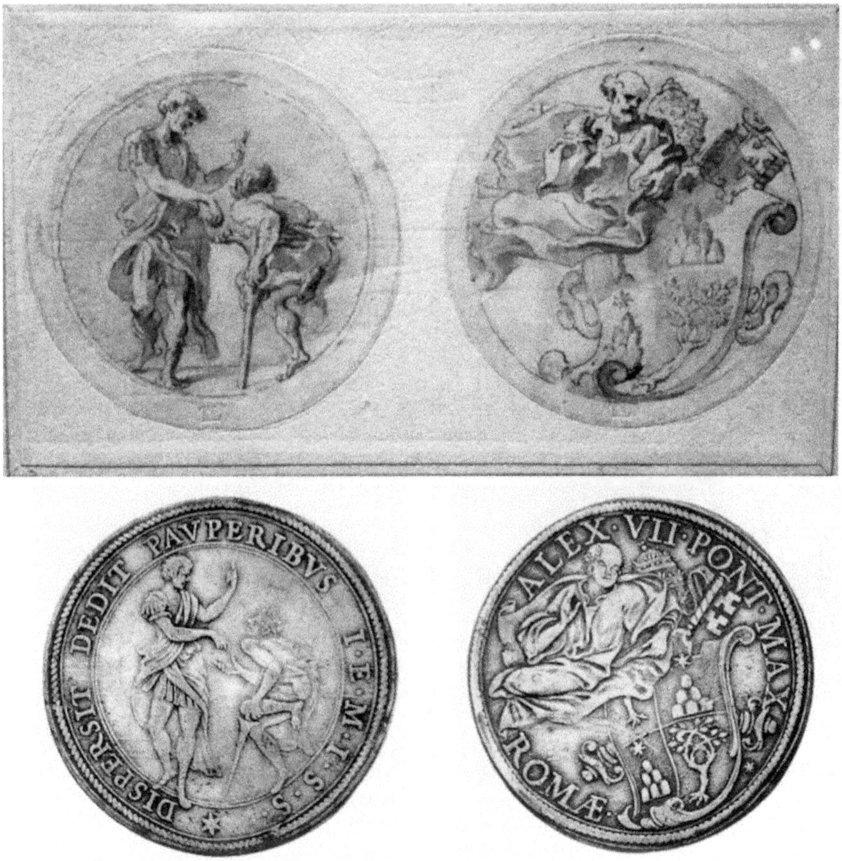

Figure 4.9 Bernini, drawing of a silver *scudo* for Alexander II, 1658. Photo: drawing, author; coin, from Charles Avery, *Bernini: Genius of the Baroque*, London, 2006, fig. 393

lost the ability to empathize with the destitute and the infirm. Nothing could be further from the truth, for Innocent XII remains famous not only for having been the pope who with the *Romanun decet pontificem* bull of June 22, 1692 juristically abolished papal nepotism[97] but, as cardinal of Naples and bishop of Rome, contributed immense funds for poor relief,[98] and in his will left the poor as his sole heirs.[99] In fact, he cared so much for the fate of the indigent and of the San Michele hospice he had helped to create that he visited the complex sixty-four times during his lifetime.[100] The truth of the matter is that the "uncontrollable hordes" of famished individuals who flooded all major cities in Italy,[101] as in the rest of Europe, during the many famine years from the sixteenth through the seventeenth century and beyond, created problems that left little leeway to the authorities who attempted to control the phenomenon. Suffice it to say that by the mid-eighteenth century in Rome there lived about two million people of which over four hundred thousand were mendicants.[102] Thus, on the one hand the popes encouraged private organizations to provide poor-relief and, on the other, they created

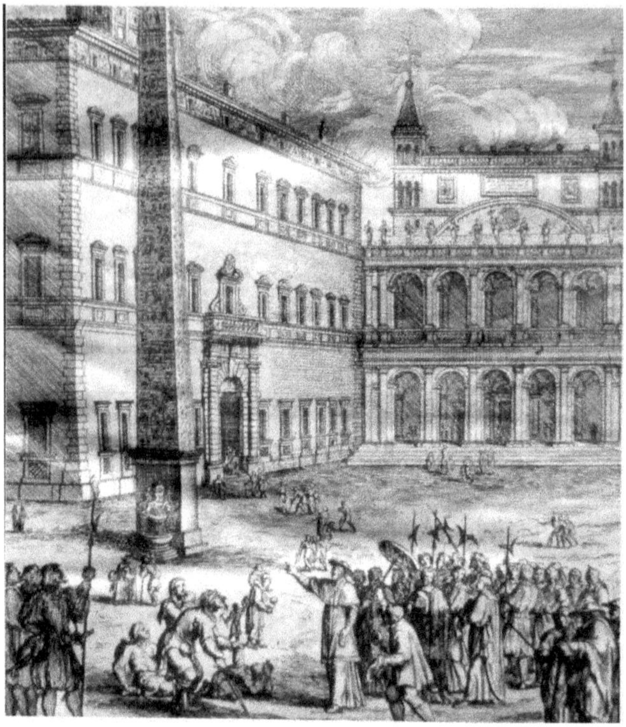

Figure 4.10 *Innocent XII Founding the Apostolic Hospice of the Poor and the Invalid,* from *La mendicita' provveduta*, Rome, 1693

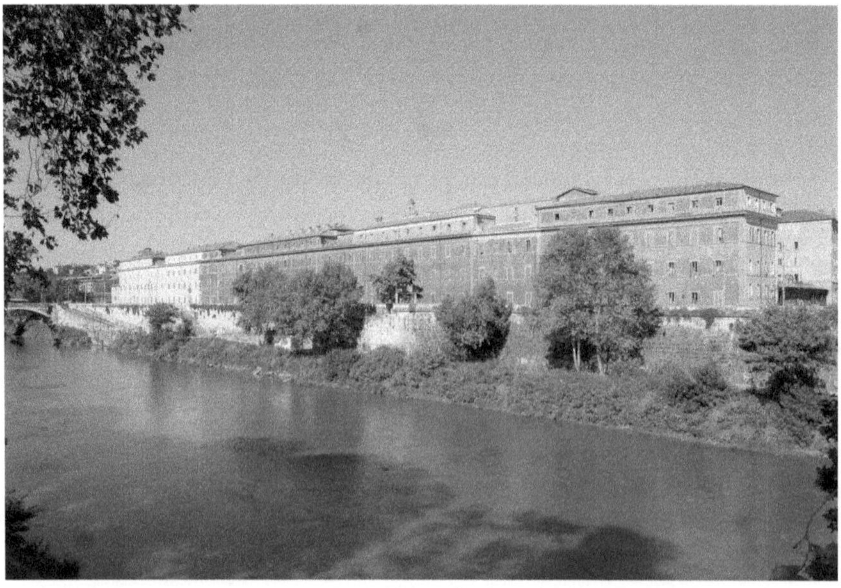

Figure 4.11 San Michele a Ripa. Photo: author

public institutions that made available social aid for some while dissuading others by threatening harsh disciplinary measures. These laws affected even the *difettosi*, the *impotenti*, the *inabili* who, nominally at least, were ranked among the deserving poor.[103] In this regard, what the papal experiments in Rome evince is that by the eighteenth century, even in the heart of Christendom, the inability to control problems of this magnitude had generated a general shift towards greater severity in the treatment of the more vulnerable members of society.

Notes

1 *Charity* is the former translation of the Greek *agape*, as in the King James Bible. Nowadays it is more frequently translated as *Love*. See *The Jerusalem Bible*, p. 305: "In short, there are three things that last: faith, hope and love; and the greatest of these is love."

2 Ibid., p. 305, n. 13. Mt 22:37–40: "But when the Pharisees heard that he had silenced the Sadducees they got together and, to disconcert him, one of them put a question, 'Master, which is the greatest commandment of the Law?' Jesus said, '*You must love the Lord your God with all your heart, with all your soul*, and with all your mind. This is the greatest and the first commandment. The second resembles it: *You must love your neighbour as yourself*. On these commandments hang the whole Law, and the Prophets also.'"

3 Quoted by Vauchez, *The Spirituality of the Medieval West*, p. 62.

4 Liverani, "Saint Peter's and the City of Rome," p. 21; Brown, *Through the Eye of a Needle*, p. 70. To be sure, the area around the Vatican was on the margins of the city, and a location where the poor had gathered even before the creation of St. Peter's Basilica: "It was a no-man's-land, a cemetery area in which beggars lived."

5 *The Book of Pontiffs (Liber Pontificalis)*, Raymond Davis (tr.), Liverpool, 1989, p. 46.

6 Ibid., p. 61.

7 Ibid., p. 49.

8 Ibid., p. 53.

9 Ibid., p. 149. For the images of the beggars in front of a temple, see Helas.

10 Ac 3:1–10.

11 On the authorship of *The Acts of the Apostles*, see *The Jerusalem Bible*, p. 195.

12 Mt 16:18: "So now I say to you: You are Peter and on this rock I will build my Church."

13 See *The Jerusalem Bible*, p. 159, note g.

14 Ml 1:2–8.

15 The translation here adopted for the saying is taken from the King James Bible. *The Jerusalem Bible* translates it as "the blind and the lame shall not enter the Temple."

16 Mt 15:29–31, Mt 21:14–15, Lk 7:22–23, Ac 3:1–10, Ac 14:8–9.

17 Anthony Molho, "The Brancacci Chapel: Studies in its Iconography and History," *Journal of the Warburg and Courtauld Institutes*, 40 (1977): 50–98, concisely recaps the issues at stake on the subject of papal authority from the fourth through to the fifteenth century. He underlines the fact that it was only in 385 that the first official claim between papal authority and that possessed by Peter in the early Christian days was enunciated. In 418 Pope Zosimus linked his authority to that of Peter, while at the 431 Council of Ephesus Peter's primacy was upheld in virtue of the keys he had been given to "bind and lose sins." See especially Molho, pp. 51–53.

18 For the Sixtus IV reliefs see Pietro Zander, *Il ciborio degli apostoli*, Città del Vaticano, 2010; Pier Luigi Silvan entry in *Roma 1300–1875: L'arte degli anni santi*, Marcello Fagiolo and Maria Luisa Madonna (eds.), Milan, 1984, pp. 357–363; and Vittorio Lanzani, "'*Ubi Petrus': L'antica immagine della Confessione vaticana*,'" in *Pellegrini alla tomba di Pietro*, Giovanni Morello (ed.), Milan, 1999, p. 56. On the Petrine iconography of the healing of the lame see Debold Kritter, *Studien zum Petruszyklus in der Brancaccikapelle*, Berlin, 1975, pp. 54–64. For the Raphael cartoon see John Shearman, *Raphael's Cartoons in the Collection of Her Majesty the Queen and the Tapestries for the Sistine Chapel*, London, 1972, p. 66.

19 These glosses were the standard commentaries on the Scriptures that from the Church Fathers well into the Middle Ages had accrued through the centuries and were typically placed in the margins of the Vulgate Bible.
20 Shearman, p. 66.
21 Francis Martin (ed.), *Ancient Christian Commentary on Scripture: New Testament, V, Acts*, Downers Grove, 2006, pp. 38–40.
22 Ibid., p. 39.
23 *The Old Testament Pseudepigrapha*, pp. 487–490.
24 Andrea Alciati, *A Book of Emblems. The* Emblematum Liber *in Latin and English by Andrea Alciati (1492–1550)*, John F. Moffitt (tr. and ed.), Jefferson, NC, and London, 2004, p. 187, Emblem 160, "Mutual Aid: The blind man carries a lame man on his back, and he receives in exchange from his partner the gift of his eyes. Hence, in mutual concord one lends to the other that which he lacks: one exchanges the eyes, and the other exchanges his feet." The emblems reproduced in this text are from the 1549 edition by Bernadino Daza Pinciano.
25 Edward A. Maser (ed.), *Baroque and Rococo Pictorial Imagery: The 1758–60 Hertel Edition of Ripa's Iconologia with 200 Engraved Illustrations*, New York, 1971, n. 52.
26 See Chapter 1, note 88. For a different interpretation of the respective roles of the blind and the lame in this story, see Nichols, *The Art of Poverty*, pp. 77–80, where the author inverts their symbolic meaning. Although Epiphanius's parenthetic remark about the lame man having been placed on the shoulders of the blind man seems to really not make any distinction as to which the blind man and the lame man represent (see *The Old Testament Pseudepigrapha*, p. 494), the rabbinic tradition, in its choice of word order, seems to indicate that the lame represents the spirit and the blind the body: "What did he (the king) do? He made the lame man ride upon the blind and he judged them as one. So the Holy One, blessed be he, brings the spirit and placing it in the body, he also judges them as one." See *The Old Testament Pseudepigrapha*, p. 493. Furthermore, that the lame should be taken as the counterpart of the soul is supported by both the pagan and the biblical tradition. Cicero, *De Oratore*, III, 221, annotates, "as the face is the image of the soul, so are the eyes its interpreters, in respect of which the subjects under discussion will provide the proper limits for the expression of joy or grief." Matthew (6:22–23) clarifies, "the lamp of the body is the eye. It follows that if your eye is sound, your whole body will be filled with light. But if your eye is diseased, your whole body will be in darkness. If then, the light inside you is darkness, what darkness that will be!" On his part, Arator, *On the Acts of the Apostles (De Actibus Apostolorum)*, Richard J. Schrader (tr. and ed.), Atlanta, 1987, p. 66, declares: "The eyes are the noblest part joined to the head: Christ creates them as a gift, He who is the Head and Brightness of the universe. In their extremity the feet are the lowest part of all; the cure of an apostolic voice heals them on the road, since the feet which carry peace to all lands are called beautiful."
27 Peter Higginson, "Poverty and Papal Piety in Rome *c.* 1600: Painting, Pastoralism and Spectacle," in *Others and Outcasts in Early Modern Europe: Picturing the Social Margins*, Tom Nichols (ed.), Aldershot, 2007, p. 89, fig. 4.2 reproduces Nicolas Dorigny's engraving after the painting. Cigoli's work was judged by the Fabbrica di San Pietro – the institution in charge of the work done in St. Peter's – to be the best painting of the cycle and the artist was rewarded with a golden chain. See also Miles L. Chappell and Chandler W. Kirwin, "A Petrine Triumph: The Decoration of the Navi Piccole in San Pietro under Clement VIII," *Storia dell'arte*, 21 (1974): 143.
28 Higginson, pp. 88–91.
29 *Acta Sanctorum*, Augusti II, Antwerp, 1735, p. 496, no. 56, *De recognitione*, 15. George Kaftal, "The Fabulous Life of a Saint," *Mitteilungen des Kunsthistorischen Istitutes in Florenz*, 17 (1973): 123–128; *Acts* 6.5–8.3; "De recognitione corporum SS. Laurentii et Stephani," *Analecta Bollandiniana*, 15 (1886): 192.
30 *Acta Sanctorum*, Augusti; Henri Leclercq, "Laurent," in Fernand Cabrol and Henry Leclercq (eds.), *Dictionnaire d'archéologie Chrétienne et de liturgie*, Paris, 1929, 8:2; Anna Benvenuti and Elena Giannarelli, *Il diacono Lorenzo tra storia e leggenda*, Florence, 1998.
31 Antonella Greco, *La cappella di Niccolò V del Beato Angelico*, Rome, 1980, p. 20; Renate Colella, "Die Kapelle Papst Nikolaus' V: zu ihrer Geschichte und Funktion inner halb des Vatikanischen

Palastes," in *Architectural Studies in Memory of Richard Krautheimer*, Cecil Striker (ed.), Mainz, 1996, pp. 37–41; Renate Colella, "Hagiographie und Kirchen politik – Stephanus und laurentius in Rom," in *Pratum Romanum: Richard Krautheimer zum 100. Geburtstag*, Renate Colella and Richard Krautheimer (eds.), Wiesbaden, 1977, pp. 75–96; Ann I. Venchi, "Il messaggio teologico della cappella Niccolina," in *Il Beato Angelico e la cappella Niccolina: storia e restauro*, Francesco Buranelli (ed.), Novara, 2001, pp. 45–62 and 63–76.

32 Greco, p. 71; Tiernay. For the fundamental texts of Cajetan, Almain and Mair see James H. Burns and Thomas M. Izbicki (eds.), *Conciliarism and Papalism*, Cambridge, 1997. In the context of the chapel of Nicholas V see Renate Colella, *Päpstiliche Suprematie und Kirhliche Reform, die Fresken Fra Angelicos in der Kapelle Papst Nikolaus'V – ein Päpstliches Programm in Spät Konsiliarer Zeit* (Ph.D. thesis, Munich, 1993); Casimiro Bonfigli, *Niccolò V: papa della rinascenza*, Rome, 1997, pp. 133–136.

33 Pietro Palazzini (ed.), *Dizionario dei Concili*, 6 vols., Rome, 1963–1968, I, p. 149.

34 Ludwig von Pastor, *Geschicte der Päpste*, I, Freiburg, 1886; Guerrino Pelliccia and Giancarlo Rocca (eds.), *Dizionario degli istituti di perfezione*, Rome, 1974–2003; Giuseppe Coluccia, *Niccolò V umanista, papa e riformatore*, Venice, 1998, pp. 115–130.

35 Anna Cavallaro, "La pittura a Roma nel tempo di Nicolò V (1447–1453)," in *La storia dei Giubilei*, Gloria Fossi and Claudio Strinati (eds.), 4 vols., Rome, 1998, II, p. 76. In keeping with the pacifying nature of his papacy, Nicholas V chose scenes from the lives of St. Stephen and St. Lawrence, thus tactfully sidestepping the issues raised in the fourteenth century by Marsilius of Padua and William Ockham, who claimed that the very existence of the papacy was not a creation of divine providence. See Previté-Orton (ed.), *The Defensor Pacis of Marsilius of Padua*, p. xx; Palazzini, I, p. 149. Had Nicholas V chosen to tackle the issue in a more polemical way, he would have required that two scenes from the life of Christ be represented in his chapel: Christ's charge to Peter to "Feed my sheep" and "The Handing of the Keys to Peter." These, indeed, had been the traditional event that stressed Christ's choice of Peter as the "rock" on which to build the Christian Church. See Molho, p. 53.

36 Molho's statements, p. 53, with reference to the Florentine Brancacci Chapel are just as pertinent to the chapel of Nicholas V: "The fact that the two principal biblical references used to support claims of papal superiority were excluded from the Chapel's iconographic programme suggests that the sponsor's and iconographer's intention was to avoid raising the enormously controversial question of the superiority of the Church over the State, and to focus the contemporary viewer's attention on the different range of problems, all of which referred to the internal administration of the Church, or to the undisputed position of the Papacy at the apex of the ecclesiastical hierarchy."

37 Quoted by Molho, p. 53.

38 Colella, as in note 31.

39 *Acta Sanctorum*, Augusti II, esp. pp. 491–493; De Voragine, *The Golden Legend*, II, pp. 65–66.

40 Colella, as in note 31.

41 Among the many studies on the subject, see John Henderson, "The Art of Healing: Hospital Wards and the Sick in Renaissance Florence"; Ludovica Sebregondi, "Carità palese e carità occulta: le vesti confraternali nell'esercizio delle opere di mesericordia"; Friedhelm Scharf, "La retorica figurativa e il significato politico-sociale degli affreschi del Pellegrinaio in S. Maria della Scala a Siena"; and Tom Nichols, "Images of Almsgiving and Poverty in Venetian Art of the Sixteenth Century" – all are published in *Armut und Armenfürsorge in der italinischen Stadtkultur zwischen 13. und 16. Jahrhundert: Bilder, Texte und Soziale Praktiken*, Philine Helas and Gerhard Wolf (eds.), Frankfurt am Main, 2006.

42 Rosa, "Poveri ed emarginati," p. 20. The following pages are derived from my article "Blindness, Lameness and Mendicancy in Italy (from the 14th to the 18th Centuries)."

43 Fiorani, "Religione e povertà," p. 103. See also Manuela Zorzi, "Anni Santi, 'mendicità provveduta' e l'Ospizio Apostolico dei Poveri Invalidi," in *L'arte per i giubilei e tra i giubilei del Settecento*, Eliza Debenedetti (ed.), Rome, 1999, p. 26 and p. 33, n. 21. For the statistics see Francesco Cerasoli, "Censimenti della popolazione di Roma dall'anno 1600 al 1739," *Studi e documenti di storia di diritto*, XII, Rome, 1891, p. 14. See also Biblioteca Apostolica Vaticana (hereafter referred to as BAV), Chigi H.II, 46.

44 Fiorani, "Religione e povertà," p. 103.
45 Archivio Segreto Vaticano, IV–V, t.9, fol. 205r.
46 Paolo Simoncelli, "Origini e primi anni di vita dell'ospedale romano dei poveri mendicanti," *Annuario dell'Istituto Storico Italiano per l'età moderna e contemporanea*, XXV–XXVI, 1973–1974 (1976), p. 129.
47 Archivio Segreto Vaticano, arm. IV–V, t. 105C, p. 95.
48 Ibid.
49 See Catherine Loisel, *Ludovico Carracci*, Paris, 2004, pl. 9, and p. 72. Despite the new attribution proposed by A. Sutherland Harris, "Ludovico, Agostino, Annibale: ... *l'abbiam fatto tutti noi*," *Accademia Clementina: atti e memorie*, 33–34 (1994): 69–84, and Loisel's reiteration, the Reunion des museés nationaux still ascribes the image to Annibale Carracci.
50 Camillo Fanucci, *Trattato di tutte le opere pie dell'alma città di Roma*, Rome, 1601, pp. 65–66. My translation.
51 Fatica, p. 167.
52 Simoncelli, p. 130. The site had been abandoned for the same reason by both St. Dominic and the nuns who had originally been assigned to this convent. St. Dominic moved to the convent of Santa Sabina, on the Aventine Hill, while the nuns moved to the convent of Santa Caterina da Siena a Magnanapoli. See Giulio Pisano, "L'ospizio-ospedale di S. Sisto e la Compagnia dei Mendicanti di S. Elisabetta," *Roma*, VI (1928): 241–258.
53 Simoncelli, p. 130.
54 Carlo Bartolomeo Piazza, *Euseuologio Romano, overo Delle Opere Pie di Roma*, Rome, 1698, p. 478. See also B. Pullan, "'Difettosi, impotenti, inabili': Caring for the Disabled in Early Modern Italian Cities," in *Poverty and Charity: Europe, Italy, Venice, 1400–1700*, Norfolk, 1994, chapter 6, p. 3.
55 Angela Groppi, "Birbanti e poveri benestanti: attitudini e pratiche assistenziali nei confronti della vecchiaia nella Roma pontificia (sec. XVI–XVIII)," in *Povertà e innovazioni istituzionali in Italia: dal medioevo ad oggi*, Vera Zamagni (ed.), Bologna, 2000, p. 266: "Nel 1596 all'indomani della visita dell'Ospedale eseguita da Clemente VIII, le autorità di S. Sisto decidono che s'haveranno da ritener solamente quelli poveri miserabili, & privi d'ogni altro aiuto, li quali, ò per vecchiezza; ò per cecità, ò per stroppiatura notabile delle membra, non potranno procacciarsi il vitto né col mendicare, né in altra maniera.'" The quotation is derived from the Archivio di Stato di Roma, Ospizio apostolico di S. Michele, b. 166, c.7, *Decreti di congregazioni particolari per l'Ospizio Apostolico dal 1692 al 1699*.
56 See, for example, BAV, Urb. Lat. 1054, fol. 117r, 14 March 1590: "È uscito bando contro i Vagabondi di q[ues]ta città, et Zingari ordinando, che fra 8 giorni debbano havere sgombrato di Roma, et suo distretto pena la galera, et in campagna non possino i padroni pigliare alcuno a' loro servitio continuo, che non habbiano fedi autentiche di non essere banditi, ne condennati, et contra i disobbedienti si provederà senza servare spesa [?] giuditiaria, et in ogni altro miglior modo." See also Pullan, "'Difettori, impotenti, inabili,'" p. 8: "Almost invariably, however, the authorities in any city had sooner or later to fall back on some system of licensed or authorized begging, which allowed a restricted number of approved local poor – usually blind persons or cripples – to come into direct contact with the public."
57 Henderson, "'Mal Francese,'" p. 505.
58 My thanks to Inge Weustink for her translation of the Latin inscriptions on the tomb. The relief, executed by Giovanni Antonio Paracca, called Valsoldo, represents some of the major projects undertaken or completed during the papacy of Sixtus V, such as, from top center clockwise, the initiation of a bridge over the Tiber between the towns of Borghetto and Otricoli, the dome of St. Peter's, the erection of the obelisk in St. Peter's square, the Lateran Palace (or the Ospizio di San Sisto?), Christian Charity (with two children) and, possibly, Religion (holding two books with the model of a church or chapel). For the latter figure see Alexandra Herz, "The Sistine and Pauline Tombs: Documents of the Counter-Reformation," *Storia dell'arte*, 43 (1981): 241–262, esp. p. 256. For the works executed for Sixtus V, see *Della Trasportatione dell'Obelisco Vaticano e delle Fabriche di Nostro Signore Papa Sisto V Fatte dal Cavallier Domenico Fontana Architetto di Sua Santita*,

Rome, 1590. See also Steven Ostrow, *Art and Spirituality in Counter-Reformation Rome: The Sistine and Pauline Chapels in S. Maria Maggiore*, Cambridge, 1996.

59 Fanucci, quoted by Simoncelli, p. 151. I have partially availed myself of Pullan's translation for a portion of this passage as it appears in Pullan, "'Difettosi, impotenti, inabili,'" p. 3. Nichols, "Secular Charity, Sacred Poverty," p. 139, quotes a comparable description of the "pestering" beggars in Venice in February 1528, as well as Luigi da Porto's lament with regard to the city of Vicenza.

60 Luigi Cajani, "Gli statuti della compagnia dei ciechi, zoppi, e stroppiati della visitazione (1698)," in *Ricerche per la storia religiosa di Roma*, Rome, 1979, III, pp. 287–288. See also Jean Delumeau, *Vie économique et sociale de Rome dans la seconde moitié du XVIe siècle*, Paris, 1957, p. 416, who, in turn, quotes from Emmanuel Pierre Rodocanachi, *Les corporations ouvrières à Rome depuis la chute de l'empire romain*, 2 vols., Paris, 1894, I, p. XXV, n. 1.

61 Ibid., p. 282.

62 In Italy, for example, as early as 1377 there was a brotherhood of the blind (Santa Maria dei Ciechi) in Padua, one for the lame (*zotti*) founded in 1392 in Venice that also enrolled the blind and amputees, and in the fifteenth century there were also confraternities for the blind and the lame in Frankfurt, Zurich and Strasburg. See Cajani, pp. 296–297.

63 Piazza, p. 479.

64 Pisano; Cajani, pp. 282–283. See also Mariano Armellini, *Le chiese di Roma dal secolo IV al XIX*, Rome, 1891, pp. 360–361: "[la compagnia] posta sotto la protezione di s. Elisabetta, sotto il qual nome era conosciuta dal popolo; e di qui il detto romano per designare una raccolta di poveri infelici: la compagnia di S. Elisabetta" ("the congregation was placed under the tutelage of St. Elizabeth, under whose name it was known by the people; this gave rise to the Roman epithet to designate a group poor wretches: the congregation of St. Elizabeth").

65 In a notarial document of September 2, 1639, St. Elizabeth is even referred to as the Virgin Mary's *cognata* (sister-in-law) instead of her cousin. See Cajani, p. 283.

66 See Gaston Duchet-Sychaux and Michel Pastoureau, *The Bible and the Saints*, Paris and New York, 1994, p. 136. For the life of St. Elizabeth of Hungary, see De Voragine's *The Golden Legend*, II, pp. 302–318 and *Butler's Lives of the Saints*, IV, pp. 386–391.

67 Duchet-Sychaux and Pastoureau, p. 136. Admittedly, the woodcut here reproduced is not by an Italian artist – it is taken from William Caxton's 1483 edition of Voragine's *Golden Legend*. Nonetheless, as images in this book have shown time and again, the lame was the "poor" and the "mendicant" *par excellence*.

68 The representation of the lame as symbolic of all of the poor is a recurring motif that testifies to those who most frequently were compelled to beg to provide for their needs. See for example Cesare Ripa, *Iconologia*, Siena, 1613, under *Hippocrisia*, p. 341, in which the recipient of hypocritical almsgiving is depicted as a lame man on hand crutches.

69 For Caccia's print see *The Illustrated Bartsch*, XLVIII, 2 (50), formerly XII, *Italian Chiaroscuro Woodcuts*, 1983, p. 62, and for Beatrizet's, ibid., XXIX, 31 (255), formerly XV (part 2), *Italian Masters of the Sixteenth Century*, 1982, p. 275.

70 Piazza, p. 479.

71 Cajani, p. 287.

72 BAV, Urb. Lat. 1080, also quoted by Cajani, p. 287. My translation. On occasions such as these, when the beggars were coerced into one of the official hospices and those who did not submit to this deprivation of freedom were sent out of the city, there were those who took an ironic view of these *bandi*, as did Vincenzo Gugnoni da Medula in a poem included in his *Historia bellissima dove s'intende l'amara partenza, che fanno li guidoni di Roma* (BAV, Capponi V 682, int. 68): "Already the *bandi* have gone out/as everyone has heard and seen/that the blind and the lame/must run to San Sisto/whoever is sorrowful and wretched from pain/accept perhaps, that this is the ointment/in the form of a resolution/that only those with license can beg/painful bitter departure." In Rose Marie San Juan, *Rome: A City out of Print*, Minneapolis and London, 2001, who also publishes the original Italian text, p. 49 and p. 263, n. 63.

73 Cajani, p. 301: "Ritrovandosi in quest'alma città di Roma molti poveri, e povere che vanno mendicando come ciechi stroppi, e zoppi, et altri inabili per altre infermità per lo più senza guida alcuna . . . ci siamo noi altri poveri ciechi, e stroppi radunati insieme per stabilire, e fondare una compagnia spirituale a similitudine dell'altre compagnie di Roma come in altre città sogliono farsi" ("There being in this hallowed city of Rome many poor men and women who go about begging, like the crippled-blind, the lame and other disabled individuals owing to other infirmities, [who] for the most part [are] without any guide . . . we the poor blind and lame gathered to create and found a spiritual congregation similar to those that are commonly initiated in Rome and other cities.")

74 Ibid., p. 282–313. See Pullan, "'Difettosi, impotenti, inabili,'" pp. 9–13.

75 Simoncelli, p. 148, quotes from a document issued in 1596 under Clement VIII relating to the Ospedale di San Sisto, which specifies that the license to beg in the streets of Rome issued by this hospice had to be placed on the left shoulder. The same instruction is found in a *bando* of 1627: "The license to beg will be granted only to the poor and wretched elderly, or blind, or crippled, or weak, and unable to sustain themselves in any other manner except by begging. To these will be given the printed license, underwritten by one of the Lord Deputies, and together with the ordinary mark, with the obligation to carry it in such a way arranged and uncovered on the left shoulder so that it is seen by all clearly." San Juan, p. 52 and p. 265, n. 83. For the drawing of a lame mendicant attributed to Annibale Carracci see http://en.wahooart.com/@@/8DNVXU-Annibale-Carracci-Crippled-beggar (last accessed October 11, 2015).

76 Ibid., p. 285 and p. 306.

77 Ibid., p. 283.

78 Ibid. For Oliviero Gatti see Spike (ed.), *The Illustrated Bartsch*, XLI, formerly XIX (Part 1), *Italian Masters of the Seventeenth Century*, p. 18. Brown, *Through the Eye of a Needle*, p. 86: "In Augustine's Hippo, the regular poor box was called 'the Quadriga.' It was seen as a four-horse chariot that swung low to sweep the alms of the faithful (as it had once swept the prophet Elijah himself) far beyond the stars to heaven."

79 Cajani, p. 306. The seven basilicas are: St. Peter's, St. John Lateran, Santa Maria Maggiore, Santa Croce in Gerusalemme, St. Paul Outside the Walls, St. Lawrence Outside the Walls and St. Sebastian.

80 Ibid.

81 Gaetano Moroni, "Confraternita di S. Elisabetta e sua Visitazione dei poveri ciechi e storpi in s. Sisto," in *Dizionario di erudizione*, Venice, 1852, LV, p. 15.

82 Cajani, p. 284.

83 Ibid., p. 299.

84 Ms. Vittorio Emanuele 630, Biblioteca Nazionale di Roma, fols. 107v–113v.

85 On the eighth-century forgery that went by the name of *The Donation of Constantine* and on the philological proof that the document was a hoax see Lorenzo Valla, *On the Donation of Constantine*, Glen Warren Bowersock (tr.), Cambridge, 2007 (*De falso credita et ementita Costantini donatione declamatio*). With this document it was believed that Constantine transferred to Pope Sylvester his authority over Rome and the western part of the Roman Empire.

86 Cajani, p. 311. Ibid., pp. 289–290: "La sua [the confraternity's] unica preoccupazione sono quei mendicanti i quali, pur essendo veri poveri, non si iscrivono nella compagnia perché 'vogliono vivere nella loro libertà senza alcun timore' e vanno in giro per le strade e per le chiese chiedendo l'elemosina con urla e lamenti, disobbedendo ai superiori e creando disordine. 'Per togliere via questi mali abusi' li si esorta quindi ad entrare nella compagnia, acquistando così anche la possibilità di lucrarne le indulgenze." ("The confraternity's only concern was those mendicants who, although truly poor, did not enroll in the confraternity because 'they want to live in freedom without fear' and go about town and churches begging for alms with shouts and moans, [thus] disobeying the authorities and creating disorder. 'To eliminate these bad abuses' they were encouraged to enroll in the congregation, thereby acquiring also the possibility of benefitting from the indulgences [it received].")

87 *Editto Sopra li Vagabondi, Mendicanti, and altri simili, che stanno nelli Portici, e Scale delle Chiese*: Archivio Segreto Vaticano, Armadio IV–V, t. 9, 17 maggio 1628, p. 284: "Avvertiamo e richiediamo tutti, e ciascuno dei sopradetti Vagabondi, Baroni, Mendichi finti, and altri, che non abbiano licenza . . . [che] dovranno lasciare quei posti dove riparano . . . sotto pena di carcere, e della frusta/da eseguirsi subito per quelli che saranno d'età capace, e per gli altri minori, di 25. Staffilate da darseli in publico, dell'esilio da Roma, e suo Distretto in perpetuo."

88 Michel Foucault, *Madness and Civilization:A History of Insanity in the Age of Reason*, New York, 1988 [orig. 1965], French edition 1961.

89 Fatica, p. 178. See *La medicità provveduta nella città di Roma coll'Ospizio Pubblico fondato dalla Pietà, e Beneficenza di Nostro Signore Innocenzo XII Pontefice Massimo Con le risposte all'Obiezioni contro simili fondazioni*, Rome, 1693, p. 29.

90 *La medicità provveduta*, p. 31. The creation of the Lateran hospice was also commemorated on the reverse of a 1692–1693 papal medal for Innocent XII that depicts the Lateran complex from the north, papal palace on the left, and above it a scroll with an inscription quoting a passage from Isaiah 58.7: EGENOS. VOGOSQ. INDUC/IN DOMUM TUAM ("Take into thy house the destitute and the homeless"). See Nathan Whitman, *Roma Resurgens: Papal Medals from the Age of the Baroque*, Ann Arbor, 1981, p. 156, no. 142.

91 A.I., "Ospizio di San Giovanni in Laterano," in *Le immagini del SS mo Salvatore: fabbriche e sculture per l'Ospizio Apostolico dei Poveri Invalidi*, Bruno Contardi and Giovanna Curcio (eds.), Rome, 1988, pp. 103–110.

92 Alberto Balzani, *L'Ospizio Apostolico dei Poveri Invalidi detto "Il S. Michele" dal 1693 al 1718*, Rome, 1969. See also Bruno Contardi, "La mendicità provveduta," in *Le immagini del SS.mo Salvatore*, pp. 17–39.

93 *La medicità provveduta*, p. 97.

94 Fatica, p. 182.

95 BAV, Ottob. Lat. 3362, I, "Avviso," November 1, 1692, p. 100.

96 Ibid.: "N[ostra] S[antità] le disse, che li voleva, ò fuori di Roma, ò racchiusi nel Serraglio."

97 Fernand Mourret, *A History of the Catholic Church*, 8 vols., Newton Thompson (tr.), St. Louis and London, 1947, VI, p. 271: "At the very outset of his pontificate he gathered about himself a large number of the poor and said: 'Here are my nephews.' To put an end to nepotism, he published (June 23 [*sic*], 1692) a constitution by which, in conformity with the holy canons, which forbids bishops to enrich their relatives with the goods of the Church, he declared that he was imposing an inviolable rule, not only for himself, but for all succeeding popes. This rule provided that no pope under any pretext whatever, not even as recompense for services, should dispose of any goods or office of the Roman Church in favor of his relatives or friends."

98 Battista Mondin, *Dizionario enciclopedico dei papi*, Rome, 1995, pp. 400–404.

99 Artaud De Montor, *The Lives and Times of the Popes* (orig. *Les vies des papes*), 10 vols., New York, 1910, 6, pp. 158–159: "In his will Innocent left the poor his sole heirs, and commanded that his property of every kind should be sold, and that the proceeds in full amount should be distributed among the poor of the city." When his architect Carlo Fontana once told the pope that he had been to the hospice to visit the "rascals" ("li birbi nel suddetto ospizio") the pope, incensed, apparently responded, "*You* are a rascal, get out of our way!" ("Un birbo siete voi, levatevici davanti!"). Quoted by Fatica, p. 102.

100 Gaetano Moroni, *Dizionario di Erudizione Storico-Ecclesiastica*, Venice, 1851, L, p. 7 and Whitman, p. 158.

101 Pullan, "'Difettosi, impotenti, inabili,'" p. 3.

102 Nicola La Marca, *Saggio di un ricerca storico-economica sull'industria e l'artigianato a Roma dal 1750 al 1849*, Rome, 1969, pp. 35–50. Quoted by Nasto, p. 27, n. 21.

103 Pullan, "'Difettosi, impotenti, inabili,'" p. 2.

5 Exit the lame

> Our poetry does not emerge from a living world, nor exist in the storm and confluence of such objects and feelings. Instead we force either our theme or our treatment of both and we have done so for so long and so often and from our tenderest years that if we attempted any free development, it would scarcely prosper; for how can a cripple get up and walk?
>
> (Johann Gottfried Herder, *Correspondence on Ossian and the Songs of Ancient Peoples* (1773), p. 75)

Even before travelling to Italy, in his *Reflections on the Painting and Sculpture Of the Greeks* (1765) Johann Joachim Winckelmann (1717–1768) expressed his disapproval of Bernini's art. Basing himself on Bernini's claim, as reported in Filippo Baldinucci's biography of the artist, that Nature contained all the beauty necessary for an artist to create a beautiful work of art, Winckelmann found Bernini at fault for not upholding the Greek ideal of the Beautiful. Indeed, the sculptor purportedly did not accept the theory that the ancients had ennobled their works by adding a certain grace that was lacking in Nature[1] and branded as an absurd invention ("a fable") the story of Zeuxis's ideal portrait of Helen of Troy that, according to Pliny, he had obtained through a selective process of the best features of five Crotonian girls.[2] This affront to the Greek ideal of the Beautiful so incensed Winckelmann that in a letter of July 1756 to his friend Berendis he sarcastically wrote: "the moderns are jackasses in comparison to the ancients . . . and Bernini is the biggest jackass of them all, the French excepted."[3]

In the changing cultural and esthetic climate of eighteenth-century Europe, the Baroque love of "curvatures, protrusions, segmentations, acute angles, cartouches, helixes, contortions, frowns, fluttering cloaks, mountainous garments, extreme emotions, floral designs, festoons, gold leafing and polychrome marbles"[4] eventually gave way to a renewed Classical ideal of the Beautiful that is frequently associated with what Winckelmann considered the most eminent characteristic of Greek art: "noble simplicity and quiet grandeur" ("*edle Einfalt und stille Größe*").[5] In fact, the trend that was associated in the seventeenth century with writers such as Giovan Pietro Bellori (1613–1696), who had begun giving greater praise to the more Classically minded artists of the Baroque period, continued in the next century. The ideas upheld by people such as Pierre-Jean Mariette (1694–1774) and Charles-Nicolas Cochin (1715–1790), as well as the impact that the discovery of Herculaneum (1738) and Pompeii (1748) had on contemporary society, culminated in the eighteenth century in an artistic world where there would be little room for images that represented an un-idealized humanity or find a justification for depicting disabilities. In truth, the one important image of the period that comes immediately to mind when thinking of the disabled in eighteenth-century art is Jacques-Louis David's *Belisarius Receiving Alms* (1780–1781) (Figure 5.1), a work that the French artist produced after his return from Italy. Having spent time in the French Academy in Rome (1775) and, more importantly, having met in Naples the theorist Quatremère de Quincy (1755–1849), David felt as if he had finally been enabled to truly understand ancient art – according to David, the meeting had had the effect of a "cataract operation" on him.[6] In this monumental painting (288 × 312 cm) the painter depicted an ennobled, magniloquent image of a soldier recognizing his former general, Belisarius, whose adverse fortune in old age forced him, blind and destitute, to revert to begging. Of course, the poor, the disabled and the outcasts in general were as prevalent in eighteenth-century societies as they had been in those of the seventeenth century, yet they tend to disappear from the artists' horizon. In the new century, in other words, the "barons" as well as the physically impaired, who had captivated the attention of Callot and other artists in the seventeenth century, lost most of their appeal for neo-Classical artists.[7]

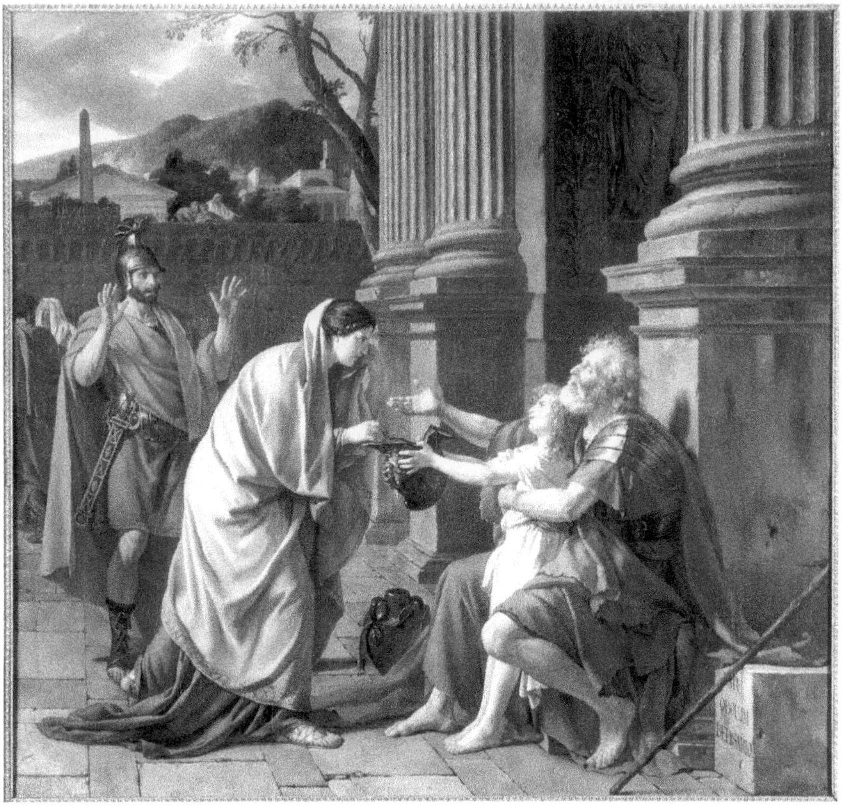

Figure 5.1 Jacques-Louis David, *Belisarius Receiving Alms*, 1780–1781, Palais des Beaux-Arts, Lille. Photo: © RMN-Grand Palais/Philipp Bernard

Certainly, the human and economic conditions in eighteenth-century Italy had not really changed from preceding centuries. If one is to believe Charles de Brosses (1709–1777), count of Tournay and baron of Montfalcon who travelled through Italy in 1739–1740, in the Papal States, for example, signs of improvement were still a long way off: "Imagine what kind of population this is, of which one third is made up of priests, another of people who hardly ever work and a final one of people who do absolutely nothing."[8] Often quoted because of the witty picture he paints of the inactivity and related indigence of the Roman masses, Brosses's sarcastic statement was a lucid, harsh assessment of the papal government's inability to confront the challenges of contemporary times. The quotation, in fact, is preceded by the following observations: "The [papal] sovereigns who, after Sixtus V, have done wonders for the embellishment of the city, have done nothing for the cultivation of the countryside, where one cannot perceive, literally, a single home nor a single shrub. The government is so bad that one cannot conceive of a worse one. Machiavelli and [Thomas] Moore applied themselves to formulating a concept of a Utopia; here [in Rome] one finds the concrete reification of its exact opposite."[9] The pope, in de Brosses's view, was at the head of a society that did not develop its agricultural potential, nor its commerce and industry. To any foreign observer it was clear that the vicars of Christ were surrounded by a system based on nepotism in which relatives tried to obtain the most for themselves before being replaced by the next group of familial "thieves" ("*voleurs*") with the election of the next pope. Such a government, in de Brosses's view, encapsulated all that ought to be shunned by a modern state.

With regard to the unemployed masses, a sagacious analysis was provided by two members of the Neapolitan intelligentsia: the economists Giuseppe Palmieri (1721–1793), who reminded his contemporaries that "manca più tosto lavoro alla gente che gente al lavoro" ("if anything, it is rather the people who are deprived of work and not positions waiting to be filled by the people"),[10] and Antonio Genovesi (1712–1769), who claimed that "the best and most effective means of diminishing the number of poor people is that of promoting industry."[11] Comparably revealing are the views of an enlightened and dispassionate observer such as Goethe to whom the proverbial southerners' laziness seemed mostly an inaccurate cliché. Sojourning in Naples, on May 28, 1787 he noted in his journal: "the only ones [beggars] I saw were very old men, no longer capable of work, and cripples. The longer and closer I looked, the fewer real idlers I could observe, either of the lower classes or the middle, either young or old, men or women, either in morning or during most of the rest of the day."[12] It was the authorities' lack of a general and viable plan of economic growth and industrialization that penalized the populace of the peninsula, since those who controlled the fate of the nation – be they high-ranking clergymen or land-owning aristocrats – especially in central and southern Italy, were more interested in preserving their established privileges and lifestyle than in "fixing" the problem.[13]

In fact, despite the efforts made by enlightened intellectuals and statesmen to eradicate poverty and mendicancy, the picture that scholars have delineated of eighteenth-century European societies in general, and Italian society in particular, is one of continuity with the preceding century. From northern to southern Italy the decrees and laws issued by the ruling classes proved to be nothing more than a recurring leitmotif of good intentions beached on the shores of stark reality.[14]

In Turin, for example, where the Ospedale di Carità was the major institution providing poor-relief, the sixteenth- and seventeenth-century discrimination between local and immigrant poor continued unabated.[15] What distinguishes poor-relief in the eighteenth century was a new form of state control that took its lead from the efforts made by the French crown to eradicate the problem of poverty and begging, as well as its determination to enclose the poor.[16] The edict of 1716, for instance, not only outlawed begging and almsgiving, ordering all mendicants to report within three days to the Ospedale di Carità, but also decreed that all outsiders leave the city and return to their place of origin. Failure to comply could result in imprisonment and punishment.[17] This was no different from an edict of 1541 that had stipulated begging was banned on penalty of being "irremissibly whipped."[18] What characterized the contemporary attitude was that now the program was designed to be executed throughout the kingdom with "a pyramidic [*sic*] structure of control emanating from the capital."[19] Still, as a "Register of the poor detained begging" of 1740 makes abundantly clear, not only the influx of the immigrant poor into Turin continued relentlessly – of the 1,911 detainees, 88 percent came from other places – but the highest percentage of these were the young (those aged 10–19 comprised 40.7 percent, followed by those aged 20–29 amounting to 12.6 percent of the internees).[20] The local poor, on the other hand, were propagandistically exploited by the Savoy dynasty in a ceremony reminiscent of the one that took place in Papal Rome described in Chapter 4, to celebrate the monarchy and its reforms.[21] In the end, Victor Amadeus's project of unifying the relief system failed, as evinced by the fact that in 1723, six years after its inception, the *congregazioni*, which were meant to carry out his reform of poor-relief throughout the kingdom, existed basically only on paper.[22] A "change," so to speak, is noticeable in the threatening warnings of the subsequent edicts, as they were now being aimed at the "vagabond," rather than at the "beggar from outside" or "able-bodied beggar."[23]

In Napoleonic Piedmont a shift in poor-relief had taken place by the beginning of the nineteenth-century, as the revolutionary/Republican ideology of the new state did not tolerate a religious or moral approach to poverty.[24] Despite the extensiveness and degree of centralization created in the wake of the French *bureaux de bienfaisance*, the hospitals and the *dépôts de mendicité*, there was a strong emphasis on putting the poor to work.[25] Thus in the hospices and hospitals where the poor were relegated, so long as they met the requirement of *family* and *residency* – that is the "homegrown" poor – *employment* was considered the solution to help defeat idleness.[26] Unfortunately, even this solution, which is a preface to the evolution of the masses from being made up of the idle poor to the poor working class, inevitably failed, as the funds available were insufficient to rectify a problem of immense dimensions. For instance, an edifice called *Ergastolo*, which had been built in 1779 two miles from Turin for spiritual exercises and converted in 1787 into a structure to keep about four hundred idle poor busy in different kinds of working activities, proved vastly inferior to the real need, since in 1809 the actual number of mendicants in the Dipartimento di Po amounted to 4,067 men and 5,395 women.[27] In fact, a year after its inauguration, in 1810, the supervisory committee of this *dépôt* had already lamented the serious financial straits in which it navigated; and in 1814 Count Cerruti, Secretary of the Interior, asked the mayor of Turin to suggest the most appropriate ways of vacating the Egastolo and of releasing the detainees according to their personal circumstances.[28] What is of interest in the context of this study is that, out of the 396 detained mendicants in the last quarter of 1812, the highest percentage was made up of invalid and crippled ("infermi e storpi") individuals (36 percent).[29]

As in Turin, also in Genoa, poor-relief in the late eighteenth and early nineteenth centuries began to be seen almost solely as giving the unemployed a job within the *Albergo dei poveri* and, consequently, as a means of eradicating begging.[30] Chief among the Albergo's goals, at least as stipulated in the 1776 regulations, was its educational function, moral and professional, and the banishment of idleness in the city.[31] Significantly, and this is in clear opposition to what took place in the Department of Po just discussed, no infirm or aged individual, nor anyone who was not productive, was to be accepted in the Albergo.[32] Thus, what one begins to witness in these institutions is that the productive capacity of their guests subsumes all other factors previously considered. The organizations, in other words, become equally, if not more, focused on profit, as in charitable assistance.[33]

In Bologna, too, comparable trends can be observed, even if some enlightened, indeed revolutionary, principles of reform in line with the resurgence of Republican feelings engendered by Napoleon's occupation of this papal city (1796) are more clearly voiced. Thus, although out of a population of about 70,000 persons 16,000 were mendicants (approximately 22.8 percent), in a plea sent to Clement XIV in 1771 the local authorities understood that the situation was not the result of the beggars' sheer inclination to laziness but much more of the lack of working opportunities.[34] And again, while on the one hand an anonymous author of a manuscript written in 1773 suggested that "universal detainment" ("l'universale reclusione") be avoided and that the poor be encouraged to work, with only the idle being detained, on the other hand, Floriano Canetoli, in his *Opuscoli di democratica istruzione* (1797), voiced more radical concepts.[35] Indeed, this author claims that "the rich are the parasitic ivy of the immense [social] edifice" and that "the poor are always creditors of their fellow men … always contributing more than they receive."[36] Furthermore, Canetoli claims that, if the political transformations underway were to succeed, it was necessary to "strip the people of their ignorance and make them aware of their rights," after which "the happy period of their regeneration" would begin.[37] Likewise, Giuseppe Gioannetti (1768–1843), in the daily "Quotidiano bolognese," wrote that there could not be any freedom without the eradication of poverty.[38] These more progressive members of the Bolognese society believed that the contemporary attempt to transform the poor into salaried workers only sidestepped the problem without really solving it. For these defenders of the embryonic working class, even a contract between two parties of different economic means – the entrepreneur and the worker – still gave rise to a "theft" ("*furto*") at the expense of the weaker party without really changing their condition.[39] Although towards the end of the three years of the Jacobinic government (1796–1799) in Bologna edicts were promulgated that coerced the homeless poor to congregate in a private hospice provided by the public administration, beginning in 1808 a "*casa di lavoro*" was built that to some extent was part of a number of changes that began the transformation of the poor into the proletariat.[40]

In *fin de siècle* Rome, which under the tutelage of the French army from February 1798 to June 1799 had become the "Prima Repubblica Romana," the French ideals of equality and loyalty to the state were meant to supplant what was considered by the French the chief "monstrosity" of the ecclesiastical state: Christian charity.[41] According to this view, the Church was guilty of having corrupted the Roman populace and, through the dysfunctional creation of its pious organizations, had given rise to the devastating effects on the development of a market economy.[42] Although this Republican experiment was short lived, an attempt was made to substitute the old system of Catholic charity with a lay, national form of beneficence. In fact, there was no better place than Rome for the secularization process so dear to the revolutionary ideals of the French to take place.[43] In this new context, in which liberty was correlated with the duty of serving the nation, the basic division among the people was between active citizens and inactive non-citizens, and their value was assessed according to their usefulness to the country.[44] Therefore, it is no surprise that, with a law of March 22, 1798, the Ministry of Justice ordered the suppression of begging and vagabondage. A new solution to the problem, however, was proclaimed on April 13, when all beggars and vagabonds had to leave the territory of the Roman Republic if within two days they failed to obtain a certificate that testified to their availability *to work on a farm*.[45]

The Republican government exalted the nation's duty to aid all of the disabled poor, but now beneficence was no longer left to the individual. The spirit of brotherhood dictated that poor-relief be solely administered by the government.[46] In the summer of 1798 all of the hospitals were nationalized[47] and the vast network of the age-old lay organizations that had served as a bulwark against the millennial problem of pauperism, such as the Confraternity of St. Elizabeth mentioned in Chapter 4, were suppressed.[48] By so doing, the government had displaced not only the Church but also all private citizens in the "flow of the gift economy." Furthermore, the social "glue" formerly provided by Christian charity was to be replaced by productive work and free commerce.[49]

In Naples the conceptual transformation of the indigent from the Poor of Christ to an individual potentially subversive of society's values does not seem to follow the timing or the experiences of other European towns.[50] Most of all, what characterizes poor-relief in the capital of the kingdom of Naples is the lack of a governmental plan to confront the serious issues raised by the swelling crowds of the indigent and beggars.[51] And it is perhaps in Naples, the last of the major Italian cities to coerce the poor into a hospice, that the immigration of the poor from the provinces to an urban setting was most acute. In fact, the lack of consideration that the country poor received from the authorities in contrast to the city poor – which according to people such as Bencivenni Pelli (1764) and Giambattista Vasco (1769) needed urgent attention – could be resolved at least partly, in Antonio Genovesi's view, by a redistribution of the land.[52] This idea, as one can well imagine, encountered strong opposition from both the aristocracy and the religious authorities who were the owners and direct beneficiaries of the *latifundia*, the great landed estates.[53]

Significantly, when the Ospizio di San Pietro e Gennaro *extra moenia* (1656) was built, and as its name implies, it was created *outside* of the city walls.[54] The creation of this Ospizio marks the end of the vice-regency's laissez-faire attitude. In 1667, Viceroy Pedro Antonio de Cardona issued an edict that ordered all mendicants and vagabonds of the city to report to the authorities so as to be escorted to said hospice.[55] The eight hundred destitute individuals who turned up – 90 percent of whom came from outside of Naples – were placed in five different venues.[56] However, a comparable edict had to be issued once again in 1671, as the conditions within the structure must not have been very appealing to its inmates,[57] and the city had to wait until 1751 before Ferdinando Fuga began building the *Albergo Reale dei Poveri*, pointedly also called *Reclusorio*.[58]

A final look at the southern extremity of the kingdom of Naples, Sicily, will complete the picture of the state of the poor and poor-relief in what became in 1860 part of the fledgling Italian state. Perhaps here, as nowhere else, the dire condition of the masses living on farms may be witnessed. While in his *Lettere* written between 1775 and 1777, the archeologist, numismatist and traveler Domenico Sestini (1750–1832) reported that the rural population of the island lived in severe conditions feeding "almost always on wild wheat, fava beans, lupini beans, prickly pears and carobs,"[59] Paolo Balsamo (1764–1816) claimed they sustained themselves by day with a bit of cheese and in the evening with a soup made of cauliflower or beets garnished with oil and salt.[60] Given the meager diet, it is not surprising that when famine ravaged the island, as in 1764, these farmers would migrate to the towns, only to be expelled after having received some basic assistance.[61]

In Palermo an *Albergo dei poveri* was created by the Bourbons in 1732; a structure that, however, depended very much on private funding. These funds went primarily to cover the cost of the personnel and were frequently insufficient. If one considers that all of the nobility of this city in 1779 donated 15 *onze* at a time when the annual income of the rector of that institution was 80 *onze* and that of a barber 24 *onze*, it is evident that the *albergo* could not expect to care for many.[62] In fact, a more concrete assistance to the poor and the infirm continued to be provided by the confraternities and the *monti di pietà* (pawnshops).[63]

Overall, the picture that emerges from the data pertaining to a selection of major Italian cities is that the poor were probably no better off, or better treated, in the eighteenth and the beginning of the nineteenth centuries than they had been in the seventeenth century. Generally speaking, at the dawn of the modern era the factors that stand out most with regard to the poor were an effort by central governments to extend their social solutions state-wide, an attempt to eradicate idleness by putting the indigent to work within the large *alberghi*, a recurring discrimination between the urban and the country poor who, not having domicility in the cities where the hospices were built, still represented the dangerous "vagabond,"[64] and, concomitantly, a determination to eradicate begging.[65] Perhaps, as Giovanni Assereto points out, life in the large eighteenth-century *alberghi*, deplorable as they might be to our way of thinking, was probably seen by the poor themselves as acceptable and maybe even desirable.[66] Nevertheless, the poorer members of society, as well as the disabled, still had to confront the same issues they had encountered in the past and continued to face the same prejudices. Within this context, as mentioned earlier, the orthopedically impaired, who were a significant component of the large mass of the deprived, no longer seem to attract the same attention they had received in Renaissance and Baroque art.

A good example of how the disabled slowly disappeared from the artists' visual field in the latter part of the seventeenth and the beginning of the eighteenth centuries is represented by Daniel Seiter's (1642/47–1705) painting of *The Blessed Amadeus Giving Alms to the Poor* (1698) in the Vercelli Cathedral, Piedmont (Figure 5.2). In this painting the Viennese-born painter, who trained and worked in Italy, replaced the prominent role reserved for the lame in traditional images of this theme – as the one individual capable of subsuming all recipients of alms seen in Chapter 2 – by a dignified man who reaches out to accept the

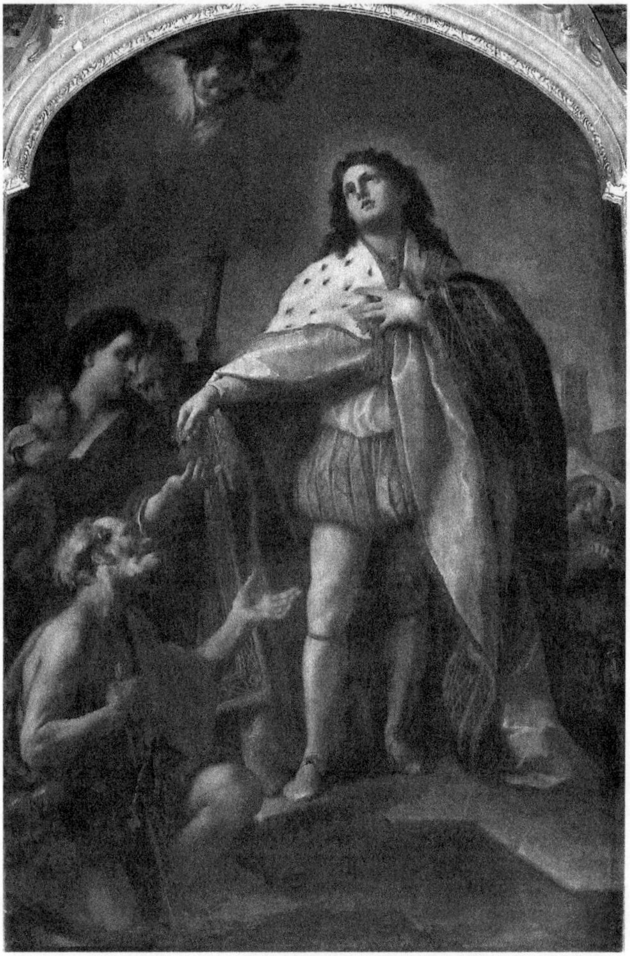

Figure 5.2 Daniel Seiter, *The Blessed Amadeus Giving Alms to the Poor*, 1698, Vercelli Cathedral. Photo: author

monetary gift of Amadeus IX, duke of Savoy (1435–1472). The elderly poor man may be depicted barefoot, semi-divested and with a short cane, but no sign of physical impairment is deemed appropriate in this royal commission. This is in sharp contrast to another princely commission painted just about a century earlier, Annibale Carracci's *Christ in Glory between Sts. Peter and John the Evangelist, St. Mary Magdalen, St. Edward of England, St. Hermenegild, and Odoardo Farnese* (ca. 1600)[67] (Plate 23). Unlike Seiter's painting, Carracci's work prominently features, if on a smaller scale, an orthopedically impaired pauper in the exact center of the painting below the silhouette of St. Peter's basilica. Needed to identify Odoardo's namesake, King Edward of England (the Confessor), who was patron saint of cripples and beggars,[68] the disabled man depicted in Carracci's canvas is represented with contorted legs while dragging his body across a landscape on hands and knees with the aid of mini-crutches. Both Seiter and

Carracci depict these indigent individuals sympathetically, but, while Seiter simply refers to the poor man's social and economic status through his humble attire and beseeching gesture, Carracci focuses on the man's physical ailment as the predominant feature by which to define his social condition.

Just like Seiter, Giuseppe Bonito (1707–1789) painted his allegory of *Charity* (1742) in the sacristy of the Pio Monte di Pietà, Naples, with an eye to representing a decorous, idealized humanity (Figure 5.3). Standing at the foot of a church portico but depicted *di sotto in su* (foreshortened), a charming, youthful girl with a cornucopia under her left arm doles out coins to a number of poor people who reach out to her. Most prominently placed and handsomely rendered at the bottom of the composition is a bare-chested young man with a headband and open hand pleading for a donation. To appreciate the psychological and artistic gap that exists between the two historical periods under discussion, compare this personification of the poor to the similar character appearing in Giovanni Serodine's *St. Lawrence Distributing Alms* (ca. 1615) in the Museo Archeologico di Casamari (Plate 24). Once again, unlike the later eighteenth-century artist, Serodine finds no better way to strike a chord in the viewer's bosom than by placing most noticeably in the foreground a young man with twisted left leg placed out of kilter behind his

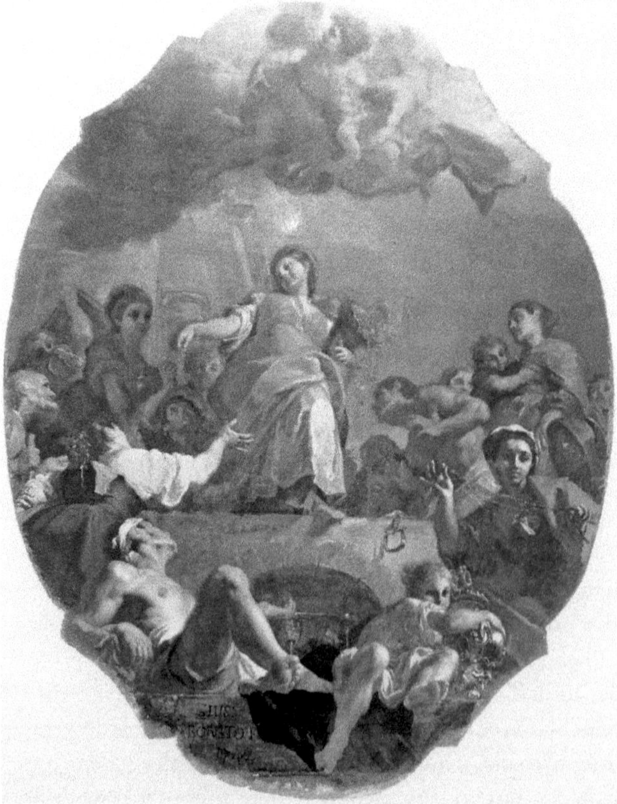

Figure 5.3 Giuseppe Bonito, *Charity*, Banco di Napoli, 1742

right; a physical trait that must have surely resulted in a syncopated, uneven gait, which is not only reminiscent of but perhaps inspired by Callot's *Captain of Rogues* (Figure 3.8). Both Bonito and Serodine paint their subjects compassionately, but while the former deemed it preferable to leave out any sign of physical ailments, the latter employs the beggar's orthopedic impairment to record a social interaction between the almsgiver and the receiver that perhaps reflected more closely what the artist's contemporaries witnessed in real life.

Analogously to Seiter and Bonito, one notices a similar tendency in Giovanni Gottardi (1733–1812), an artist born in Faenza who studied and worked primarily in Rome. His rendition of the famous biblical passage of St. Peter's *Healing of the Lame Man* (1765) (Figure 5.4), painted for the church of San Antonio Abate in Parma, also gives us an inoffensive, sterilized interpretation of the lame man's orthopedic condition by eliminating any veristic representation of his ailment, depicting just a cane by his side to indicate his lameness. No such pictorial exercise in visual euphemism troubled artists in

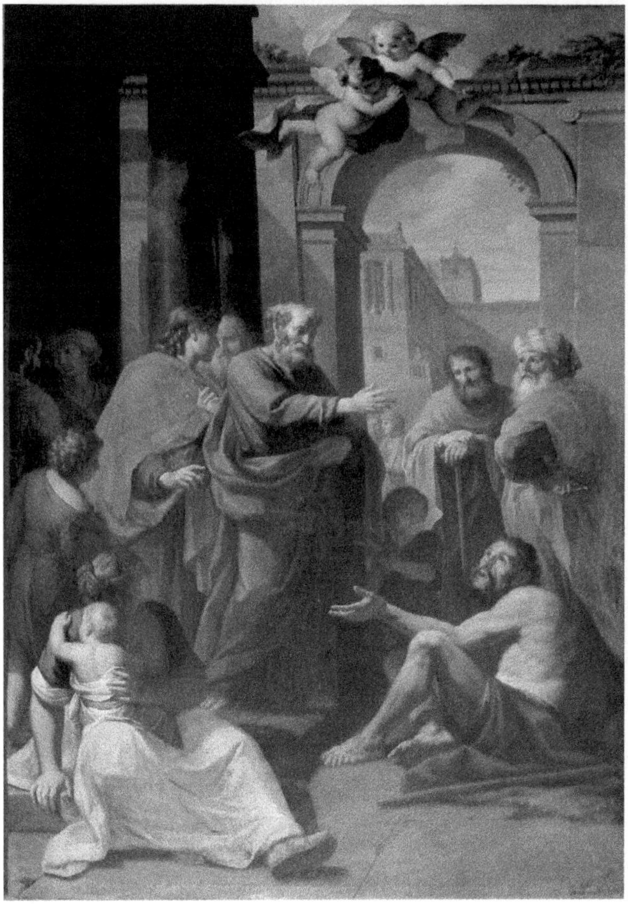

Figure 5.4 Giovanni Gottardi, *St. Peter Healing the Lame Man*, 1765, Church of San Antonio Abate, Parma. Photo: author

the previous century. A painting depicting *St. Bernardine Healing the Infirm* (Figure 5.5), executed between 1647 and 1653, formerly attributed to Mattia Preti and more recently to Gregorio Preti and Francesco Cozza, evinces how the artist – and one must believe the patron, as well – is untroubled by the prominent inclusion of an unkempt beggar who is in need of a crutch and wooden prosthesis placed beneath his left knee. In fact, the painter redoubles the visual impact by including next to the lame man a child who is forced to rely on hand trestles to drag his body from place to place.

Naturally, this is not to say that depictions of the orthopedically impaired disappeared altogether in the course of the eighteenth century. They may be few and far between, but, of course, one does find them in contexts that require their presence, as in religious paintings that focus on miracles. Sebastiano Conca's *Healing of the Cripple at the Pool of Bethesda* (1731) is one such grand example (Plate 25).

Painted for the chapel of the Spedale Santa Maria della Scala in Siena, the fresco is a worthy successor of majestic backdrops for late Baroque royal masques. Framed by a monumental

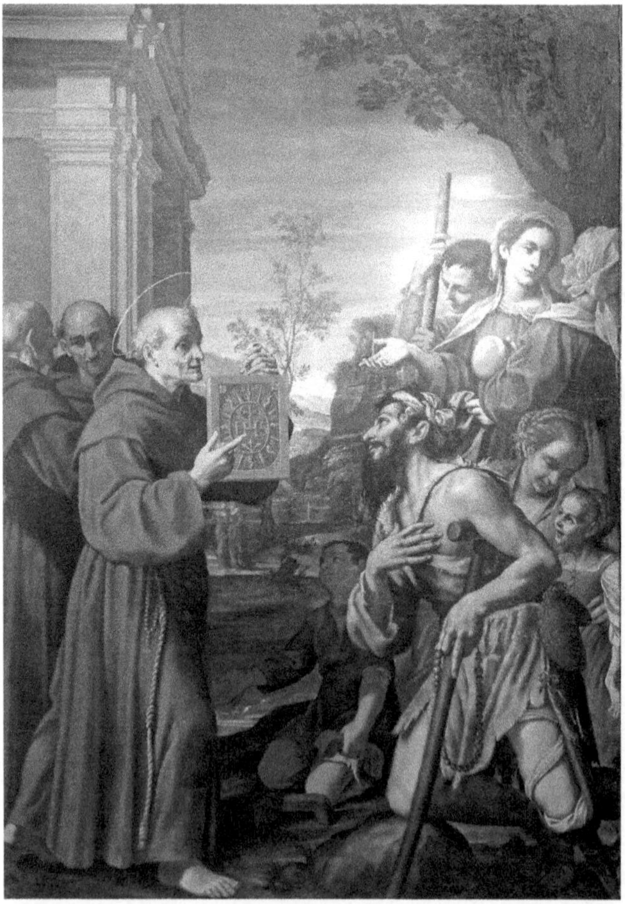

Figure 5.5 Gregorio Preti or Francesco Cozza, *St. Bernardine Healing the Infirm*, 1647–1653, Correggio (RE). Photo: Museo il Correggio, Fototeca (fot. G. Garuti)

columned portico, the scene features the descending figure of an angel as evidence of God's benevolent disposition towards an ailing humanity:

> Now at the Sheep Pool in Jerusalem there is a building, called Bethzatha in Hebrew, consisting of five porticos; and under these were crowds of sick people – blind, lame, paralyzed – waiting for the water to move; for at intervals the angel of the Lord came down into the pool, and the water was disturbed, and the first person to enter the water after this disturbance was cured of any ailment he suffered from. One man there had an illness which had lasted thirty-eight years, and when Jesus saw him lying there and knew he had been in this condition for a long time, he said, "Do you want to be well again?" "Sir," replied the sick man "I have no one to put me into the pool when the water is disturbed; and while I am still on the way, someone else gets there before me." Jesus said, "Get up, pick up your sleeping-mat and walk."The man was cured at once, and he picked up his mat and walked away.[69]
>
> (John 5:1–15)

In the lower part of the fresco, surrounded by a curvilinear, four-sided portico – just to be true to the biblical passage a fifth portico is seen in front of a temple painted in the background, while some sheep are shown approaching the body of water – the protagonists of the narrative share front stage. On the right, Christ, with right hand outstretched, has just spoken his miraculous words ("Get up, pick up your sleeping-mat and walk") and immediately, on the left, the man who had been waiting thirty-eight years for his cure is seen walking away with mat, blanket and crutches. All around the pool numerous "blind, lame, paralytic" are sprawled waiting for their opportunity to be the first to enter the pool after the angel has stirred the water. Some infirm are being carried physically, one old man is transported on a cart, while three lame individuals are leaning on their crutches. The rendition of this biblical story was perhaps never portrayed in a more effective yet grand, theatrical manner.

In Rome, where by now the neo-Classical artistic trends championed by Winckelmann and "brought to life" by Antonio Canova (1757–1822) held sway, in 1818 Domenico del Frate (1765–1821) painted a fresco in the Galleria Clementina of the Vatican Museums that is part of a series of scenes highlighting the major events of Pius VII's papacy. *Pius VII's Creation of the Ospizio di S. Maria degli Angeli* (1818) (Plate 26), shows the pope inaugurating another hospice for the indigent in a building that was formerly part of the Baths of Diocletian complex and for which he allotted the conspicuous yearly sum of 50,000 *scudi*.[70] Comparable to other depictions that propagandize papal support for the destitute, in this fresco Pius VII is shown paying personal attention to his flock. Backed by a retinue of three Carthusian monks, since the hospice was created within the complex of their monastery in Santa Maria degli Angeli, the pope gestures towards the entrance of the building while the crowd of poor men, women and children look at the pope weary-eyed and dejected.[71] Not surprisingly, as we have seen time and again, it is a lame man with crutch under his shoulder that the artist has chosen to represent the many infirm and disabled people who hoped to find shelter and solace in the papal structure.[72]

At the tip of the "boot," in the town of Bagheria, which is located 8 kilometers east of Palermo, Villa Palagonia sports some of the most whimsical decorative statuary ever conceived (1715–1749). Quite understandably, the sculpture and architecture of the place did not impress Goethe during his April 9, 1789 visit and he includes a description of it in his *Italian Journey* only to disparage the owner and his lack of taste. In his words: "Our entire day has been taken up with the madness of the Prince of Pallagonia [*sic*]. His follies turned out to be quite different from anything I had imagined after hearing and reading about them."[73] And in describing the sculptures that decorate the perimeter walls, to give his reader "a better idea of what Prince Pallagonia has perpetrated in his madness," he lists some of the creatures that populate the place: "Beggars of both sexes, men and women of Spain, Moors, Turks, hunchbacks, deformed persons of every kind, dwarfs, musicians, Pulcinellas, soldiers in antique uniforms, gods and goddesses, persons dressed in French fashions of long ago, soldiers with ammunition pouches and leggings, mythological figures with grotesque accessories; for instance: Achilles and Chiron with Pulcinella."[74] Naturally, the visual impact could only generate disgust on Goethe's part: "the repulsive appearance of these deformities, botched by inferior stonecutters, is reinforced by the crumbly shell-tufa of which they are made, but a better material would, no doubt, have made the worthlessness of the form still more conspicuous."[75] Therefore, it should come as no surprise if among the members of this motley crew one should find a hunchbacked, lame man who supports his body with two crutches and a wooden peg under his left knee (Figure 5.6). Given that for Goethe there was "no instinctive feeling for art here, as there is in Rome, to set a standard,"[76] it must have seemed perfectly fitting for him to see such a sculpture included in this "Villa of the Monsters," as it is sometimes called.

A few days after having visited Villa Palagonia, on April 13, 1789, Goethe began one of his letters by writing: "To have seen Italy without having seen Sicily is not to have seen Italy at all, for Sicily is the clue to everything."[77] Exactly a month later, on May 13, having just about fully "circumnavigated" most of the island on land, he sailed from Messina to Naples. Had he continued his tour of the island by going further west, he would have come across the beautiful town of Cefalù with its majestic Norman cathedral. In this church nowadays one can appreciate a turn-of-the-century funerary monument to one of the town's most famous citizens: Bishop Gioacchino Castelli (1708–1788). Known for his incredible sensitivity to the needy, so much so that he sold all that he owned to give to the poor and refused any preferential treatment by paying out of his own pocket for the same meager meals that were served to the seminarians, Castelli was eventually commemorated by his compatriots with a statuary group executed in 1788 by Leonardo Pennino (1765–1850) (Plate 27).[78] Pennino, a sculptor from Palermo working in Rome, portrayed the bishop in the very act of donating garments to a half-divested, emaciated lame man who, needless to say, continued to encapsulate in most people's imagination the whole category of the poor and dejected. Evidently, although their presence diminished in time, images of individuals with limited mobility in late eighteenth- and early nineteenth-century Italy continued to resonate with traditional, universal tones.

A last example of the dwindling attention the lame received in the eighteenth century art is rather telling. When Jacopo Bellini set about to design a Renaissance *campo* (a Venetian square) around 1450–1455, besides depicting the imposing church with its belfry in center background and porticated palace fronts on either side of the square, he included a number of people that, starting from the left of the drawing, include a group of three young men,

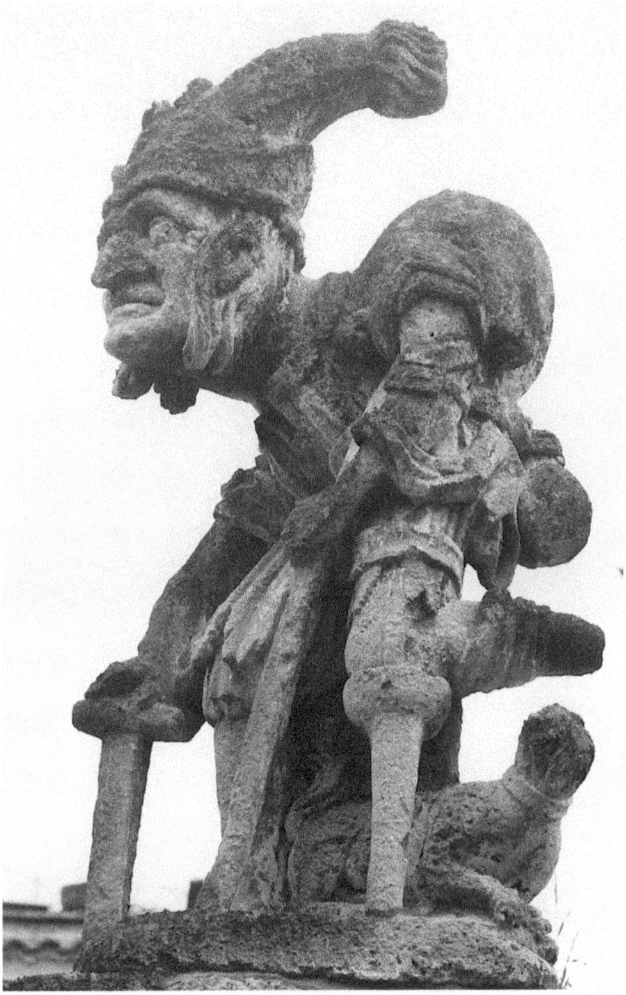

Figure 5.6 Hunchbacked, Lame Man, 1715–1749, Villa Palagonia, Bagheria. Photo: author

a gentleman with hat and cape, a mother and child, a knight, a porter, and some friars (Figure 5.7). In the very center of this Venetian cityscape Bellini felt compelled to include a lame man walking with the aid of two crutches and, at far left, a crippled man moving about the square on hand trestles and shin pads. It is clear that the artist inserted these disabled individuals in the representation of a typical square because they were part and parcel of the Venetian cityscape.

The same may be said of Federico Zuccari's drawing executed about a century and a half later, around 1595, in which the artist records an event that took place in 1547–1548, when his brother Taddeo frescoed the walls of Palazzo Mattei in Rome. In a posthumous attempt to glorify his brother, Federico depicted and inscribed the names of a number of famous artists who stopped to admire Taddeo's work (Plate 28).

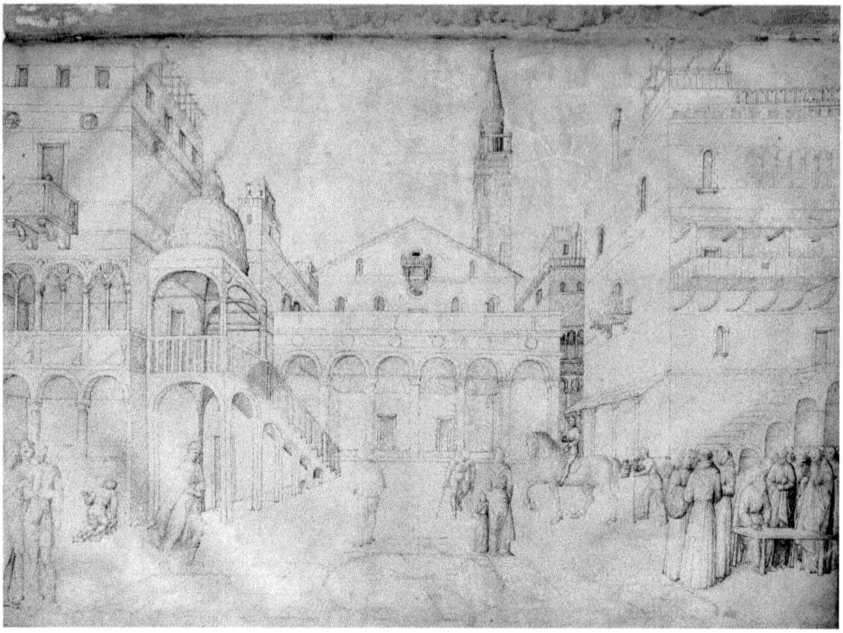

Figure 5.7 Jacopo Bellini, *A City Square*, 1450–1455, Cabinet des dessins, Musée du Louvre, Paris. Photo: © RMN-Grand Palais/Gérard Blot

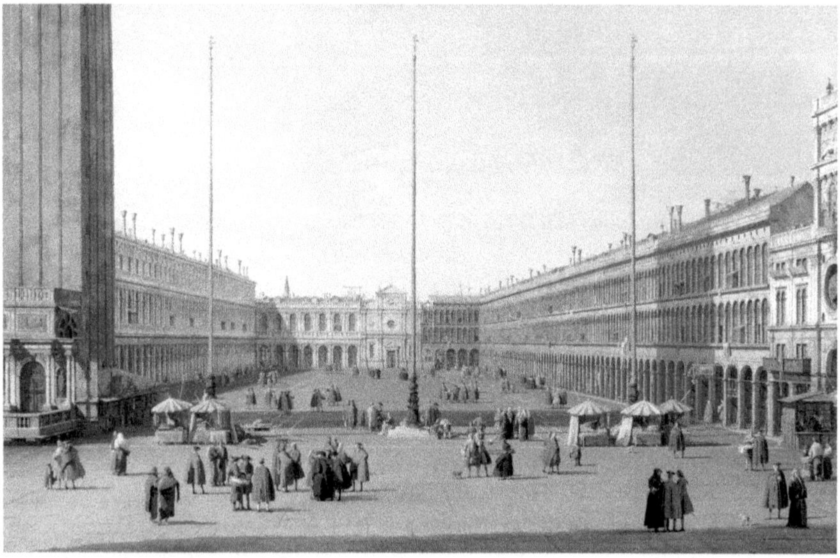

Figure 5.8 Canaletto (Giovanni Antonio Canali), *Piazza San Marco*, (1697–1768)/Detroit Institute of Arts, USA/Founders Society purchase, Edsel B. Ford fund/Bridgeman Images

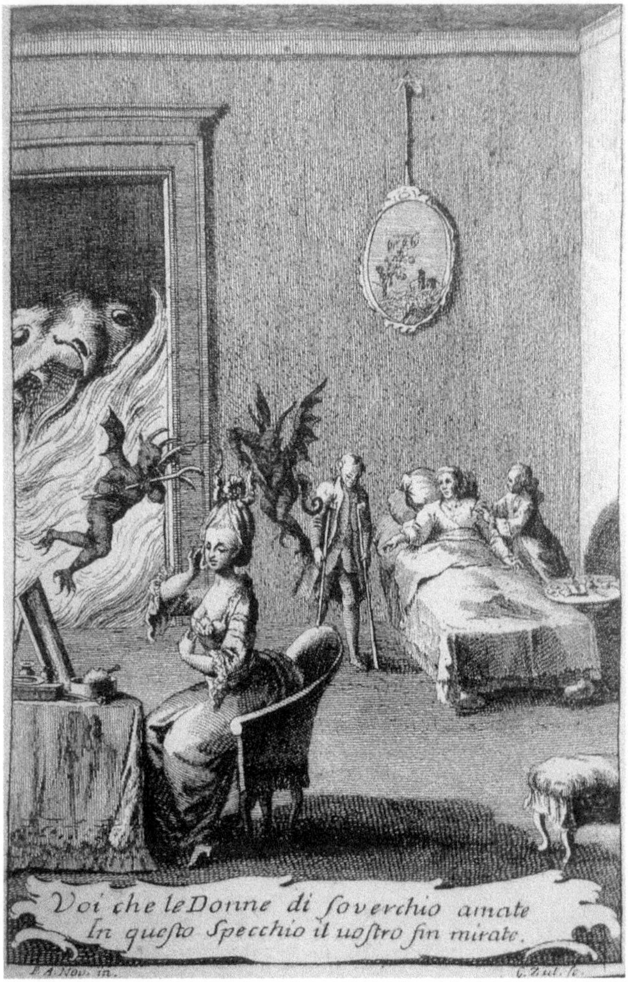
Voi che leDonne di ſoverchio amate
In queſto Specchio il uoſtro fin mirate.

Figure 5.9 Giuseppe Zuliani from a drawing by Pietro Antonio Novelli, *Voi che le donne di soverchio amate*, 1774. Photo: from Massimo Favilla, Ruggero Rugolo and Luca Sassi, *Venezia '700: arte e società nell'ultimo secolo della Serenissima*, Schio, 2011, p. 79

Along with Daniele da Volterra and Siciolante da Sermoneta, on the left side of the drawing, as well as Michelangelo on his horse with his assistant Urbino next to him, on the right side of the sheet Federico represented the younger Florentine artists Francesco Salviati and Giorgio Vasari. To give his image a touch of quotidian normality, Zuccari inserted at bottom center a boy playing with a dog along with a street vendor carrying his wares in two trays. To complete this "eyewitness" report, however, at the right side of the sheet Federico must have deemed it perfectly normal to include at the feet of the gesturing Salviati and Vasari two individuals whose presence was ubiquitous in Italian city streets: a cripple and a lame man.[79]

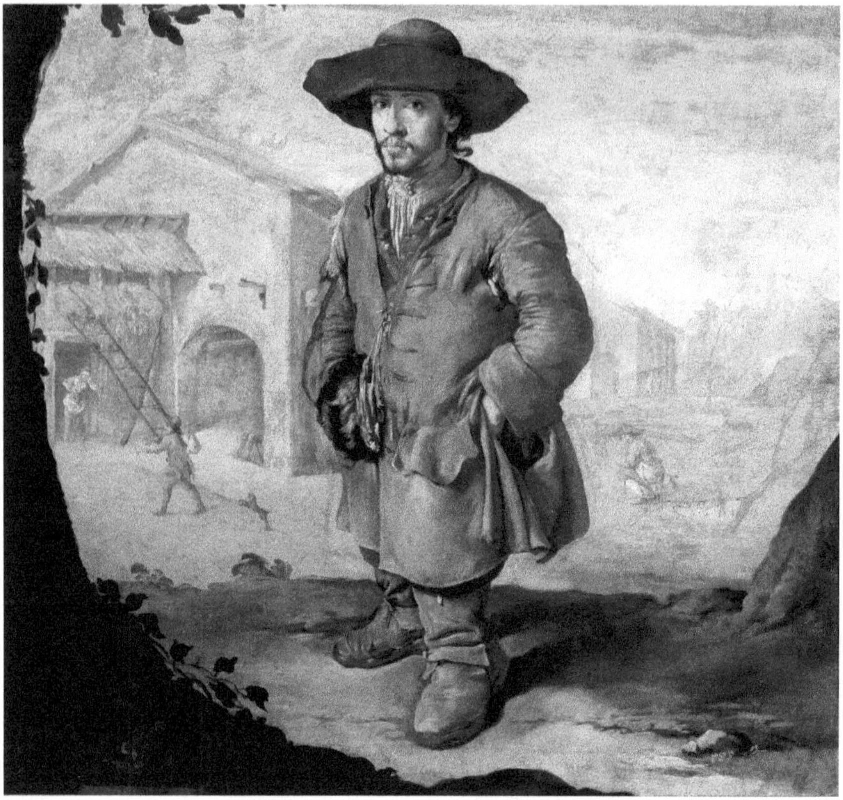

Figure 5.10 Giacomo Ceruti, *The Dwarf*, private collection, 1720s. Photo: Mondadori Portfolio/ Electa/Art Resource, NY

By contrast, if one looks at paintings by Canaletto – an artist who certanly did not refrain from including genre-like details in his works – one is hard put to find the presence of a disabled individual. Of course, they do occasionally appear in his oeuvre as, for example, the cripple in the painting representing *The Upper Reaches of the Grand Canal with S. Simeone Piccolo* of about 1738, or the lame man in *The Doge's Palace and the Riva degli Schiavoni* of the late 1730s, both in the National Gallery, London. However, they are not featured as predominantly as one might expect – see, for instance, his view of *Piazza San Marco* of about 1738–1740 (Figure 5.8).[80]This is not to say that the lame totally disappear from the Venetians' collective imagination, as witness the print of a moralizing book in which men are warned of the nefarious outcome to be expected by those who habitually frequent courtesans (Figure 5.9). The engraving includes, among the hallucinatory visions "à la Goya" the sick man is having while in bed, his worst nightmare: his becoming a lame man on crutches.[81] Nevertheless, what the above examples indicate is that in the eighteenth century interest in confronting the viewer with images of people with a compromised gait was a less compelling need than it had been for preceding generations of artists.

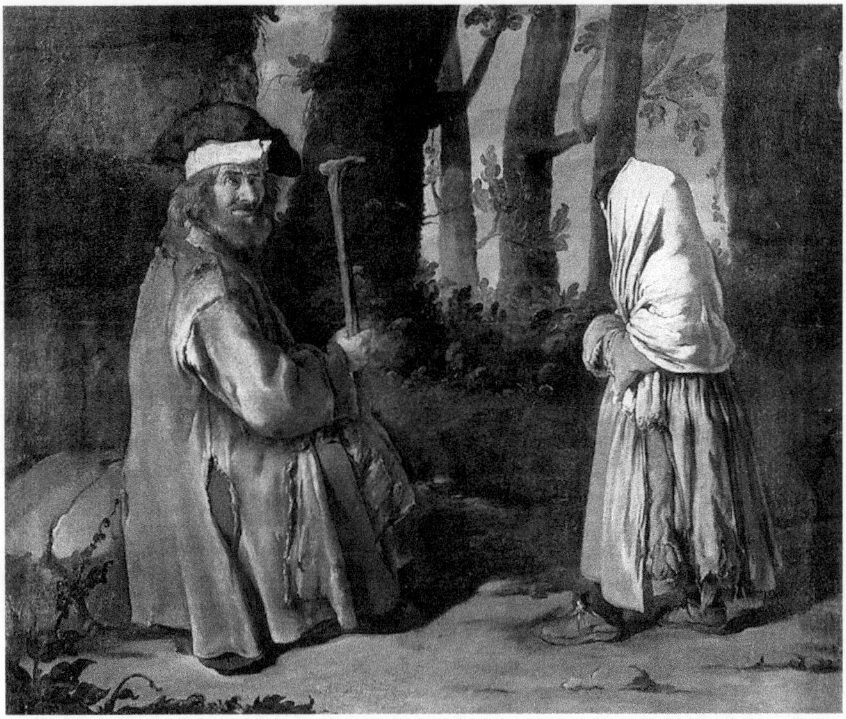

Figure 5.11 Giacomo Ceruti, *Encounter in the Wood*, Pinacoteca Tosio Martinengo, Brescia. Photo: in the public domain

The paradox, from an art historical perspective, is that, although the problems posed by disabled mendicants from Turin to Novara, Genoa, Florence and Rome remained unchanged at least through the nineteenth century,[82] the orthopedically impaired and outcasts in art received the greatest attention just when, in the course of the sixteenth and seventeenth centuries, society at large detected a negative charge in the swelling ranks of the destitute.[83] Still, although depictions of the lame tended to disappear, an interesting phenomenon took place in northern Italy. At the hands of the Milanese painter Giacomo Ceruti (1698–1767), who was active especially in Brescia, beggars received a proper homage before leaving center stage. Known especially for his depictions of *pitocchi* and the destitute, Ceruti (whose nickname was *Pitocco*, "beggar") projected an image of these outcasts with an objectivity that is totally void of any prejudicial moral censure typically witnessed in such images at the hands of other artists. Perhaps his inclination was due to a more enlightened approach to these issues by his patrons or to the influence of the writings of thinkers such as Ludovico Muratori for whom, among other things, it was evident that the attempt to solve the problem of begging by creating hospices had failed.[84] What is clear is that the people Ceruti represented in his canvases are rendered with admirable impartiality.

Take, for example, his portrait of *The Dwarf* (Figure 5.10). Although a tongue-in-cheek undercurrent may be detectable in the defecating person in the right background, there is no sign of a supercilious rendition of this individual and the crass detail, if anything, supports by way of contrast the humble, sober dignity of the man portrayed. Similarly, the strabismic yet self-assured stare of the beggar in the puzzling *Encounter in the Wood* (Figure 5.11) or the alert, penetrating gaze of the *Beggar Resting* (Figure 5.12) – both paintings executed in the 1720s – are exercises in the depiction of a dignified humanity that is left unscathed by their economic or social condition. And no other image captures better than Ceruti's *Three Beggars* (1736) (Plate 29) his sensitivity to these poor people's plight. Most of all, in this image one may clearly see how the orthopedically impaired did not appeal to eighteenth-century artists. No better opportunity would have presented itself to a painter of the previous century than to include the lame in such a picture. This is not what Ceruti does or is interested in. Instead of focusing on physical disabilities, the painter concentrates on a meticulous rendition of these beggars' threadbare garments and worn footwear, the uncomplaining acceptance of their social condition and the noble gentleness of their mien. By so doing, he turns these weakest members of society into the natural "heirs" of the disabled beggars of the previous centuries and contributes superbly to the swansong of all outcasts in Italian art, able-bodied and disabled.

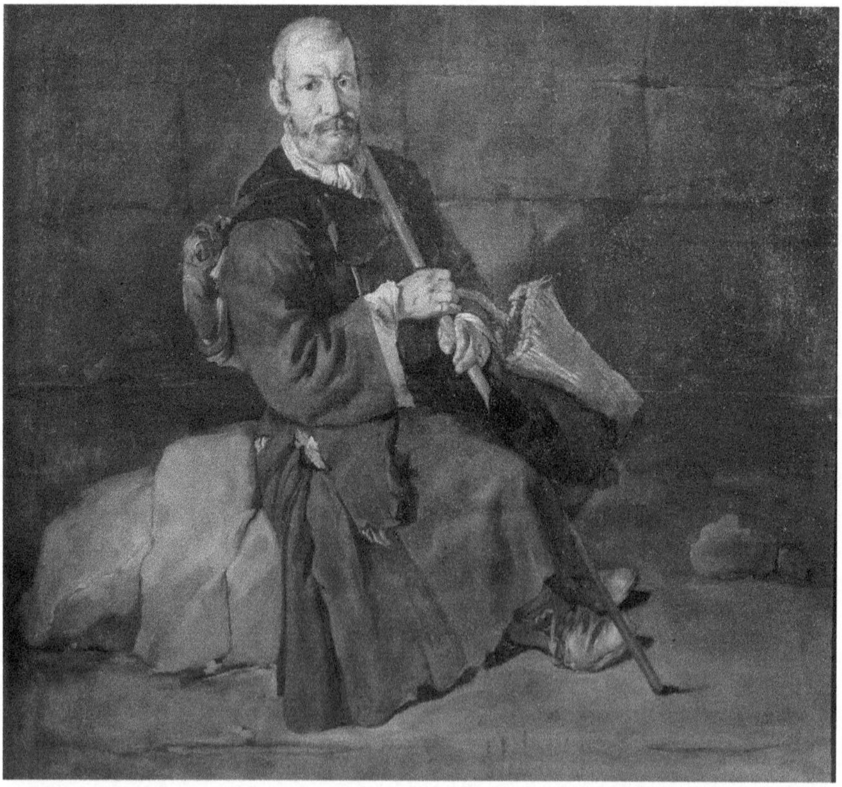

Figure 5.12 Giacomo Ceruti *Beggar Resting*, private collection. Photo: Mondadori Portfolio/Electa/Art Resource, NY

Notes

1 Johann Joachim Wincklemann, *Reflections on the Painting and Sculpture of the Greeks*, Johann Heinrich Füssli (tr.), London, 1765, pp. 16–17: "Such as would fain deny to the Greeks the advantages both of a more perfect Nature and of ideal Beauties, boast of the famous Bernini, as their champion. He was of the opinion, besides, that Nature was possessed of every requisite beauty: the only skill being to discover that." See also Gerald Heres, "Winckelmann, Bernini, Bellori: Betrachtungen zur 'Nachahmung der Alten,'" *Staatliche Museen zu Berlin, Forschungen un Berichte*, 19 (1979): 9.

2 Filippo Baldinucci, *The Life of Bernini*, Catherine Engass (tr.), University Park, 2006 (orig. 1966), pp. 76–77: "Bernini wanted his students to love that which was most beautiful in nature. He said that the whole point of art consisted in knowing, recognizing, and finding it. He, therefore, did not accept the thesis of those who stated that Michelangelo and the ancient masters of Greece and Rome had added a certain grace to their work which is not found in the natural world. Nature knows how to give to every part its commensurate beauty, Bernini said, but one must know how to recognize it when the opportunity arises .... He held that the story of the Venus that Zeuxis made was a fable: that is to say, the story that Zeuxis had made her from the most beautiful parts of many different girls, taking one part from one and another part from another. He said that the beautiful eyes of one woman do not go well with the beautiful face of another woman, and so it was with a beautiful mouth, and so on." Baldinucci is here confusing Venus with Helen of Troy. See Livio Pestilli, "On Bernini's Reputed Unpopularity in Late Baroque Rome," *Artibus et historiae*, 63 (2011): 119–142. Pliny, *Natural History*, XXXV, xxxvi, pp. 63–64.

3 In a letter written to Berendis from Rome, probably on July 7, 1756: "Die Neuern sind Esel gegen die Alten, von denen wir gleich wohl das allerschönste nicht haben, und Bernini ist der größte Esel unter den Neuern, die Fransosen ausgenommen." See Johann Joachim Winckelmann, *Briefe*, 4 vols., Berlin, 1952, I, p. 235. See also Heres, p. 9.

4 This synthesis of what Baroque art "was all about," is taken from Francesco Milizia's criticism of all those artists who strayed away from the Classical ideals of Greek art. See Giovanni Gaetano Bottari and Stefano Ticozzi, *Raccolta di lettere sulla pittura, scultura ed architettura scritte da' più celebri personaggi dei secoli XV, XVI, e XVII*, 8 vols., Milan, 1822–1825, VIII, p. 439. See also Pestilli, "On Bernini's Reputed Unpopularity," p. 140.

5 Wincklemann's *Reflections*, p. 30.

6 Hugh Honour, *Neo-Classicism*, Westford, 1981 (orig. 1968), p. 33.

7 Giuliano Briganti in his introduction to *La pittura in Italia: il Settecento*, Milan, 1990, p. 12, still considered not fully convincing the answers given by scholars to the question as to why Ceruti's paintings of low-life people, observed with a totally new objectivity from his predecessors, should have taken place. See the end of this chapter.

8 Charles de Brosses, *Lettres familières écrites d'Italie en 1739 et 1740*, 2 vols., Paris, 1858, II, p. 6: "Imaginez ce que c'est qu'un peuple dont le tiers est de prètres, le tiers de gens qui ne travaillent guère et le tiers de gens qui ne font rien du tout." Also quoted by Balzani, p. 17. The phrase was somewhat of a commonplace as the Venetian Luigi Mocenigo in 1560 stated similarly, "sono quasi tutti gli abitanti di quella città [Rome] persone senza industria, onde quasi sempre vivono in povertà" ("almost all of the inhabitants of that city [Rome] are unemployed, thus they very often live in poverty"). Ibid., p. 46.

9 Brosses, p. 6: "Les souverains qui, depuis Sixte V, on fait de choses immenses pour l'embellissement de la ville, n'ont rien fait pour la culture de la campagne, où l'on n'aperçoit, à la lettre, ni une seule maison ni un seul arbrisseau. Le gouvernement est aussi mauvais qu'il soit possible de s'en figurer un à plaisir. Machievel et Morus se sont plu à forger l'idée d'une utopie; on trouve ici la réalité du contraire."

10 See Chapter 3, note 121. Giuseppe Palmeri, *Riflessioni critiche sull'arte della guerra* (1761), cited by Fatica, p. 276.

11 My translation. Quoted by Giovanni Assereto, "Pauperismo e assistenza: messa a punto di studi recenti," *Archivio storico italiano*, Florence, 516 (1983): 258, quoting from Franco Venturi, *Settecento*

riformatore: da Muratori a Beccaria, Turin, 1969, p. 583. Genovesi deplored most of all the complex social and economic backwardness of the kingdom of Naples, especially when compared with the powerful and reforming countries such as England and Spain. Venturi, p. 574. Mario Rosa, "Chiesa, idee sui poteri e assistenza in Italia dal Cinque al Settecento," *Società e storia*, 10 (1980): 802, undescores Genovesi's solution for eradicating "the spirit of idleness" in the kingdom of Naples, that is, the development of agriculture, commerce and industry, as the only means of placing the kingdom in the larger context of European developments in the eighteenth century.

12 Johann Wolfgang Goethe, *Italian Journey [1786–1788]*, Wystan Hugh Auden and Elizabeth Mayer (trs.), Harmondsworth, 1982, p. 318.

13 Pullan, "Poveri, mendicanti e vagabondi," p. 1046. See Chapter 3, p. 86. Idem, "La nuova filantropia nella Venezia cinquecentesca," in *Nel regno dei poveri: arte e storia dei grandi ospedali veneziani in età moderna 1474–1797*, Venezia, 1989, p. 33: "Si può più correttamente sostenere che la carità aveva la funzione di promuovere l'interesse collettivo delle classi dirigenti e di perpetuarne il sistema di governo." ("One may more precisely claim that charity promoted the collective interest of the ruling classes and perpetuated their regime.")

14 For the historical panoramic view here advanced I am much indebted to the essays published as the proceedings of a conference on "Pauperismo e assistenza negli antichi stati italiani" held in Cremona on March 28–30, 1980 edited by Giorgio Politi, Mario Rosa and Franco della Peruta, published as *Timore e carità: i poveri nell'Italia moderna*, Cremona, 1982 (hereafter *Timore e carità*).

15 Sandra Cavallo, "Conception of Poverty and Poor-Relief in Turin in the Second Half of the Eighteenth Century," in *Domestic Strategies: Work and Family in France and Italy 1600–1800*, Stuart Woolf (ed.), Cambridge and Paris, ca. 1991, pp. 148–199.

16 Ibid., pp. 150 and 154. The various pamphlets published on the *sbandimento della mendicità* (the suppression of begging) were all derived from the Jesuit Father André Guevarre's *La Mendicité abolie par un bureau de charité à Toulouse*, Toulouse, 1692. See Cavallo, pp. 154–155. In the eyes of Muratori, one of the most prominent exponents of the Italian Enlightenment, the trend to leave almsgiving solely to the state and the total "enclosure" of the mendicants was an error, for this would undercut the necessary social awaress and Christian desire to help others. In other words, this would create a moral void that would lead to a calloused "out of sight, out of mind" situation: "Tolto da gli occhi del Popolo il vivo aspetto de'i Limosinanti, cala anche subito in lor cuore la voglia o l'impulso di sovvenirli." ("Just as soon as the beggars' presence is removed from the people's sight, so is their desire or impulse to help the mendicants removed from their heart.") Ludovico Antonio Muratori, *Della carità cristiana, in quanto essa è Amore del Prossimo*, Modena, 1723, p. 345.

17 Cavallo, ibid.

18 Ibid., p. 157.

19 Ibid., p. 159.

20 Ibid., pp. 160–161.

21 Ibid., pp. 163–164. The procession of the indigent from the Ospedale through the streets of Turin occurred on April 7, 1717, when all the inmates were dressed in a habit of blue cloth, the invalids being carried on carts, and Father Guevarre delivered a sermon "in which he exhorted the people to give thanks to God, the King and the charity of the clergy, the magistrates and the nobility for their support for the holy work." Subsequently all of the poor were served a meal in Piazza Castello and, at the end of the ritualistic thanksgiving of the King on the part of the poor, the latter were escorted back to the hospital.

22 Cavallo, p. 165.

23 See Stuart J. Woolf, "Problems in the History of Pauperism in Italy, 1800–1815," in *Timore e carità*, pp. 317–329, esp. pp. 326–327.

24 Alberto Monticone, "Lavoro, risorse e nuova società nell'età della restaurazione," in *La storia dei poveri: pauperismo e assistenza nell'età moderna*, Alberto Monticone (ed.), Rome, 1985, pp. 255–256.

25 Antonio Genovesi himself, *Delle lezioni di commercio o sia d'economia civile*, Naples, 1768, p. 268, emphasizes this concept: "In ogni paese vi è, dove più, dove meno, sempre un dato numero di poveri, e di mendicanti. Se si potessero far entrare nella massa de' lavoratori e de' renditori, si

farebbero due beni. I. Si accrescerebbe la rendita generale della nazione. II. E si farebbe un gran servizio al buon costume." ("In every country – in some more, in others fewer – one always finds a number of poor people and mendicants. If they could only be enlisted in the mass of workers and solvent debtors, two positive goals would be achieved. I. The country's general prosperity would increase. II. Good customs would be engendered.")

26 Woolf, p. 327: "In later years progress and poverty would be reconciled through the work ethic." However, it is important to remember that putting the poor to work was not unheard of in the previous century. See Assereto, "Pauperismo e assistenza," p. 260, who in turn cites Daniela Lombardi, "Poveri a Firenze: programmi e realizzazioni della politica assistenziale dei Medici tra Cinque e Seicento," in *Timore e carità*, pp. 165–184.

27 Daniela Maldini, "Il *Dépot de Mendicité* del Dipartimento di Po: analisi di una struttura assistenziale nel Piemonte napoleonico," in *Timore e carità*, p. 336. The word "ergastolo" is derived from the Greek εργαστήριον (workshop, laboratory, factory) and the Latin suffix *–ŭlum*, *ergastŭlum*. In Italian *ergastolo* means a sentence to lifetime incareration, or a structure utilized for such detention. See Giacomo Devoto and Gian Carlo Oli, *Vocabolario illustrato della lingua italiana*, 2 vols., Milan, 1976, I, p. 937.

28 Maldini, "Il *Dépot de Mendicité*," p. 344.

29 Ibid., p. 340.

30 Giovanni Assereto, "Aspetti dell'assistenza pubblica a Genova nei primi anni dell'Ottocento," in *Timore e carità*, pp. 348–349.

31 Ibid., p. 351.

32 Ibid., p. 352.

33 Ibid., p. 353–354.

34 Piero Camporesi, *Il pane selvaggio*, Milan, 2004 (orig. 1980), p. 70, quoting from Enzo Piscitelli, "Le classi sociali a Bologna nel secolo XVIII," *Nuova Rivista Storica*, 38 (1954): p. 105.

35 Daniele Menozzi, "Pauperismo e assistenza nel triennio giacobino: il caso di Bologna," in *Timore e carità*, pp. 298 and 303.

36 Ibid., p. 303. My translation.

37 Ibid. My translation.

38 Ibid., p. 304.

39 Ibid., p. 312.

40 Ibid., p. 315.

41 Veit Elm, "La riforma assistenziale della Prima Repubblica Romana (1798–1799)," in *Popolazione e società a Roma dal medioevo all'età contemporanea*, Eugenio Sonnino (ed.), Rome, 1998, p. 563.

42 Ibid., p. 564.

43 Ibid.

44 Ibid., p. 565.

45 Ibid., p. 566. My italics. By January 1799, after the Neapolitan invasion was repelled, a project was advanced that suggested the conscription of all the idle in the army. Ibid., p. 567.

46 Ibid., p. 569.

47 Nasto, p. 22, points out how on January 24, 1800 the sign in front of the Lateran Palace, which had read *Hospitium Apostolicorum Pauperum Invalidorum*, was replaced by one that stated, "Ospizio Nazionale," and adds that the obsolete system was disolved and, at the turn of the century, the poor and the vagabonds crowded the Roman streets.

48 Ibid., pp. 569–570. Cajani, p. 294.

49 Elm, pp. 571–572.

50 Giovanni Muto, "Forme e contenuti economici dell'assistenza nel mezzogiorno moderno: il caso di Napoli," in *Timore e carità*, p. 237.

51 Ibid.

52 Mario Rosa, "Pauperismo e riforme nel Settecento italiano: linee di ricerca," in *Povertà e carità dalla Roma tardo-antica al '700 italiano*, P. Brown, O. Capitani, F. Cardini and M. Rosa, Padua, 1983, pp. 102–104.

53 Ibid., p. 107.
54 Marino Beregno, "Conclusioni," in *Timore e carità*, p. 491.
55 Assereto, "Pauperismo e assistenza," p. 257.
56 Ibid.
57 Ibid., pp. 257–258.
58 Assereto, "Pauperismo e assistenza," p. 262. Rosa, "Pauperismo e riforme," p. 100, defines the *Albergo dei Poveri* in Naples as "il grandioso fallimento del progetto carolino" ("the grand failure of Charles VII's project"). Idem, "Chiesa, idee sui poteri e assistenza," p. 802, claims that the *Alberto dei Poveri* was "la risposta in ritardo di un grandioso e fallimentare *renfermement* d'antico regime" ("the delayed answer of a grand, catastrophic *renfermement* typical of the *Ancien Régime*").
59 Calogero Valenti, "I poveri in Sicilia nella seconda metà del Settecento," in *Timore e carità*, p. 287.
60 Ibid.
61 Ibid., pp. 288–289.
62 Ibid., p. 289.
63 Ibid., pp. 291–292.
64 Beregno, p. 491.
65 Assereto, "Aspetti dell'assistenza pubblica a Genova," p. 349.
66 Assereto, "Pauperismo e assistenza," p. 271.
67 See also Robertson, *The Invention of Annibale Carracci*, pp. 113–114.
68 Duchet-Suchaux and Pastoureau, pp. 131–132. The twelfth-century legend held that St. John the Evangelist, wanting to put Edward's charity to the test, disguised himself as a beggar and asked for alms. Not having any money, Edward gave the beggar a gold ring, which was then returned seven years later to an English pilgrim by St. John when he appeared to him in Palestine and asked him to instruct Edward that his time had come and he would soon be called among the elect.
69 *The Jerusalem Bible*, pp. 154–155.
70 Gaetano Moroni, *Dizionario di erudizione storico-ecclesiastica*, Venice, 1851, LIII, p. 160. For a useful recap of Pius VII's life and papacy see http://www.treccani.it/enciclopedia/pio-vii_%28Enciclopedia_dei_Papi%29/ (last accessed March 24, 2016).
71 The caption at the bottom of the fresco states: "Pius VII opened a building at the Baths of Diocletian for the poor who subsist on begging and he assigned a piece of land for food [to feed them] in the year 1817." My thanks to Inge Weustink for her translation from the Latin.
72 See *Compendio storico su Pio VII*, Milan, 1824, p. 139, and Gaetano Giucci, *Storia della vita e del pontificato di Pio VII*, 2 vols., Rome, 1857. Not surprisingly, Giucci's comments, II, p. 165–166, continue to propagate even in the nineteenth century the usual annoyance displayed by the well-to-do towards the poor in all historical periods: "Fra le molte provvidenze adottate da Pio [*sic*] per assicurare la pubblica quiete è a ricordarsi quella che salvò la capitale dalle noiose insistenze dei poveri che, o per vero o per simulato bisogno, ingombravano le strade, penetravano nei negozi, assediavano le case, turbavano la tranquillità delle chiese .... Sorse in tal modo il grandioso stabilimento di santa Maria degli Angeli alle terme diocleziane, ove oltre i vecchi che trovano in esso stanza e alimento s'istruisce un numero ingente di giovanetti d'ambo i sessi, ch'ivi ricevono cirstiana educazione e si addestrano alle arti e mestieri." ("Among the many measures adopted by Pius [VII] to ensure public peace there is the one that rescued the capital from the annoying begging of the poor who, be it for true or simulated need, used to clutter the streets, penetrated into shops, besieged the homes, [and] upset tranquillity in the churches .... Thus came about the grandiose edifice of Santa Maria degli Angeli by the baths of Diocletian where, besides the elderly, who received room and board, a large number of boys and girls obtained a Christian education and were trained in the arts and crafts.")
73 Goethe, p. 237.
74 Ibid., p. 239.
75 Ibid. Interestingly, centuries earlier the Greek physician Galen argued against Goethe's opinion that inferior materials underscored a carver's lack of talent: "Come, then, let us make you skillful in

Nature's art so that we may call you no longer uncultivated person, but natural philospher instead. Disregard differences of material and look only at the naked art itself, keeping in mind when you inspect the structure of the eye and the foot that the one is an instrument of vision and the other of locomotion." *On the Usefulness of the Parts of the Body*, 2 vols., Margaret Tallmadge May (tr.), Ithaca, 1968, p. 189, I, 175.

76 Ibid., p. 231.

77 Ibid., p. 246.

78 Giuseppe Misuraca, *Serie dei vescovi di Cefalù*, Rome, 1960, pp. 59–61. See also Giovanni Castelli, *Orazione ne' funerali di Monsignor Gioachino Castelli*, Palermo, 1789, at http://cattedraledicefalu.com/orazione-funebre-per-mons-gioacchino-castelli/ (last accessed on September 30, 2014).

79 Cristina Acidini, "Elementi di una biografia eccezionale," in *1564/2014 Michelangelo: incontrare un artista universale*, p. 33, plate on p. 31. Catalogue of exhibition held at the Capitoline Museums, Rome, May 27 to September 14, Florence, 2014.

80 Tom Nichols, "Secular Charity, Sacred Poverty: Picturing the Poor in Renaissance Venice," *Art History*, 30 (2007): 152, rightly points out how in the Renaissance images of poor citizens dependent on charity "found little expression in official art picturing Venice as an ideal state."

81 The caption reads: "You who frequently make love to women/In this mirror see reflected your demise." ("Voi che le Donne di soverchio amate/In questo specchio il vostro fin mirate.") See Massimo Favilla, Ruggero Rugolo and Luca Sassi, *Venezia '700: arte e società nell'ultimo secolo della Serenissima*, Schio, 2011, p. 79. The engraving by Giuseppe Zuliani was based on a drawing by Pietro Antonio Novelli, *La vanità delle donne*, in Diunilgo Valdecio pastore arcade, *Lo scoglio dell'umanità [...] per cautelarsi contro le male qualità delle donne cattive*, Venice, 1774.

82 See Daniela Maldini, "Pauperismo e mendicità in Torino nel periodo napoleonico," *Studi Piemontesi*, 8:1 (1979): 50–64; Alfredo Papale, "L'istituto De Pagave ed il pauperismo a Novara nell'Ottocento," *Bollettino storico per la provincia di Novara*, 75:1 (1984): 93–140; Edoardo Grendi, "Pauperismo e Albergo dei poveri nella Genova del Seicento," *Rivista storica italiana*, 87:4 (1975): 621–665; Daniela Lombardi, "I gesuiti, il principe e i modello francese nella politica di assistenza di fine Seicento," in *La Toscana di Cosimo II: Atti del convegno*, Florence, 1993, pp. 521–539. See also Charles James Ribton-Turner, *A History of Vagrants and Vagrancy and Beggars and Begging*, London, 1887, pp. 552–553.

83 Francesco Porzio, "Aspetti e problemi," p. 20.

84 Lodovico Antonio Muratori, *Della carità cristiana, in quanto essa è Amore del Prossimo*, Modena, 1723. See Rosa, "Pauperismo e riforme," p. 95. See also Porzio, "Aspetti e problemi," p. 35. However, Elisabetta Selmi, "Cultura e committenza artistica: il 'caso' di Giacomo Ceruti," in *La società bresciana e l'opera di Giacomo Ceruti*, Brescia, 1988, p. 229, advises caution in relating the painter's intentions to his patrons': "è problematico individuare comuni intenzioni nei rapporti tra il pittore ed i suoi committenti" ("it is problematic to identify common intentions in the rapport between the painter and his patrons").

Coda

> The study of paralysis is a splendid arena for viewing this struggle of the individual against society, for the disabled are not a breed apart but a metaphor for the human condition. The disabled represent humanity reduced to its bare essentials.
>
> (Robert F. Murphy, *The Body Silent*, p. 5)

As we have seen, representations of people whose mobility was partially or totally impeded have taken on different meanings in the course of history; meanings that could range from the unsightly, in antiquity, to the embodiment of Christ, in the Middle Ages, to the threatening representative of a world of cheats and lazy beggars, in the sixteenth and seventeenth centuries. And even though it is clear that this investigation remains a biased view of the phenomenon, since what typically caught the eye of artists were lame people from the lower classes, and records pertaining to them reflect the opinions of the upper echelon,[1] at every point of the way one finds that the images the artists recorded in painting or in other media clearly captured the dominant spirit of the age. This is not to say that images themselves did not influence the way people looked at the lame, the disabled and the mendicants, for images can mold the way people regard others. However, not only is this opinion more difficult to sustain without documentary proof, but it is even more likely, to paraphrase St. Augustine's comments about miracles quoted in Chapter 2, that these images would never have been produced had they not reflected the way "normal," able-bodied society perceived lameness.[2]

Thus it is clear that images of the lame typically reveal more about the context in which the orthopedically impaired lived than the actual difficulties and challenges those individuals had to confront on a daily basis.[3] Actually, the presence in art works of people whose ambulatory ability was adversely affected by congenital causes or external agents is not only pervasive because it reflects a common ailment in all societies but also because it represents the vulnerability of the human condition. Anyone, at any moment, may be affected by a number of factors that could impede the fluid gait of the able-bodied, even if only temporarily. Indeed, as scholars in Disability Studies have pointed out, everyone is a "TAB," a temporarily able-bodied individual. People who live long enough will eventually become disabled one way or another.[4]

The afterlife of the orthopedically impaired in Italian art starting with neo-Classicism was destined to wane. However, there was one, outstanding resurgence of such imagery at the beginning of the twentieth century. It involved a young amputee, Enrico Toti, whose condition was used by the fledgling Italian state during World War I to advance its patriotic cause and by the ensuing Fascist regime to propagate its "ideal of a belligerent masculinity."[5]

Born in Rome in 1882 of a humble family, at age 15 Enrico Toti enlisted in the navy and subsequently worked on two cruisers.[6] In 1905, at age 23, he was hired as a stoker by the Ferrovie dello Stato, Italy's state-owned railroad company. As a result of a dramatic incident while greasing a machine, in 1908 Enrico had his left leg amputated, but this did not diminish his desire to live life to the fullest.[7] In 1911, when Italy was celebrating the fiftieth anniversary of its unification and the cities of Rome and Turin were hosting the World's Fair (*Esposizione Universale*), Toti decided to embark on a bicycle tour of Europe, taking as his point of departure the monumental Arch of the Fair in Rome.[8] The feat gave him some notoriety and successively, in 1913, he decided to embark on a comparable deed in Africa, but the British authorities in Sudan put an end to his plans and persuaded him to return home.[9]

In 1915, the year after World War I broke out, Italy ended its alliance with the Central Powers led by Germany and entered the war on the side of the Entente (France, Britain and Russia). Toti tried to enlist in the Italian Army but was refused because of his disability. He subsequently succeeded in being accepted as a civilian volunteer dispatcher attached to a number of units. Still desiring to give his support to the national cause against the Austro-Hungarians who were attacking the country in the northeast, Toti managed to become a member of the Bersaglieri bicycle corps (Figure C.1). Unwilling to be treated differently from the rest of his comrades-in-arms, he joined them in the trenches. Then, during the sixth battle by the Isonzo River, on August 6, 1916, he took part in a charge and, fatally wounded, died hurling his crutch at the enemy.[10]

For the Italian government, which had illusorily hoped the war would be a brief affair and that the cost in human lives would be contained,[11] Enrico Toti's selfless sacrifice and iconic last gesture was the ideal propagandistic event needed to ignite the patriotic spirit. Not surprisingly, Toti became a national hero and artists as well as illustrators did their part in sustaining the government's political and military efforts.

Thus, sympathizing with the anti-Austro-Hungarian powers, the year before Italy entered the international conflict (May 24, 1915), the front page of *La Domenica del Corriere* featured an image of military comradeship at the front (Plate 30).[12] Instead of depicting a battle scene, Achille Beltrame (1871–1945) opted to represent an act of reciprocal aid, with two wounded French soldiers leaving the "lunar" battlefield – one blindfolded, supplying the "legs" to the friend he is carrying on his back, the other, unable to walk, providing the guiding "eyes." Beltrame, of course, had done his homework and created an image of assured impact on the readers, since it was clearly based on the Renaissance print of *Mutual Aid* discussed in Chapter 4 (Figure 4.2). Predictably, a month after Toti's death, the same newspaper immortalized his heroic deed (Plate 31).[13] Beltrame represented Toti towering over his fellow soldiers as they charge fearlessly towards the Austrian trenches, launching the symbol of his seemingly physical disability, his crutch, towards the fleeing enemy. Conceived to sustain the morale of the soldiers at the front and even more to muster public support for a war that claimed the lives of half a million Italian soldiers, in this newspaper cover Toti represented the apotheosis of the disabled at the service of the nation.[14]

When on May 24, 1922 – on the eighth anniversary of Italy's declaration of war – Toti's mortal remains were brought back to Rome from the military cemetery in Monfalcone,

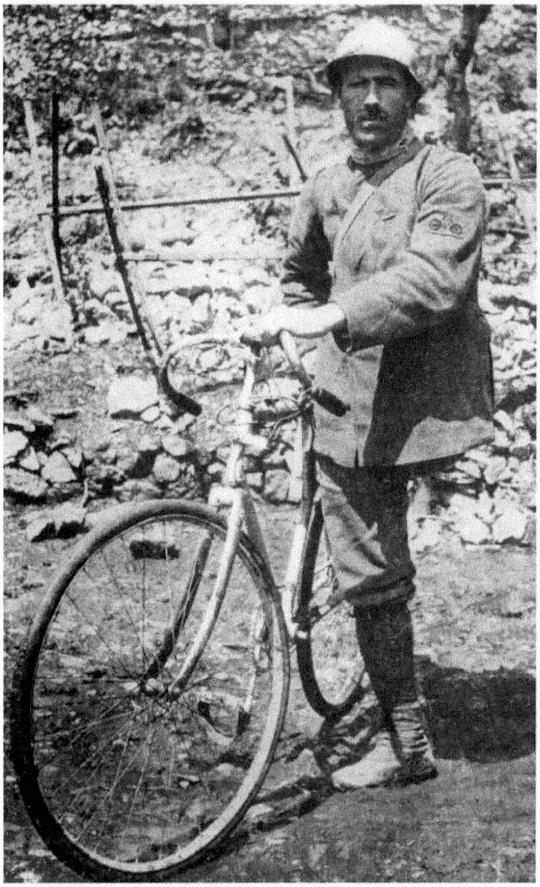

Figure C.1 Enrico Toti with his bicycle, near Vermegliano, June 1916. Photo: in the public domain

near the battlegrounds where he had died, serious clashes took place between groups of fascists–nationalists and liberals–socialists. This happened because the former political exponents tried to symbolically appropriate the remains of the national hero by joining the convoy, "despite their informal interdiction from entering working-class Roman districts, such as San Lorenzo and Testaccio."[15] The fact that this event resulted in four deaths and many wounded is an indication of the political and propagandistic charge Toti's name and deed had taken on for both the Italian Liberal Government and the rising Fascist party that would see its founder, Benito Mussolini, designated head of the government only a few months later, on October 28, 1922.[16]

Two weeks after Toti's remains were interred in the Verano cemetery on June 4, 1922, a monument to the courageous young man was erected in the presence of King Victor Emanuel III in Rome's most popular park, Villa Borghese, on the Pincian Hill (Plate 32). Not surprisingly, Enrico Toti's intrepid feat gave rise to a statue that aptly projects a nationalistic, virile ideology, perfectly suited to both the Italian Liberal Government and its later Fascist transmutation.[17] The sculptor chosen for the task was Arturo Dazzi (1881–1966), a Tuscan artist who is perhaps best known for his 1932 giant statue of a man representing the Fascist Era, formerly topping the fountain in Piazza della Vittoria in Brescia and subsequently removed to a warehouse by the local authorities in 1945 because if its strong association with the Fascist regime. Dazzi's representation of a stern, cold, yet idealized representation of the male form is a premonition of the type of art that would be produced during the Fascist regime. This ideal in art is perhaps best expounded in an article of 1927:

> The fascist concept of war ... induces us to glorify, not bewail, our fallen [soldiers], it encourages us to represent them erect, proud, with drawn sword, with the [victor's] laurel in hand, and not like falling corpses as, unfortunately, one sees in many monuments dedicated to our heroes, who instead deserve a much different commemoration! ... We demand that the symbols that represent them portray them proud, with vibrant muscles, with a noble and purposeful look.[18]

Quite prophetically, Dazzi's statue portrayed Toti in the "garb" of a Classical, athletic nude figure, stoutly leaning on a rock with his left arm and truncated thigh, while his right leg is outstretched to create the kind of "heroic diagonal" often seen in Roman battle sarcophagi.[19] The frowning, determined young man is caught, just like so many baroque sculptures in the city, at the apex of the action, with his right arm fully extended behind him ready to defiantly hurl the crutch at the enemy. Perhaps there is no greater example of the glorification (and exploitation) of the orthopedically disabled body in Western art.

* * *

In 1569 a Venetian patrician, Lorenzo Priuli, penned his last will and testament. In it, the testator instructed his eldest heir to become guardian of a small hospital for twelve elderly people and explicitly warned him "to allow [into the hospital] people of good morals, who do not have sons or wives, and who are Venetians, that is citizens, because I absolutely do not want that [room] to be made available ... for people from other towns, even if they have been living in Venice for thirty or more years."[20] To be a foreigner in the country where one resides, in the sixteenth as in the twenty-first century, is not advantageous. To be poor and a foreigner in the country one lives in is certainly inauspicious.

At times history does seem to repeat itself. Recently, in the Veneto region the three center-left mayors of Padua, Treviso and Venice signed a pact to oust beggars that goes by the acronym Pa-tre-ve (for Padova, Treviso and Venezia) (Figure C.2).[21] In an interview with the daily *La Repubblica*, the mayor of Treviso, Giovanni Manildo, stated:

> We are fighting most of all against organized begging and for the safety of our citizens. There are people who come from outside [Treviso] and ask for alms in an aggressive way. They are organized and travel from Mestre [mainland Venice] by train or by car. On market days they place themselves in the best of locations [in town]. A woman felt threatened in Piazza Giustiniani. The measures taken in the past by the Lega Nord [right wing, anti-immigration party] mayors are insufficient and don't serve any purpose. Since 2009 eight hundred fines of 50 euros each have been issued but no one has paid them.

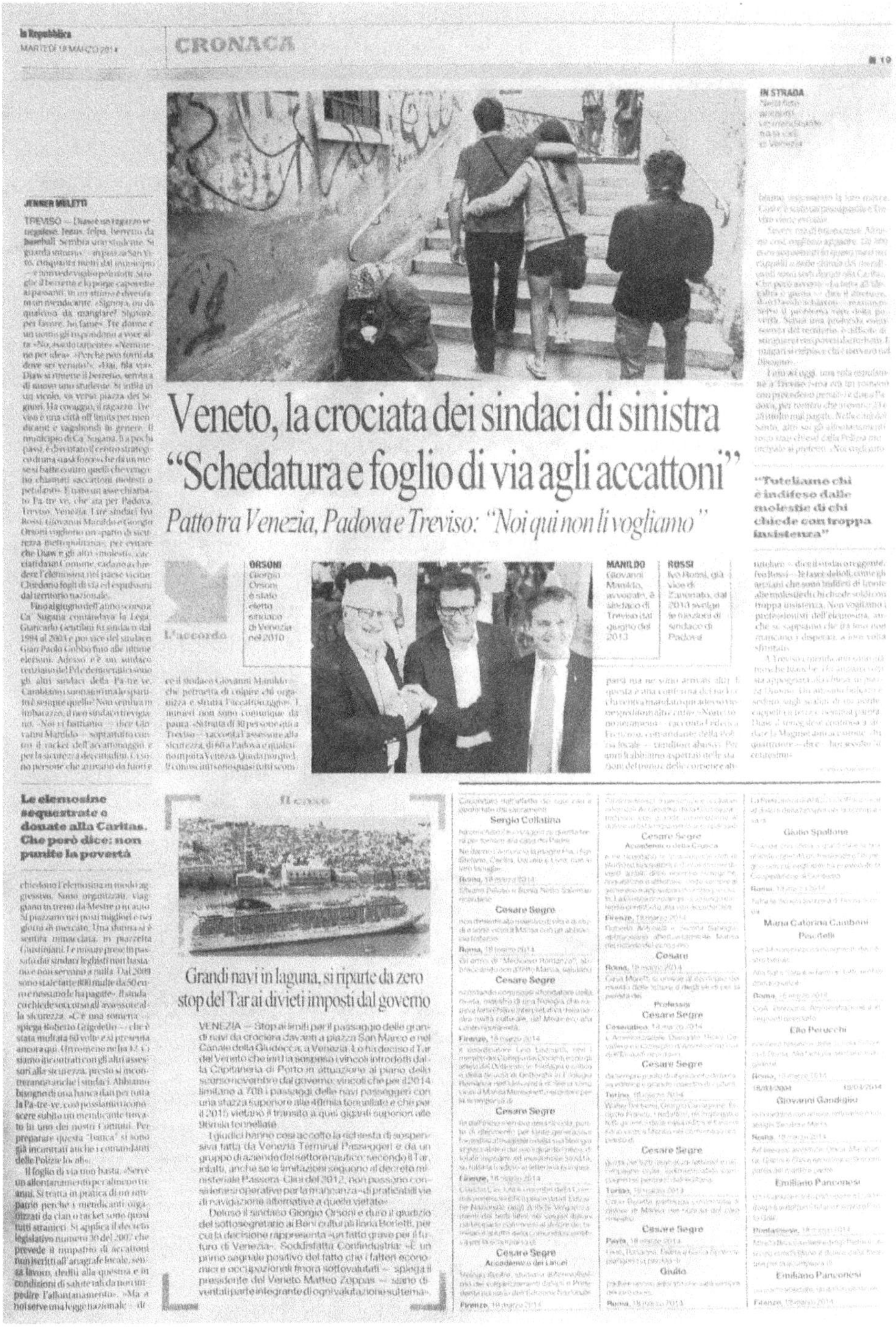

la Repubblica

CRONACA

Veneto, la crociata dei sindaci di sinistra
"Schedatura e foglio di via agli accattoni"

Patto tra Venezia, Padova e Treviso: "Noi qui non li vogliamo"

"Tuteliamo chi è indifeso dalle molestie di chi chiede con troppa insistenza"

Le elemosine sequestrate e donate alla Caritas. Che però dice: non punite la povertà

Grandi navi in laguna, si riparte da zero
stop del Tar ai divieti imposti dal governo

Figure C.2 Pact of three center-left mayors of Padua, Treviso and Venice (Pa-tre-ve). Photo: from *La Repubblica*, March 18, 2014

Safety Deputy Roberto Grigoletto expands on the story by telling how a Romanian woman, who was apparently fined sixty times, still hangs around town. What is necessary, the deputy claims, is a data bank for the Pa-tre-ve area so one may immediately identify a vagrant who has been found begging in one of their counties. The expulsion papers handed to these mendicants in the past years are insufficient. "What is needed," he adds, "is their expulsion [from the region] for at least three years. It is practically a process whereby these people are sent back to their homeland since most of the beggars, who are controlled by organized crime or the cartel, are primarily foreigners."[22] According to the same spokesman, all one needs to do is enforce a law issued in 2007 that ruled the coerced repatriation of beggars not registered in the local record bureau, who are without work, bent on begging and healthy enough to be returned to their country of origin.[23] Mayor Manildo of Treviso insists that what is needed is a nation-wide law that will help zero in on those who organize and exploit beggars. The numbers of the local, modern-day mendicants are not excessive, according to Deputy Grigoletto: thirty individuals in Treviso, sixty persons in Padua and a few more than that in Venice. "Here [in Treviso] the 'usual suspects' have just about disappeared but others have arrived. It proves that there is a cartel: those who were sent here are now dispatched to other cities."[24] As the journalist points out, the public servants of these affluent towns are stern but care to appear clement, since the 800 euros they sequestered in recent months from the beggars was donated to the Catholic poor-relief agency, *Caritas*. However, Father Davide Schiavon, director of the local *Caritas* branch, prudently warns: "Fighting illegality is a just cause but it does not eradicate the real problem of poverty. Without a thorough knowledge of the territory, it is difficult to distinguish the truly poor from the cunning. And perhaps one is likely to punish those who are really needy."[25]

Among these alien, modern-day "vagabonds," of course, there are a number of simulators who, just as in the Renaissance, "work the town" by feigning lameness and physical ailments. For example, on October 24, 2002, Rome's daily *Il Messaggero* published an article complemented by photographs that recorded "a day in the life" of a false lame mendicant in the streets of Rome (Figure C.3). The impostor is shown walking on his way to "work" carrying a chair

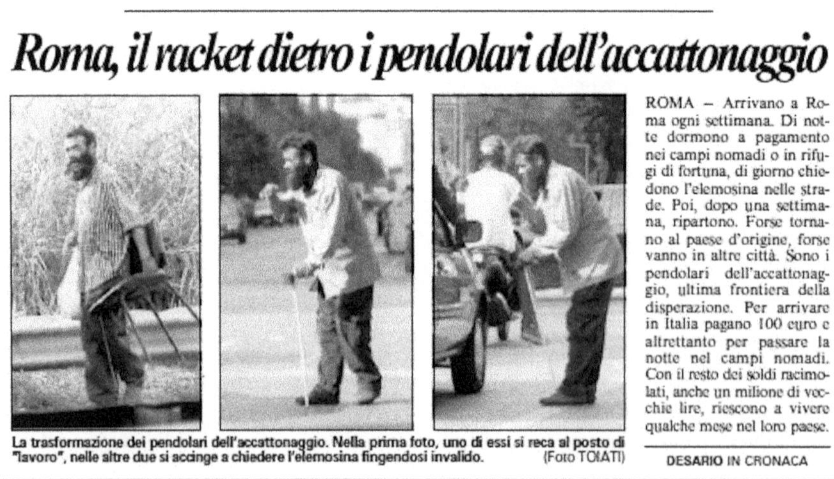

Roma, il racket dietro i pendolari dell'accattonaggio

ROMA – Arrivano a Roma ogni settimana. Di notte dormono a pagamento nei campi nomadi o in rifugi di fortuna, di giorno chiedono l'elemosina nelle strade. Poi, dopo una settimana, ripartono. Forse tornano al paese d'origine, forse vanno in altre città. Sono i pendolari dell'accattonaggio, ultima frontiera della disperazione. Per arrivare in Italia pagano 100 euro e altrettanto per passare la notte nel campi nomadi. Con il resto dei soldi racimolati, anche un milione di vecchie lire, riescono a vivere qualche mese nel loro paese.

DESARIO IN CRONACA

La trasformazione dei pendolari dell'accattonaggio. Nella prima foto, uno di essi si reca al posto di "lavoro", nelle altre due si accinge a chiedere l'elemosina fingendosi invalido. (Foto TOIATI)

Figure C.3 Fake Mendicant, *Messaggero*, October 24, 2002

and a plastic bag. Then again he is photographed "on the job," begging for alms while leaning on a cane as he limps his way around cars stopped at a traffic light.

The general belief that these pseudo, physically impaired beggars are for the most part foreigners is supported not just by journalists but also by the police and representatives of *Caritas* (Figure C.4).[26] Nevertheless, whatever their nationality, even though Italy is obviously more affluent than centuries ago and the number of indigent people in the country is certainly inferior to that witnessed in the course of history, there are still a number of orthopedically impaired beggars who populate the city streets especially around tourist attractions or churches. Often the reaction of mainstream society at the sight of an orthopedically impaired mendicant, when dubiously lame, has not changed. Skepticism, if not total insensibility, in the past as in today's Italy continues to be the common denominator in these social encounters.

* * *

Although legislature on disability in Italy has not established milestones comparable to the Americans with Disabilities Act (ADA) of 1990, matters have changed. The most important advance in this field has been the promulgation of law no. 13/1989 on architectural barriers – a law that Italy's Corte Costituzionale (Supreme Court) defined as the "Copernican Revolution" on disability.[27] Even if only on a symbolical level, in this country as elsewhere in the West there has also been a tangible modification in the way people speak about the subject, which is reflected in the vocabulary currently in use. Thus, there has been a substitution

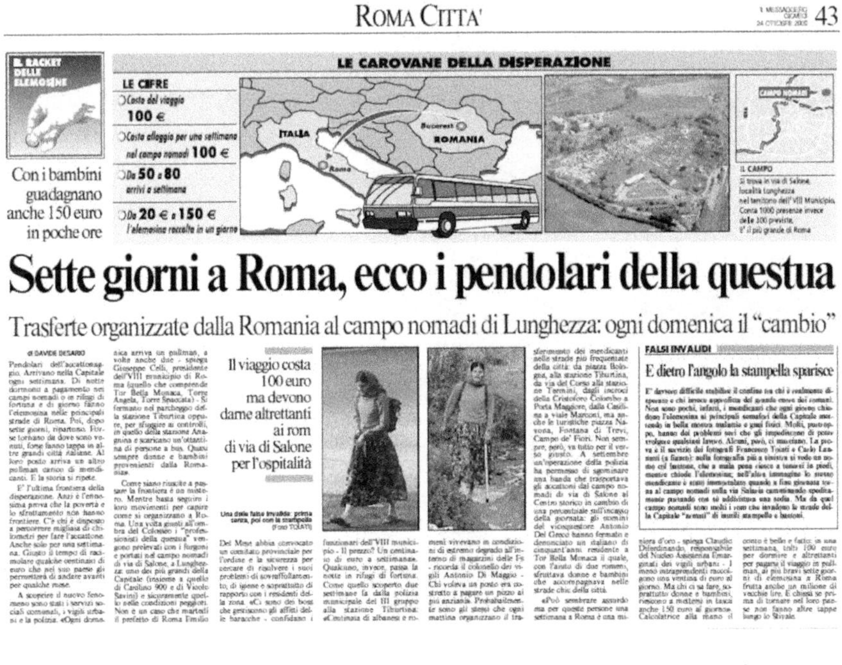

ROMA CITTA' 43

LE CAROVANE DELLA DISPERAZIONE

LE CIFRE
Costo del viaggio 100 €
Costo alloggio per una settimana nel campo nomadi 100 €
Da 50 a 80 arrivi a settimana
Da 20 € a 150 € l'elemosina raccolta in un giorno

Con i bambini guadagnano anche 150 euro in poche ore

IL CAMPO
Si trova in via di Salone, località Lunghezza nel territorio dell'VIII Municipio. Conta 1000 presenze invece delle 300 previste. E' il più grande di Roma

Sette giorni a Roma, ecco i pendolari della questua

Trasferte organizzate dalla Romania al campo nomadi di Lunghezza: ogni domenica il "cambio"

Il viaggio costa 100 euro ma devono darne altrettanti ai rom di via di Salone per l'ospitalità

FALSI INVALIDI

E dietro l'angolo la stampella sparisce

Figure C.4 Flow of the new poor from Eastern Europe to Italy, *Messaggero*, October 24, 2002

of socially charged terminology now considered offensive (such as "zoppo/lame," "storpio/crippled," "handicappato/handicapped," "disabile/disabled") with what the contemporary Western world deems more appropriate ("portatore di handicap/people with disability," "diversamente abile/differently able"). It is not just a matter of being politically correct. Rather, it is an effort to change deep-seated, collective prejudices and misunderstandings of the human condition that, no doubt, will take time to permeate most members of society.

Indicative of the change is the way the disabled have gained greater visibility and have taken on a more active role in society. A good example is a political poster of Valentina Valenti used to publicize her campaign for the May 2006 administrative elections in the region of Lazio. The image wisely contrasts her physical impairment – proudly displayed in a photo of her sitting on a wheelchair – with Valentina Valenti's undiminished capability to represent the citizens of Rome, as the phrase under her name makes abundantly clear: "abile a rappresentarti" ("able to represent you") (Figure C.5).

As elsewhere in the West, in Italy there are many associations for the disabled such as the Associazione Nazionale Disabili Italiani (ANDI) and the Lega Arcobaleno. There is a sports model of strength and determination in the face of adversity, Alex Zanardi, a former Formula 1 pilot who, despite an accident in 2001 that cost him the loss of both legs, has gone on to become a Paralympic champion of handcycle. There is a comedian, David Anzalone, who has

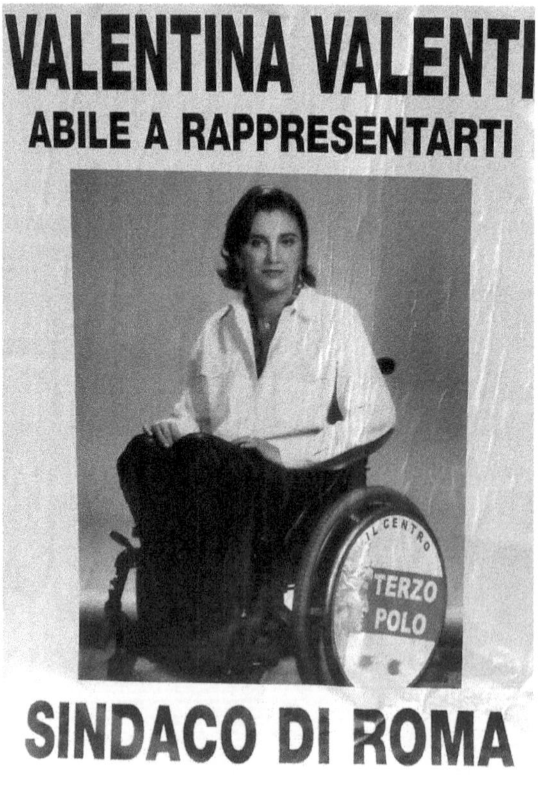

Figure C.5 Valentina Valenti, Administrative Elections, Rome, May 27–28, 2006. Photo: author

turned his wit and disability to advantage, and has mildly jolted public opinion by turning upside-down a number of commonplaces about the disabled, as the title of his book implies: *A Handicapped and a Stinker* (*Handicappato e Carogna*).[28] However, in the visual arts, modern Italian artists have not produced anything comparable to Marc Quinn's giant nude sculpture of *Alison Lapper Pregnant* exhibited in Trafalgar Square in 2005 (Figure C.6).[29] Although visitors to the Venice Biennale in 2013 were able to see the even larger inflatable version of Quinn's marble statue appropriately entitled *Breath*, the representation of disabilities has not concerned Italian artists the way it has their Anglo-American counterparts.[30] Indeed, no such artistic statements are currently being produced in Italy by disabled artists or artists sympathetic to their cause. In fact, the one thing that has not happened is that the disabled have not taken "the bull by the horns" and confronted the society they live in with paintings, sculptures, photographs, artifacts or performances that jolt the able-bodied out of their torpor and force them to come to terms with the prejudices and misunderstandings of certain human conditions that concern everyone. It may not be the solution to the many obstacles confronting the disabled in contemporary society. Nevertheless, the visual arts could do much to help the able-bodied overcome the mental – more than the architectural – barriers that obstruct the progress of the orthopedically impaired.

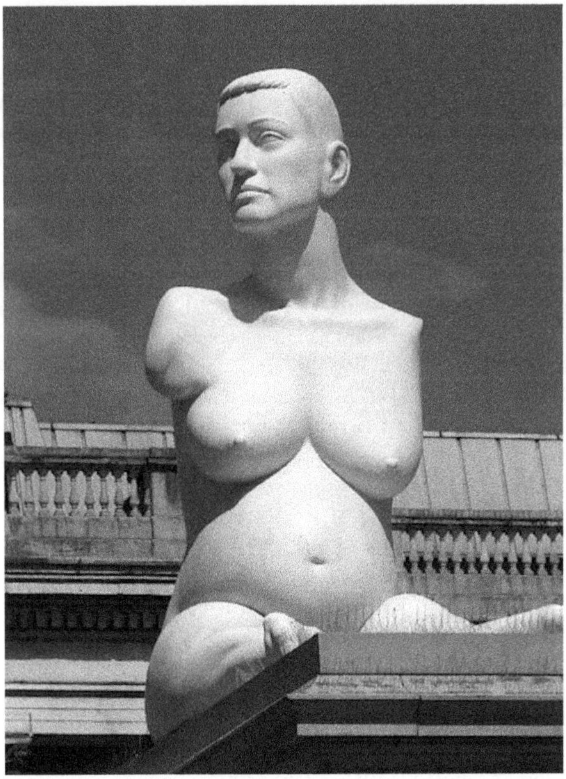

Figure C.6 Marc Quinn, *Alison Lapper Pregnant*, Trafalgar Square, London, 2005. Photo: in the public domain

Notes

1 See the Introduction, note 8.
2 See Chapter 2, p. 36.
3 A similar idea is expressed in Millett-Gallant, pp. 14–15, who cites performance theorist Peggy Phelan for whom "images often depict the desires of those who produce them rather than offering self-directed visibility of the subject depicted in them."
4 Garland-Thomson, p. 14, and p. 141, n. 14. See the Introduction, note 11.
5 For a recap of Toti's life see http://en.wikipedia.org/wiki/Enrico_Toti; see also http://www.carabinieri.it/Internet/Editoria/Carabiniere/2004/08-Agosto/Storia/073-00.htm (both last accessed March 25, 2016). A biography of Toti written under the influence of a strong patriotic spirit engendered by the outcome of World War I is Luigi Re's *Enrico Toti: profilo*, Piacenza, 1923. A second biography, written during the Fascist era's exploitation of Toti's deed, is Milla Vignini Paloschi's *Enrico Toti. La centuria di ferro: la pattuglia dei combattenti*, Milan, 1940, no. 78. For a recent, more balanced and objective reassessment of the national hero, see Lucio Fabi, *Enrico Toti: una storia tra mito e realtà*, Cremona, 2005. On the way the mutilated soldier's body was manipulated by the Italian State after World War I and Fascist appropriation of such imagery, see, for example, Martina Salvante, "Italian Disabled Veterans between Experience and Representation," in *Men After War*, Stephen McVeigh and Nicola Cooper (eds.), New York, 2013, pp. 111–129.
6 Salvante, "Italian Disabled Veterans," p. 114.
7 Ibid., p. 115.
8 Fabi, p. 26.
9 Salvante, "Italian Disabled Veterans," p. 115.
10 On the conflicting reports about Toti's heroic deed, see Fabi, pp. 89–100.
11 Nicola Tranfaglia, *La prima Guerra mondiale e il fascismo*, Turin, 1995, p. 61: "The losses were immense: 62,000 dead and 170,000 wounded soldiers as of November 30, 1915. Most of all, there was a strong sensation among the army officers, the politicians and the rest of the country, that the illusion that the war would be short lived did not hold up to reality, that it would be necessary to fight many other battles and accumulate many more human losses before making a breakthrough and [forcing] the enemy to retreat." My translation.
12 The Milan daily *Corriere della Sera* on Sundays published the supplement *Domenica del Corriere*. The issue in question is dated November 1–8, 1914.
13 The issue is dated September 24–October 1, 1916.
14 As one might expect, there are numerous monuments dedicated to Toti all over Italy and, as late as 1955, Toti's deed was kept alive in David Carbonari's film *Bella non piangere!* His role was played by Ettore Manni. For the gradual inclusion of the World War I veterans' movement within the Fascist Party's apparatus, see Martina Salvante, "The Italian Associazione Nazionale Mutilati e Invalidi di Guerra and Its International Liaisons in the Post Great War Era," in *The Great War and Veterans' Internationalism*, Julia Eichenberg and John Paul Newman (eds.), London and New York, 2013, pp. 164–166 and ff.
15 Fabi, pp. 148–157.
16 Salvante, "Italian Disabled Veterans," p. 117.
17 The elaboration of mourning via monuments had occurred already prior to the rise of Fascism. Once Mussolini had obtained the seat of power, there was a change in emphasis on these monuments that went from commemoration to celebration. See Bruno Tobia, "Dal Milite ingonto al nazionalismo monumentale fascista (1921–1940)," in *Guerra e pace*, Walter Barberis (ed.), Turin, 2002, pp. 598–599. The fascists' attempt at controlling "l'universo simbolico dello Stato" has recently been investigated in a line of research that has been appropriately labeled "Nation building." In the region of Lazio alone, between 1919 and 1922 more than thirty monuments were dedicated to the fallen soldiers. See Manuela Riosa, "Comitati locali e potere politico: i caratteri della committenza," in *La memoria perduta: i monumenti ai caduti della Grande Guerra a Roma e nel Lazio*, Vittorio Vidotto, Bruno Tobia and Catherine Brice (eds.), pp. 17 and 22. Renato Monteleone and Pino

Sarasini, "I monumenti italiani ai caduti della Grande Guerra," in *La Grande Guerra: esperienza, memoria, immagini*, Diego Leoni and Camillo Zadra (eds.), Bologna, 1986, p. 633: "con l'avvento del fascismo la rappresentazione *eroica* del combattente s'impone definitivamente su quella *dolorante* che in precedenza era stata un modello alternativo (benché infrequente)" ("with the advent of Fascism the *heroic* representation of the fighting soldier definitively replaced that of the *suffering* [soldier] that previously had been an alternative model (if infrequent), so charged with significant ethical and political implications"). See also Vittorio Vidotto, "La Vittoria e i monumenti ai caduti," in *Mélanges de l'École Française de Rome. Italie et Méditerranée*, 112:2 (2000): 505–513.

18 Monteleone and Sarasini, "I monumenti italiani," p. 633. The article citation was first published by L.A. Maggiorotti, "L'espressione del dolore nella pittura bellica," *Esercito e Nazione*, Rome, 1927, I, p. 39.

19 Monteleone and Sarasini, "I monumenti italiani," p. 637, observe that, while in funerary or sepulchral monuments the composition at times develops horizontally, normally these emphasize vertical or diagonal lines: "il monumento assume, allora, una proiezione ascensionale che tende a produrre effetti visivi abbastanza simili a quelli di una trionfale lievitazione."

20 Brian Pullan, "La nova filantropia nella Venezia cinquecentesca," in *Nel regno dei poveri: arte e storia dei grandi ospedali veneziani in età moderna 1474–1797*, Bernard Aikema and Dulcia Mejers (eds.), Venice, 1989, p. 20, citing from Francesco Semi, *El parlar s'ceto e neto de Capodistria: testi antichi e moderni, glossario*, Venice, 1983, pp. 278–280.

21 See Jenner Meletti's article in *La Repubblica*, dated March 18, 2014, p. 19.

22 Ibid.

23 Ibid.

24 Ibid.

25 Ibid.

26 According to a report in *Il Messaggero*, October 24, 2002, many of these mendicants came from Romania and stayed for roughly a week in Rome under dire living conditions, after which they returned home with enough money to last them for a few months. This was before January 1, 2007, when Romania was admitted as a member of the European Union, at which time it became easier to cross the borders from that nation into countries belonging to the EU. Since then, the phenomenon has perhaps escalated. A follow-up on this topic, also in *Il Messaggero*, appeared on October 25, 2002. For a glimpse at the front pages of these two issues see under the pertinent dates in the paper's website, http://shop.ilmessaggero.it/home_sd.php?page=layoutStorico (last accessed March 24, 2016).

27 For a recap of the major legislative steps taken with regard to disability, see Rolando Alberto Borzetti's "L'handicap nella società," http://www.didaweb.net/handicap/leggi.php?a=110 (last accessed on May 31, 2014). The law states that it is not people who are disabled but the way edifices are built that creates difficulties or barriers for individuals with physical impairments. Thus it is the legislators' and administrators' main responsibility to keep a vigilant eye on the planning and construction of new structures to make sure that architectural barriers are eliminated so as not to constitute a handicap for the physically impaired. An important document on the subject that takes into consideration the new International Classification of Functioning, Disability and Health (ICF) is the volume published by Istat (the National Institute for Statistics), *La disabilità in Italia: il quadro della statistica ufficiale*, Alessandro Solipaca (ed.), Rome, 2009, available online at http://www3.istat.it/dati/catalogo/20100513_00/arg_09_37_la_disabilita_in_Italia.pdf (last accessed March 24, 2016).

28 David Anzalone, *Hadicappato e carogna*, Milan, 2008.

29 See Adam Broomberg and Oliver Chanarin, "Beauty Unseen, Unsung," *The Guardian Weekend*, September 3, 2005 and Juman Farouky's article "Rubbing Shoulders with Lord Nelson," *Time*, October 31, 2005. Alison Lapper went on to publish her autobiography in *My Life in My Hands*, London, 2005. Marc Quinn's *Breath*, the 36-foot inflatable version of the marble statue of Alison Lapper, was exhibited at the 2013 Venice Biennale, where it met with some criticism by the Venetian Patriarchate. See Nick Squires's article in *The Telegraph* and Carol Vogel's in *The New York Times*, both published on May 30, 2013.

30 For example, nothing has been produced in the peninsula that could be seen on a par with images taken from Mary Duffy's live performance of 1995 or Joel-Peter Witkin's photographs of the *First Casting for Milo* (2004) and *Portrait of Greg Vaughn* (2004). In the first two works, in which Mary Duffy divested herself and in Witkin's photograph of the *First Casting for Milo*, both artists offer to the viewer's gaze two disabled bodies purposely posed to recall the famous statue of the *Venus de Milo*. Comparably conceived is Witkin's *Portrait of Greg Vaughn*, in which the photographer recreates a modern-day counterpart of the Classical sculptural type of the nude ephebe. In these works the artists investigate fundamental questions about the disabled body that span the gap from the personal to the political and the corporeal. From an art historical perspective viewers are forced to ponder why it is that Western societies consider mutilated Classical sculptures beautiful objects yet find the disabled human body esthetically deficient. See Millett-Gallant's stimulating analyses in *The Disabled Body in Contemporary Art*, chapter 1, "Disarming Venus," pp. 25–49 and chapter 3, "Performing Amputation," pp. 83–111.

Bibliography

A.I., "Ospizio di San Giovanni in Laterano," in *Le immagini del SS. mo Salvatore: fabbriche e sculture per l'Ospizio Apostolico dei Poveri Invalidi*, Rome, 1988, pp. 103–110.

Acidini, C., "Elementi di una biografia eccezionale," in *1564/2014 Michelangelo: incontrare un artista universale*, Florence, 2014, pp. 25–33.

Acta Sanctorum, Augusti II, Antwerp, 1735.

Agostino, Giovanni Crisostomo, Gregorio di Nazianzo, Gregorio di Nissa, Servire i poveri gioiosamente, Rosadoni, L. (tr.), Turin, 1971.

Agrippa, C., *De incertitudine et scientiarum et artium (Of the Vanitie and Uncertaintie of Artes and Sciences)*, Sanford, J. (tr.), London, 1569.

———, *De incertitudine et vanitate scientiarum declamation invectiva, ex postrema Authoris recognitione*, Cologne, 1584.

Ahlquist, G.W. and Cook, W.R., "The Representation of the Posthumous Miracles of St. Francis of Assisi in Thirteenth-Century Italian Painting," in *The Art of the Franciscan Order in Italy*, Cook, W.R. (ed.), Leiden, 2005, pp. 211–256.

Alberti, L.B., *De re ædificatoria*, in *Ten Books on Architecture*, Bartoli, C. (tr. into Italian) and Leoni, J. (tr. into English), London, 1965.

———, *Momus*, Knight, S. (tr.), Brown, V. and Knight, S. (eds.), Cambridge and London, 2003.

———, *On Painting*, Sinisgalli, R. (tr.), Cambridge, 2011.

Alciati, A., *A Book of Emblems: The* Emblematum Liber *in Latin and English by Andrea Alciati (1492–1550)*, Moffitt, J.F. (tr. and ed.), Jefferson, NC, and London, 2004.

Alexandre-Bidon, D. and Lett, D., *Children in the Middle Ages: Fifth–Fifteenth Centuries*, Gladding, J. (tr.), Notre Dame, 1999.

Amato, P.F. (ed.), *Le piante di Roma*, Rome, 1962.

Amundsen, D.W., *Medicine, Society, and Faith in the Ancient and Medieval Worlds*, Baltimore and London, 1996.

Anzalone, D., *Hadicappato e carogna*, Milan, 2008.

Apuleius, *Apologia*, Butler, H.E. (tr.), Oxford, 1909.

Arator, *On the Acts of the Apostles (De Actibus Apostolorum)*, Schrader, R.J. (tr. and ed.), Atlanta, 1987.

Archivio Luoghi Pii Elimosinieri (Azienda Servizi alla Persona "Golgi-Redaelli"), Statuti 3, Buganza, S., Vanoli, P. and Zardin, D. (eds.), Milan, 2011, pp. 107, 138–139.

Archivio Segreto Vaticano, IV–V, t. 9, fol. 205r.

———, IV–V, t. 105C, p. 95.

Aristophanes, *Clouds*, Henderson, J. (tr.), Cambridge and London, 1998.

Aristotle, *Constitution of Athens*, in *The Complete Works of Aristotle*, Barnes, J. (ed.), 2 vols., Princeton, 1985.

———, *Generation of Animals*, in *The Complete Works of Aristotle*, Barnes, J. (ed.), 2 vols., Princeton, 1985.
———, *History of Animals*, in *The Complete Works of Aristotle*, Barnes, J. (ed.), 2 vols., Princeton, 1985.
———, *Politics*, in *The Complete Works of Aristotle*, Barnes, J. (ed.), 2 vols., Princeton, 1985.
Armellini, M., *Le chiese di Roma dal secolo IV al XIX*, Rome, 1891.
Assereto, G., "Aspetti dell'assistenza pubblica a Genova nei primi anni dell'Ottocento," in *Timore e carità: i poveri nell'Italia moderna*, Politi, G., Rosa, M. and della Peruta, F. (eds.), Cremona, 1982, pp. 347–357.
———, "Pauperismo e assistenza: messa a punto di studi recenti," *Archivio storico italiano*, 516 (1983): 253–271.
Augustine, *Concerning the City of God against the Pagans*, Bettenson, H. (tr.), Middlessex, 1972.
Avery, C., *Bernini: Genius of the Baroque*, London, 2006.
Bagnoli, M., "Fonti per la storia delle pitture della cripta," in *Il restauro della cripta di Anagni*, Bianchi, A. (ed.), Rome, 2003, pp. 77–78.
Bainton, R.H., *Here I Stand*, London, 1950.
Baldinucci, F., *The Life of Bernini*, Engass, C. (tr.), University Park, 2006.
Balzani, A., *L'Ospizio Apostolico dei Poveri Invalidi detto "Il S. Michele" dal 1693 al 1718*, Rome, 1969.
Baracchini, C. and Castelnuovo, E. (eds.), *Il Camposanto di Pisa*, Turin, 1996.
Barocchi, P. (ed.), *Scritti d'arte del Cinquecento*, 3 vols., Milan and Naples, 1971–1977.
Battaglia, S., *Grande dizionario della lingua italiana*, Turin, 2002.
Baumann, P., "Margins/Outsiders," in *Encyclopedia of Comparative Iconography: Themes Depicted in Works of Art*, 2 vols., Roberts, H.E. (ed.), Chicago, 1998, II, pp. 545–551.
Bellori, G.P., *The Lives of the Modern Painters, Sculptors and Architects*, Sedgwick Wohl, A. (tr.), Cambridge, 2005.
Belting, H., *Likeness and Presence: A History of the Image before the Era of Art*, Chicago and London, 1994.
Benati, D., "Annibale Carracci e il vero," in *Annibale Carracci*, Benati, D. and Riccòmini, E. (eds.), Milan, 2006, pp. 27–29.
Benvenuti, A. and Giannarelli, E., *Il diacono Lorenzo tra storia e leggenda*, Florence, 1998.
Beregno, M., "Conclusioni," in *Timore e carità: i poveri nell'Italia moderna*, Politi, G., Rosa, M. and della Peruta, F. (eds.), Cremona, 1982, pp. 491–496.
Berlin Staatliche Museen, Kupferstichkabinett 78 A 4, fol. 2r.
Berlin Staatsbibliothek, Cod. Lat. Theol. Fol. 323, fol. 12r.
Bernabò, M. (ed.), *Il Tetravangelo di Rabbula*, Florence, 2008.
Bertelli, C., "L'altare di Volvinio nella basilica milanese di Sant'Ambrogio," *Rivista dell'Istituto per la Storia dell'Arte Lombarda*, 5 (2012): 41–54.
Bianchi, A., "I dipinti," in *Il restauro della cripta di Anagni*, Bianchi, A. (ed.), Rome, 2003, pp. 79–182.
Biblioteca Apostolica Vaticana, Chigi H.II, 46.
———, Ottob. Lat. 3362, I, "Avviso," November 1, 1692, p. 100.
Blunt, A., *Artistic Theory in Italy*, London, Oxford and New York, 1973.
Boardman, J., *Athenian Black Figure Vases*, Singapore, 1980.
———, *Intaglios and Rings: Greek, Etruscan and Eastern from a Private Collection*, London, 1975.
Bohn, H.B., *Polyglot of Foreign Proverbs*, London, 1857.
Bonfigli, C., *Niccolò V: papa della rinascenza*, Rome, 1997.
Bonnefoy, Yves, *Dictionnaire des mythologies et des religions des sociétés traditionnelles et du monde antique*, 2 vols., Chicago, 1991.
Botero, G., *Della Ragion di Stato Libri Dieci, con tre libri delle cause della Grandezza e Magnificenza delle Città*, Venice, 1589.
Bottari, G.G. and Ticozzi, S., *Raccolta di lettere sulla pittura, scultura ed architettura scritte da' più celebri personaggi dei secoli XV, XVI, e XVII*, 8 vols., Milan, 1822–1825.

Braudel, F., *The Structures of Everyday Life: The Limits of the Possible (Civilization and Capitalism: 15th–18th Century)*, Berkeley and Los Angeles, 1992.

Briganti, G., *La pittura in Italia: il Settecento*, Milan, 1990.

Brion-Guerry, L., *Le thème du "Triomphe de la Mort" dans la peinture italienne*, Paris, 1950.

Brocchi, G.M., *Vita di S. Gherardo*, Lucca, 1750.

Brooke, R.B., *The Images of St. Francis: Responses to Sainthood in the Thirteenth Century*, Cambridge, 2006.

Brown, P., *Authority and the Sacred: Aspects of the Christianisation of the Roman World*, Cambridge, 1997.

———, *Poverty and Leadership in the Later Roman Empire*, Hanover and London, 2002.

———, *The Cult of the Saints: Its Rise and Function in Latin Christianity*, London, 1981.

———, *Through the Eye of a Needle: Wealth, the Fall of Rome, and the Making of Christianity in the West, 350–550*, Princeton and Oxford, 2012.

Burns, J.H. and Izbicki, T.M. (eds.), *Conciliarism and Papalism*, Cambridge, 1997.

Butler's Lives of the Saints, 4 vols., Thurston, H.J. and Attwater, D. (eds.), Westminster, MD, 1990.

Cajani, L., "Gli statuti della compagnia dei ciechi, zoppi, e stroppiati della visitazione (1698)," in *Ricerche per la storia religiosa di Roma*, Rome, 1979, pp. 281–313.

Caleca, A., "Costruzione e decorazione dalle origini al secolo XV," in *Il Camposanto di Pisa*, Turin, 1996, pp. 13–48.

Cameron, E., *Waldenses: Rejections of Holy Church in Medieval Europe*, Oxford, 2000.

Camporesi, P., *Il libro dei vagabondi*, Turin, 1773; reprinted by Garzanti, Milan, 2003.

———, *Il pane selvaggio*, Milan, 2004.

———, *The Land of Hunger*, Croft-Murray, T., Foley, C. and Mitchell, S. (trs.), Cambridge, 1996.

Caner, D., *Wandering, Begging Monks: Spiritual Authority and the Promotion of Monasticism in Late Antiquity*, Berkeley, Los Angeles and London, 2002.

Carmichael, A.G., *Plague and the Poor in Renaissance Florence*, New York, 1986.

Carracci, A., *Le arti di Bologna di Annibale Carracci*, Marabottini, A. (ed.), Rome, 1966.

Castelli, C., *Orazione ne' funerali di Monsignor Gioachino Castelli*, Palermo, 1789.

Cavallaro, A., "La pittura a Roma nel tempo di Nicolò V (1447–1453)," in *La storia dei Giubilei*, 4 vols., Fossi, G. and Strinati, C. (eds.), Rome, 1998, II, pp. 74–91.

Cavallo, S., "Conception of Poverty and Poor-Relief in Turin in the Second Half of the Eighteenth Century," in *Domestic Strategies: Work and Family in France and Italy 1600–1800*, Woolf, S. (ed.), Cambridge and Paris, ca. 1991, pp. 148–199.

Cerasoli, F., "Censimenti della popolazione di Roma dall'anno 1600 al 1739," *Studi e documenti di storia di diritto*, Rome, 1891, XII.

Chappell, M.L. and Kirwin, C.W., "A Petrine Triumph: The Decoration of the Navi Piccole in San Pietro under Clement VIII," *Storia dell'arte*, 21 (1974): 119–170.

Cicatelli, S., *Vita di San Camillo de Lellis: fondatore della religione de' chierici regolari, ministri degli infermi*, Rome, 1746.

Cicero, *De Natura Deorum*, Rackham, H. (tr.), Cambridge, MA, and London, 1979.

———, *De Legibus*, Keyes, C.W. (tr.), Cambridge, MA, and London, 1972.

———, *De Oratore*, 2 vols., Sutton, E.W. and Rackham, H. (trs.), Cambridge, MA, and London, 1976.

———, *De Senectute*, Armistead Falconer, W. (tr.), Cambridge and London, 2001.

———, *Tusculan Disputations*, King, J.E. (tr.), London and New York, 1927.

Civiltà del Seicento a Napoli, 2 vols., Naples, 1984.

Codice Campori, Biblioteca Estense, y X 2,5.

Cohn, Jr., K., *Death and Prosperity in Siena, 1205–1800: Strategies for the Afterlife*, Baltimore and London, 1988.

Colella, R., "Die Kapelle Papst Nikolaus' V. zu ihrer Geschichte und Funktion inner halb des Vatikanischen Palastes," in *Architectural Studies in Memory of Richard Krautheimer*, Striker, C. (ed.), Mainz, 1996, pp. 37–41.

———, "Hagiographie und Kirchenpolitik – Stephanus und Laurentius in Rom," in *Pratum Romanum: Richard Krautheimer zum 100. Geburtstag*, Colella, R. and Krautheimer, R. (eds.), Wiesbaden, 1977, pp. 75–96.

———, *Päpstiliche Suprematie und Kirhliche Reform, Die Fresken Fra Angelicos in der Kapelle Papst Nikolaus' V – ein Päpstliches Programm in Spät Konsiliarer Zeit* (Ph.D. thesis, Munich, 1993).

Collected Works of Erasmus: Colloquies, Thompson, C.R. (tr. and ed.), Toronto, Buffalo and London, 1997.

Colmeiro, Manuel, *Historia de la economia politica en España*, 2 vols., Madrid, 1863.

Coluccia, G., *Niccolò V umanista, papa e riformatore*, Venice, 1998.

Compendio storico su Pio VII, Milan, 1824.

Constable, G., *The Reformation of the Twelfth Century*, Cambridge, 1996.

Contardi, B., "La mendicità provveduta," in *Le immagini del SS. mo Salvatore: fabbriche e sculture per l'Ospizio Apostolico dei Poveri Invalidi*, Contardi, B. and Curcio, G. (eds.), Rome, 1988, pp. 17–39.

Cook, W., "Early Images of St. Francis of Assisi in Rome," in *"Exegisti Monumentum Aere Perennius": Essays in Honor of John Frederick Charles*, Baker, B. and Fischer, J. (eds.), Indianapolis, 1994, pp. 19–34.

———, *Images of Saint Francis of Assisi in Painting, Stone and Glass from the Earliest Images to c. 1320 in Italy: A Catalogue*, Florence, 1999, pp. 183–196.

Croce, G.C., *L'arte della Forfanteria Cantata da Gian Pitocco Fornaro, alla sua amata Signora. Opera Guidonesca dell'Accademico Calcante: Drizzata alla Baronia di Campo di Fiore*, Venice, 1618.

da Campagnola, S., *L'angelo del sesto sigillo e l'"alter Christus": genesi e sviluppo di due temi francescani nei secoli XII–XIV*, Rome, 1971.

Daley, B.E., *Gregory of Nazianzus*, London and New York, 2006.

Davidsohn, R., *Storia di Firenze*, 3 vols., Florence, 1957.

Davis, L.J., "Dr. Johnson, Amelia, and the Discourse of Disability in the Eighteenth Century," in *"Defects": Engendering the Modern Body*, Deutsch, H. and Nussbaum, F. (eds.), Ann Arbor, 2000, pp. 54–74.

———, *Enforcing Normalcy: Disability, Deafness and the Body*, London and New York, 1995.

de Brosses, C., *Lettres familières écrites d'Italie en 1739 et 1740*, 2 vols., Paris, 1858.

de la Ronciere, C.M., "Pauvres et pauvreté à Florence au XIVe siècle," in *Études sur l'histoire de la pauvreté (Moyen Âge–XIVe siècle)*, Mollat, M. (ed.), Paris, II, 1974, pp. 661–745.

De Montor, A., *The Lives and Times of the Popes* (orig. *Les vies des papes*), 10 vols., New York, 1910.

"De recognitione corporum SS. Laurentii et Stephani," *Analecta Bollandiniana*, 15 (1886).

de Voragine, J., *The Golden Legend*, 2 vols., Granger Ryan, W. (tr.), Princeton, 1993.

Decrees of the Ecumenical Councils, 2 vols., Tanner, N.P. (ed.), London and Washington, 1990.

Decreti di congregazioni particolari per l'Ospizio Apostolico dal 1692 al 1699, Archivio di Stato di Roma, Ospizio apostolico di S. Michele, b. 166, c.7.

Delehaye, H., *Les orgines du culte des martyrs*, Paris, 1933.

Della Casa, G., *Galateo*, Romano, R. (ed.), Turin, 1975.

Della Trasportatione dell'Obelisco Vaticano e delle Fabriche di Nostro Signore Papa Sisto V Fatte dal Cavallier Domenico Fontana Architetto di Sua Santita, Rome, 1590.

Delumeau, J., *Vie économique et sociale de Rome dans la seconde moitié du XVIe siècle*, Paris, 1957.

Demosthenes, *De Corona*, Vince, C.A. and Vince, J.H. (tr.), London and New York, 1926.

Deutsch, H. and Nussbaum, F. (eds.), *"Defects": Engendering the Modern Body*, Ann Arbor, 2000.

Devoto, G. and Oli, G.C., *Vocabolario illustrato della lingua italiana*, 2 vols., Milan, 1976.

Dillenberger, J., *Martin Luther: Selections from his Writings*, Garden City, 1961.

Dio Cassius, *Roman History*, 9 vols., Ernest Cary (tr.), London and New York, 1924.

Dionysius of Halicarnassus, *Roman Antiquities*, Cary, E. (tr.), London and Cambridge, 1937.

Duchet-Sychaux, G. and Pastoureau, P., *The Bible and the Saints*, Paris and New York, 1994.

Dustmann, H.O., "Das Bildnis des Amputierten in der Kunst," in *Der Körperbehinderte in Mythologie und Kunst*, Schlegel, K.F. (ed.), Stuttgart and New York, 1983, pp. 57–87.

Editto Sopra li Vagabondi, Mendicanti, and altri simili, che stanno nelli Portici, e Scale delle Chiese, Archivio Segreto Vaticano, Armadio IV–V, t. 9, 17 maggio 1628.

Edwards, M.L., "Constructions of Physical Disability in the Ancient Greek World: The Community Concept," in *The Body and Physical Difference: Discourses of Disability*, Mitchell, D.T. and Snyder, S.L. (eds.), Ann Arbor, 2004, pp. 35–50.

Elbern, V.H., *Der karolingische Goldaltar von Mailand*, Bonn, 1952.

Elm, V., "La riforma assistenziale della Prima Repubblica Romana (1798–1799)," in *Popolazione e società a Roma dal medioevo all'età contemporanea*, Eugenio Sonnino (ed.), Rome, 1998, pp. 563–572.

Elton, G.R., *Persecution and Toleration: Studies in Church History*, Oxford, 1984.

Encyclopedia of Comparative Iconography: Themes Depicted in Works of Art, 2 vols., Roberts, H.E. (ed.), Chicago, 1998.

Erasmus, *Beggar Talk*, in *Collected Works of Erasmus: Colloquies*, Thompson, C.R. (tr. and ed.), Toronto, Buffalo and London, 1997.

Eyben, E., "Family Planning in Graeco-Roman Antiquity," *Ancient Society*, 11–12 (1980–1981): 12–13.

Fabi, L., *Enrico Toti: una storia tra mito e realtà*, Cremona, 2005.

Fantelli, P.L., "I pitocchi nell'arte veneta del XVII secolo," in *La pittura nel Veneto: il Seicento*, 2 vols., Milan, 2001, II, pp. 709–724.

Fanucci, C., *Trattato di tutte le opere pie dell'alma città di Roma*, Rome, 1601.

Farmer, S., "The Beggar's Body: Intersections of Gender and Social Status in High Medieval Paris," in *Monks and Nuns, Saints and Outcasts: Religion in Medieval Society*, Farmer, S. and Rosewein, B.H. (eds.), Ithaca, NY, and London, 2000, pp. 153–171.

Fatica, M., *Il problema della mendicità nell'Europa moderna (secoli XVI–XVIII)*, Naples, 1992.

Favilla, M., Rugolo, R. and Sassi, L., *Venezia '700: arte e società nell'ultimo secolo della Serenissima*, Schio, 2011.

Fay Ablou-El-Haj, B., *The Medieval Cult of Saints: Formations and Transformations*, Cambridge, 1997.

Finn, R., *Almsgiving in the Later Roman Empire: Christian Promotion and Practice (313–450)*, Oxford, 2006.

Fiorani, L., "Religione e povertà: il dibattito sul pauperismo a Roma tra Cinque e Seicento," *Ricerche per la storia religiosa di Roma*, 3 (1979): 43–131.

Flower, H.I., "Elite Self-Representation in Rome," in *Social Relations in the Roman World*, Peachin, M. (ed.), Oxford, 2011, pp. 271–285.

Foucault, M., *Madness and Civilization: A History of Insanity in the Age of Reason*, New York, 1988.

Fouracre, P.J., "The Origins of the Carolingian Attempt to Regulate the Cult of Saints," in *The Cult of Saints in Late Antiquity and the Middle Ages: Essays on the Contribution of Peter Brown*, Howard-Johnston, A. and Hayward, P.A. (eds.), Oxford, 1999, pp. 143–165.

Fracastor, J., *La syphilis ou le mal français*, Vons, J. (ed.), Paris, 2011.

Frianoro, Rafaele (*alias* Nobili Giacinto), *Dell'origine de' bianti, pitocchi, cerretani, o vagabondi*, in Camporesi, P., *Il libro dei vagabondi*, Turin, 1773; reprinted by Garzanti, Milan, 2003, pp. 263–331.

Fridrichsen, A., *The Problem of Miracle in Primitive Christianity*, Harrisville, R.A. and Hanson, J.S. (trs.), Minneapolis, 1972.

Frugoni, C., *Francesco: un'altra storia*, Florence, 1988.

———, *Francesco e l'invenzione delle stimmate*, Turin, 1993.

Frye, N., *Anatomy of Criticism: Four Essays*, Princeton, 1971.

Galen, *On the Usefulness of the Parts of the Body*, 2 vols., Tallmadge May, M. (tr.), Ithaca, 1968.

Gandolfo, F., "Gli affreschi di San Saba," in *Fragmenta picta: affreschi e mosaici staccati del medioevo romano*, Rome, 1989, pp. 183–188.

Garland, R., *The Eye of the Beholder: Deformity and Disability in the Graeco-Roman World*, Ithaca, NY, 1995.

———, *The Greek Way of Death*, London, 1985.

Garland Thomson, R., *Extraordinary Bodies: Figuring Physical Disability in American Culture and Literature*, New York, 1997.

Garzoni, T., *La Piazza Universale di tutte le Professioni del Mondo*, Venice, 1617.

Genovesi, A., *Delle lezioni di commercio o sia d'economia civile*, Naples, 1768.

Geremek, B., "Il pauperismo nell'età preindustriale (secoli XIV–XVIII)," in *Storia d'Italia*, Turin, 1973, V, pp. 670–698.

———, *Poverty: A History*, Oxford, 1994.

———, *The Margins of Society in Late Medieval Paris*, Cambridge, 1987.

Gilbertson, L., "The Vanni Altarpiece and the Relic Cult of Saint Margaret: Considering a Female Audience," in *Decorations for the Holy Dead: Visual Embellishments on Tombs and Shrines of Saints*, Lamia, S. and Valdez del Álamo, E. (eds.), Turnhout, 2002, pp. 179–190.

Giucci, G., *Storia della vita e del pontificato di Pio VII*, 2 vols., Rome, 1857.

Glissenti, F., *Discorsi morali contro il dispiacer del morire detto athanatophilia*, Venice, 1600.

Goethe, J.W., *Italian Journey [1786–1788]*, Auden, W.H. and Mayer, E. (trs.), Harmondsworth, 1982.

Goffen, R., *Spirituality in Conflict: Saint Francis and Giotto's Bardi Chapel*, University Park and London, 1988.

Goldthwaite, R.A., "Artisans and the Economy in Sixteenth-Century Florence," in *The Medici, Michelangelo, and the Art of Late Renaissance Florence*, Luchinat, C.A. (ed.), New Haven, 2002, pp. 85–93.

Goodson, C., "Building for Bodies: The Architecture of Saint Veneration in Early Medieval Rome," in *Roma Felix: Formation and Reflections of Medieval Rome*, Carragáin, É.Ó. and Neuman de Vegvar, C. (eds.), Burlington, VT, 2007, pp. 51–79.

———, "The Relic Translations of Paschal I: Transforming City and Cult," in *Roman Bodies: Antiquity to the Eighteenth Century*, Hopkins, A. and Wyke, M. (eds.), London, 2005, pp. 123–141.

Grabar, A., *Christian Iconography: A Study of Its Origins*, Princeton, 1968.

———, *Martyrium: recherches sur le culte des reliques et l'art chrétien antique*, 2 vols., Paris, 1946.

———, *The Beginnings of Christian Art 200–395*, London, 1967.

Gracia, D., "The Ethics of Diagnosis in Early Christianity and the Middle Ages," in *The Ethics of Diagnosis*, Peset, J.L. and Gracia, D. (eds.), Dordrecht, 1992, pp. 19–27.

Grant, M., *The Twelve Caesars*, London, 1975.

Graves, R., *Claudius the God*, London, 1966.

Greco, A., *La cappella di Niccolò V del Beato Angelico*, Rome, 1980.

Gregory of Tours, *De Virtutibus Sancti Martini*, 4 vols., Krusch, B. (ed.), Monumenta Germaniae Historica, Scriptores Rerum Merovingicarum, Hannover, 1885.

Grendi, E., "Pauperismo e Albergo dei poveri nella Genova del Seicento," *Rivista storica italiana*, 87:4 (1975): 621–665.

Grigsby, B., "Medical Misconceptions," in *Misconceptions about the Middle Ages*, Harris, S.J. and Grinsby, B.L. (eds.), New York, 2008, pp. 142–150.

Groppi, A., "Birbanti e poveri benestanti: attitudini e pratiche assistenziali nei confronti della vecchiaia nella Roma pontificia (sec. XVI–XVIII)," in *Povertà e innovazioni istituzionali in Italia: dal medioevo ad oggi*, Zamagni, V. (ed.), Bologna, 2000, pp. 259–272.

Grubbs, J.E., "The Dynamics of Infant Abandonment: Motives, Attitudes and (Unintended) Consequences," in *The Dark Side of Childhood in Late Antiquity and the Middle Ages*, Mustakallio, K. and Laes, C. (eds.), Oxford, 2011, pp. 21–36.

Guevarre, A., *La Mendicité abolie par un bureau de charité à Toulouse*, Toulouse, 1692.

Hageneder, O. and Haidacher, A., *Das Register Innocenz' III*, I, Graz and Cologne, 1964.

Hahn, C., "Narrative on the Golden Altar of Sant'Ambrogio in Milan: Presentation and Reception," *Dumbarton Oaks Papers*, 53 (1999): 167–187.

———, *Passio Kiliani*, Graz, 1988.

———, "Pictorial Cycles of Non-Biblical Saints: The Seventh- and Eighth-Century Mural Cycles in Rome and Contexts for their Use," *Papers of the British School at Rome*, 67 (1999): 233–279.

———, "Picturing the Text: Narrative in the *Life* of the Saints," *Art History*, 13 (1990): 1–33.

———, *Portrayed on the Heart: Narrative Effect in Pictorial Lives of Saints from the Tenth through the Thirteenth Century*, Berkeley, 2001.

———, "Seeing and Believing: The Construction of Sanctity in Early-Medieval Saints' Shrines," *Speculum*, 72 (1997): 1079–1106.

Harrison, E.B., "Alkamenes' Sculptures for the Hephaisteion: Part I, The Cult Statues," *American Journal of Archaeology*, 81:2 (1977): 137–178.

Helas, P., "Die Bettler for dem Tempel: Zur Invenzione und Transformation eines Bildmotivs in der Italienischen Malerei der Renaissance (1423–1552)," *Iconographica*, 3 (2004): 62–99.

Helas, P. and Wolf, G. (eds.), *Armut und Armenfürsorge in der italienischen Stadtkultur zwischen 13. und 16. Jahrhundert: Bilder, Texte und Soziale Praktiken*, Frankfurt am Main, 2006.

Henderson, J., "'Mal Francese' in Sixteenth-Century Rome: The Ospedale di San Giacomo in Augusta and the 'Incurabili,'" in *Popolazione e società a Roma dal medioevo all'età contemporanea*, Sonnino, E. (ed.), Rome, 1998, pp. 483–523.

———, *Piety and Charity in Late Medieval Florence*, Oxford, 1994.

———, "The Art of Healing: Hospital Wards and the Sick in Renaissance Florence," in *Armut und Armenfürsorge in der italinischen Stadtkultur zwischen 13. und 16. Jahrhundert: Bilder, Texte und Soziale Praktiken*, Helas, P. and Wolf, G. (eds.), Frankfurt am Main, 2006, pp. 79–96.

Herder, J.G., *Correspondence on Ossian and the Songs of Ancient Peoples*, in *The Origins of Modern Critical Thought*, Simpson, D. (ed.), Cambridge, 1988, pp. 71–76.

Heres, G., "Winckelmann, Bernini, Bellori: Betrachtungen zur 'Nachahmung der Alten,'" *Staatliche Museen zu Berlin, Forschungen un Berichte*, 19 (1979): 9–16.

Herz, A., "The Sistine and Pauline Tombs: Documents of the Counter-Reformation," *Storia dell'arte*, 43 (1981): 241–262.

Hesiod, *The Homeric Hymns and Homerica*, Evelyn-White, H.G. (tr.), London and Cambridge, 1977.

———, *Theogony*, Most, G.W. (tr.), Cambridge and London, 2006.

Higginson, P., "Poverty and Papal Piety in Rome *c.* 1600: Painting, Pastoralism and Spectacle," in *Others and Outcasts in Early Modern Europe: Picturing the Social Margins*, Nichols, T. (ed.), Aldershot, 2007, pp. 87–106.

Hippocrates, Withington, E.T. (tr.), III, London and New York, 1927.

Hock, R.F. (tr.), *The Infancy Gospels of James and Thomas: With Introduction, Notes, and Original Text Featuring the New Scholars Version Translation*, Santa Rosa, 1996.

Homer, *Iliad*, Latimore, R. (tr.), Chicago and London, 1970.

———, *Iliad*, Taber Murray, A. (tr.), London and New York, 1925.

Honour, H., *Neo-Classicism*, Westford, 1981.

Hopkins, A. and Wyke, M. (eds.), *Roman Bodies: Antiquity to the Eighteenth Century*, London, 2005.

Horace, *Ars Poetica*, in *Satires, Epistles and Ars Poetica*, Rushton Fairclough, H. (tr.), London and Cambridge, MA, 1978.

Horn, C.B., "A Nexus of Disability in Ancient Greek Miracle Stories: A Comparison of Accounts of Blindness from the Asklepieion in Epidaurus and the Shrine of Thecla in Seleucia," in *Disabilities in Roman Antiquity: Disparate Bodies a capite ad calcem*, Laes, C., Goodey, C.F. and Rose, C.L. (eds.), Leiden and Boston, 2013, pp. 115–143.

Hughes, P., *A Popular History of the Catholic Church*, Garden City, 1962.

———, *A Popular History of the Reformation*, Garden City, 1960.

Il Menologio di Basilio II: (cod.Vaticano greco 1613), 2 vols, Turin, 1907.

Jacobs, F.H., *Votive Panels and Popular Piety in Early Modern Italy*, New York, 2013.

Jensen, R.M., *The Early Christian World*, 2 vols., London and New York, 2000.

———, *Understanding Early Christian Art*, London and New York, 2000.

Jurgens, W.A., *The Faith of the Early Fathers*, Collegeville, MN, 1970.

Jütte, R., *Poverty and Deviance in Early Modern Europe*, Cambridge, 1994.

Kaftal, G., *Iconography of the Saints in Central and South Italian Schools of Painting*, Florence, 1986.

———, *Iconography of the Saints in the Painting of North East Italy*, Florence, 1978.

———, *Iconography of the Saints in the Painting of North West Italy*, Florence, 1985.

———, *Iconography of the Saints in Tuscan Painting*, Florence, 1986.

———, "The Fabulous Life of a Saint," *Mitteilungen des Kunsthistorischen Istitutes in Florenz*, 17 (1973): 123–128.

Karerouni, G. and Kientz, G. (eds.), *Ribera à Rome, autour de l'Apostolado*, Rennes (Musée des Beaux-Arts) and Strasbourg (Musée des Beaux-Arts), 2014–2015.

Kee, H.C., *Miracle in the Early Christian World: A Study in Social Historical Method*, New Haven, 1983.

Kessler, H.L., "Pictorial Narrative and Church Mission in Sixth-Century Gaul," *Studies in the History of Art*, 16 (1985): 75–91.

———, "The Christian Realm: Narrative Representations," in *Age of Spirituality: Late Antique and Early Christian Art, Third to Seventh Century*, Kurt Weitzmann (ed.), New York, 1979, pp. 449–512.

Kitzinger, E., *The Mosaics of Monreale*, Palermo, 1960.

Kraemer, E., "Le type du faux mendiant dans les littératures romanes depuis le Moyen Âge jusq'au XVIIe siècle," in *Societas Scientiarum Fennica Commentationes Humanarum Litterarum*, Helsingfors, 1944, pp. 41–83.

Krautheimer, R., Corbett, S. and Frankl, W., *Corpus Basilicarum Christianarum Romae*, IV, Vatican City, 1970.

Kritter, D., *Studien zum Petruszyklus in der Brancaccikapelle*, Berlin, 1975.

Kruger, K., *Der Frühe Bildkult des Franziskus in Italien: Gestalt- und Funktionswandel des Tafelbildes im 13. und 14. Jahrhundert*, Berlin, 1992.

La Marca, N., *Saggio di un ricerca storico-economica sull'industria e l'artigianato a Roma dal 1750 al 1849*, Rome, 1969.

La medicità provveduta nella città di Roma coll'Ospizio Pubblico fondato dalla Pietà, e Beneficenza di Nostro Signore Innocenzo XII Pontefice Massimo Con le risposte all'Obiezioni contro simili fondazioni, Rome, 1693.

Lactantius, *The Divine Institutes*, Fletcher, W. (tr.), Edinburgh, 1871.

Laes, C., "Learning from Silence: Disabled Children in Roman Antiquity," *Arctos*, 42 (2008): 85–122.

———, "Raising a Disabled Child," in *The Oxford Handbook of Childhood and Education in the Classical World*, Grubbs, J.E. and Parkin, T. (eds.), Oxford, 2013, pp. 125–144.

Langdon, H., "Bari, zingare e venditori ambulanti," in *Il genio di Roma, 1592–1623*, Brown, B.L. (ed.), Milan, 2001, pp. 44–65.

Lanzani, V., "'*Ubi Petrus*': l'antica immagine della Confessione vaticana," in *Pellegrini alla tomba di Pietro*, Morello, G. (ed.), Milan, 1999, pp. 33–59.

Lapper, A., *My Life in My Hands*, London, 2005.

Le Goff, J., *Medieval Civilization 400–1500*, Julia Barrow (tr.), Oxford and Cambridge, MA, 2001.

Leclercq, H., "Laurent," in *Dictionnaire d'archéologie Chrétienne et de liturgie*, Chabrol, F. and Leclercq, H. (eds.), Paris, 1929, 8, 2.

Lewis Allen, P., *The Wages of Sin: Sex and Disease, Past and Present*, Chicago and London, 2000.

Lexicon Iconographicum Mythologiae Classicae, 8 vols., Zürich and Düsseldorf, 1981–1999.

Lise, G. and Salsi, C., "Emilia e Romagna, ovvero Mitelli e Soliani," in *Pittura votiva e stampe popolari*, Milan, 1987, pp. 194–205.

Liverani, P., "Saint Peter's and the City of Rome between Late Antiquity and the Early Middle Ages," in *Old Saint Peter's, Rome*, McKitterick, R., Osborne, J., Richardson, C.M. and Story, J. (eds.), Cambridge, 2013, pp. 21–34.

Livy, *Histories*, Frank Gardner Moore (tr.), 13 vols., Cambridge, MA, and London, 1950.

Loisel, C., *Ludovico Carracci*, Paris, 2004.

Lombardi, D., "I gesuiti, il principe e i modello francese nella politica di assistenza di fine Seicento," in *La Toscana di Cosimo II: Atti del convegno*, Florence, 1993, pp. 521–539.

———, "Poveri a Firenze: programmi e realizzazioni della politica assistenziale dei Medici tra Cinque e Seicento," in *Timore e carità: i poveri nell'Italia moderna*, Politi, G., Rosa, M. and della Peruta, F. (eds.), Cremona, 1982, pp. 165–184.

Löpelmann, M., "Il diletteuole Essamine de' Guidoni, Furfanti ò Calchi, altramente detti Guitti nelle Carceri di Ponte Sisto di Roma nel 1598: con la cognitione della lingua furbesca ò zerga commune à tutti loro," *Romanische Forschungen* 34 (1913): 653–664.

Lucian, *The Parasite: Parasitic an Art*, Morris Harmon, A. (ed.), Cambridge and London, 1995.

Lysias, "For the Disabled Man," Todd, S.C. (tr.), Austin, 2000, pp. 252–259.

———, "On the Refusal of a Pension," Lamb, W.R.M. (tr.), Cambridge, MA, and London, 1943, 22–23, pp. 529–531.

Maggiorotti, L.A., "L'espressione del dolore nella pittura bellica," *Esercito e Nazione*, Rome, 1927, I.

Mairs, N., "On Being a Cripple," in *Plaintext: Essays*, Tucson, 1986, pp. 9–20.

Maldini, D., "Il *Dépot de Mendicité* del Dipartimento di Po: analisi di una struttura assistenziale nel Piemonte napoleonico," in *Timore e carità: i poveri nell'Italia moderna*, Politi, G., Rosa, M. and della Peruta, F. (eds.), Cremona, 1982, pp. 331–346.

———, "Pauperismo e mendicità in Torino nel periodo napoleonico," *Studi Piemontesi* 8:1 (1979): 50–64.

Mâle, É., *The Gothic Image: Religious Art in France of the Thirteenth Century*, New York, 1972.

Martin, F. (ed.), *Ancient Christian Commentary on Scripture: New Testament, V, Acts*, Dowers Grove, 2006.

Maser, E.A. (ed.), *Baroque and Rococo Pictorial Imagery: The 1758–60 Hertel Edition of Ripa's Iconologia with 200 Engraved Illustrations*, New York, 1971.

Mathews, T.F., *The Clash of Gods: A Reinterpretation of Early Christian Art*, Princeton, 1993.

Mayer, W., "John Chrysostom: Extraordinary Preacher, Ordinary Audience," in *Preacher and Audience: Studies in Early Christian and Byzantine Homiletics*, Allen, P. and Cunningham, M.B. (eds.), Leiden, 1998, pp. 105–137.

McCulloh, J.M., "The Cult of Relics in the Letters and 'Dialogues' of Pope Gregory the Great: A Lexicographical Study," *Traditio*, 32 (1976): 145–184.

McTighe, S., "Perfect Deformity, Ideal Beauty, and the *Imaginaire* of Work: The Reception of Annibale Carracci's *Arti di Bologna* in 1646," *Oxford Art Journal*, 1 (1993): 75–91.

Meditations on the Life of Christ, Taney, F.X. (tr.), Asheville, NC, 2000.

Menozzi, D., "Pauperismo e assistenza nel triennio giacobino: il caso di Bologna," in *Timore e carità: i poveri nell'Italia moderna*, Politi, G., Rosa, M. and della Peruta, F. (eds.), Cremona, 1982, pp. 297–316.

Merlin Compton, T., *Victim of the Muse*, Cambridge and London, 2006.

Metzler, I., *A Social History of Disability in the Middle Ages: Cultural Considerations of Physical Impairment*, New York and London, 2013.

———, *Disability in Medieval Europe: Thinking about Physical Impairment during the Middle Ages, c. 1100–1400*, London and New York, 2006.

Milicua, J., "Da Jàtiva a Napoli (1591–1616)," in *Jusepe de Ribera, 1591–1652*, Pérez Sánchez, A.E. and Spinosa, N. (eds.), Naples, 1992, pp. 17–30.

Millett-Gallant, A., *The Disabled Body in Contemporary Art*, New York, 2000.

Misuraca, G., *Serie dei vescovi di Cefalù*, Rome, 1960

Mitchell, A.G., *Greek Vase-Painting and the Origins of Visual Humour*, Cambridge, 2009.

Mitchell, D.T. and Snyder, S.L., *Narrative Prosthesis: Disability and the Dependencies of Discourse*, Ann Arbor, 2000.

——— (eds.), *The Body and Physical Difference: Discourses of Disability*, Ann Arbor, 2004.

Molho, A., "The Brancacci Chapel: Studies in Its Iconography and History," *Journal of the Warburg and Courtauld Institutes*, 40 (1977): 50–98.

Mollat, M., *The Poor in the Middle Ages: An Essay in Social History*, Goldhammer, A. (tr.), New Haven and London, 1986.

Mondin, B., *Dizionario enciclopedico dei papi*, Rome, 1995.

Monteleone, R. and Sarasini, P., "I monumenti italiani ai caduti della Grande Guerra," in *La Grande Guerra: esperienza, memoria, immagini*, Leoni, D. and Zadra, C. (eds.), Bologna, 1986, pp. 631–662.

Monticone, A., "Lavoro, risorse e nuova società nell'età della restaurazione," in *La storia dei poveri: pauperismo e assistenza nell'età moderna*, Monticone, A. (ed.), Rome, 1985, pp. 255–296.

Moraldi, L. (ed.), *Apocrifi del Nuovo Testamento*, Turin, 1971.

Moroni, G., *Dizionario di erudizione storico-ecclesiastica*, Venice, 1852.

Morozzo Della Rocca, R., "Il potere, la sicurezza, l'ordine," in *La storia dei poveri: pauperismo e assistenza nell'età moderna*, Monticone, A. (ed.), Rome, 1985, pp. 153–182.

———, "Vecchio e nuovo nell'immagine della povertà agli inizi dell'età moderna," in Monticone, A. (ed.), *La storia dei poveri: pauperismo e assistenza nell'età moderna*, Rome, 1985, pp. 1–26.

Morton Braund, S. and James, P., "Quasi Homo: Distortion and Contortion in Seneca's *Apocolocyntosis*," *Arethusa*, 31 (1998): 285–311.

Mourret, F., *A History of the Catholic Church*, 8 vols., Thompson, N. (tr.), St. Louis and London, 1947.

Ms. Vittorio Emanuele 630, Biblioteca Nazionale di Roma, fols. 107v–113v.

Muratori, L.A., *Della carità cristiana, in quanto essa è Amore del Prossimo*, Modena, 1723.

Murphy, R.F., *The Body Silent*, New York and London, 2001.

Mustakallio, K. and Laes, C. (eds.), *The Dark Side of Childhood in Late Antiquity and the Middle Ages: Unwanted, Disabled and Lost*, Oxford and Oakville, 2011.

Muto, G., "Forme e contenuti economici dell'assistenza nel mezzogiorno moderno: il caso di Napoli," in *Timore e carità: i poveri nell'Italia moderna*, Politi, G., Rosa, M. and della Peruta, F. (eds.), Cremona, 1982, pp. 237–258.

Nasto, L., *La questione della mendicità nello stato pontificio (sec. XVIII–XIX)*, Rome and Pisa, 2001.

Nichols, T., "Images of Almsgiving and Poverty in Venetian Art of the Sixteenth Century," in *Armut und Armenfürsorge in der italinischen Stadtkultur zwischen 13. und 16. Jahrhundert: Bilder, Texte und Soziale Praktiken*, Helas, P. and Wolf, G. (eds.), Frankfurt am Main, 2006, pp. 349–370.

———, "Secular Piety, Sacred Poverty: Picturing the Poor in Renaissance Venice," *Art History*, 30, 2007, pp. 139–169.

———, *The Art of Poverty: Irony and Ideal in Sixteenth-Century Beggar Imagery*, Manchester, 2007.

——— (ed.), *Others and Outcasts in Early Modern Europe: Picturing the Social Margins*, Aldershot, 2007.

Omont, H.A. (ed.), *Évangiles avec peintures byzantines du XIe siècle*, 2 vols., Paris, 1908.

Ostrow, S., *Art and Spirituality in Counter-Reformation Rome: The Sistine and Pauline Chapels in S. Maria Maggiore*, Cambridge, 1996.

Paglia, V., *"La pietà dei carcerati": confraternite e società a Roma nei secoli XVI–XVIII*, Rome, 1980.

Palazzini, P. (ed.), *Dizionario dei Concili*, 6 vols., Rome, 1963–1968.

Palmeri, G., *Riflessioni critiche sull'arte della guerra*, Naples, 1761.

Papale, A., "L'istituto De Pagave ed il pauperismo a Novara nell'Ottocento," *Bollettino storico per la provincia di Novara*, 75:1 (1984): 93–140.

Papetti, S., "Gli ex voto: la 'Sistina dei poveri,'" in *Per grazia ricevuta: gli ex voto del Museo di San Nicola a Tolentino*, Tolentino, 2005, pp. 7–14.

Paravicini Bagliani, A., "The Corpse in the Middle Ages: The Problem of the Division of the Body," in *The Medieval World*, Linehan, P. and Nelson, J.L. (eds.), London and New York, 2001, pp. 327–341.

Paris, Bibliothèque Nationale, gr. 510, fol. 32v.

———, MS Lat. 5594, fol. 70r.

———, MS n.a.l. 1390, fol. 1r.

Pausanias, *Guide to Greece*, 2 vols., Levi, P. (tr.), Harmondsworth, 1985.

Pavone, M.A., *Iconologia francescana: il Quattrocento*, Todi, 1988.

Peachin, M. (ed.), *Social Relations in the Roman World*, Oxford, 2011.

Pelliccia, G. and Rocca, G. (eds.), *Dizionario degli istituti di perfezione*, Rome, 1974–2003.

Pender, S., "In the Bodyshop: Human Exhibition in Early Modern England," in *"Defects": Engendering the Modern Body*, Deutsch, H. and Nussbaum, F. (eds.), Ann Arbor, 2000, pp. 95–126.

Pestilli, L., "Blindness, Lameness and Mendicancy in Italy (from the 14th to the 18th Centuries)," in *Others and Outcasts in Early Modern Europe: Picturing the Social Margins*, Nichols, T. (ed.), Aldershot, 2007, pp. 107–129.

———, "Disabled Bodies: The (Mis)Representation of the Lame in Antiquity and Their Reappearance in Early Christian and Medieval Art," in *Roman Bodies: Antiquity to the Eighteenth Century*, Hopkins, A. and Wyke, M. (eds.), London, 2005, pp. 85–97.

———, "On Bernini's Reputed Unpopularity in Late Baroque Rome," *Artibus et historiae*, 63 (2011): 119–142.

———, *Paolo de Matteis: Neapolitan Painting and Cultural History in Baroque Europe*, Farnham, 2013.

———, "Simulare disabilità: mendicanti e furfanti a Roman nel Rinascimento," in *Armut und Armenfürsorge in der italienischen Stadtkultur zwischen 13. und 16. Jahrhundert: Bilder, Texte und soziale Praktiken*, Helas, P. and Wolf, G. (eds.), Frankfurt am Main, 2006, pp. 371–383.

Pfisterer, U., "*L'Elemosina di san Rocco* di Annibale Carracci e l'innovazione della *historia* cristiana," in *Programme et invention dans l'art de la Renaissance*, Hochmann, M. (ed.), Rome, 2008, 247–269.

Phelan, P., *Unmarked: The Politics of Performance*, London, 1993.

Piazza, C.B., *Euseuologio Romano, overo Delle Opere Pie di Roma*, Rome, 1698.

Pierpont Morgan Library, MS M. 736, fol. 9r.

Pisano, G., "L'ospizio-ospedale di S. Sisto e la Compagnia dei Mendicanti di S. Elisabetta," *Roma*, VI (1928): 241–258.

Piscitelli, E., "Le classi sociali a Bologna nel secolo XVIII," *Nuova Rivista Storica*, 38 (1954): 79–120.

Plato, *Laws*, in *The Collected Dialogues of Plato*, Hamilton, E. and Cairns, H. (eds.), Princeton, 1985.

———, *Lesser Hippias*, in *The Collected Dialogues of Plato*, Hamilton, E. and Cairns, H. (eds.), Princeton, 1985.

———, *Sophist*, in *The Collected Dialogues of Plato*, Hamilton, E. and Cairns, H. (eds.), Princeton, 1985.

———, *Theaetetus*, in *The Collected Dialogues of Plato*, Hamilton, E. and Cairns, H. (eds.), Princeton, 1985.

———, *Timaeus*, in *The Collected Dialogues of Plato*, Hamilton, E. and Cairns, H. (eds.), Princeton, 1985.

Pliny, *Natural History*, 10 vols., Rackham, H. (tr.), Loeb Classical Library, Cambridge, MA, and London.

Plutarch, *Lives*, Perrin, B. (tr.), III, London, 1996.

Politi, G., Rosa, M. and della Peruta, F. (eds.), *Timore e carità: i poveri nell'Italia moderna*, Cremona, 1982.

Pomponius Porphyro, *Commentum in Horatium Flaccum: De arte poetica*, Alfred Holder (ed.), Innsbruck, 1894.

Porzio, F., "Aspetti e problemi della scena di genere in Italia," in *Da Caravaggio a Ceruti: la scena di genere e l'immagine dei pitocchi nella pittura italiana*, Porzio, F. (ed.), Milan, 1998, pp. 17–41.

Porzio, G. and D'Alessandro, D.A., "Ribera between Rome and Naples: New Documentary Evidence," *The Burlington Magazine*, CLVII, October 2015, pp. 682–683.

Preto, P., "Gli emarginati," in *Mentalità comportamenti e istituzioni tra Rinascimento e decadenza 1550–1700*, Giuseppe Galasso (ed.), Milan, 1988, pp. 157–177.

Prosperi Valenti Rodinò, S. and Strinati, C. (eds.), *L'immagine di San Francesco nella Controriforma*, Rome, 1983.

Pullan, B., "Catholics, Protestants, and the Poor in Early Modern Europe," *The Journal of Interdisciplinary History*, 35:3 (2005): 441–456.

———, "'Difettosi, impotenti, inabili': Caring for the Disabled in Early Modern Italian Cities," in *Poverty and Charity: Europe, Italy, Venice, 1400–1700*, Norfolk, 1994, Ch. 6, pp. 1–21.

———, "La nuova filantropia nella Venezia cinquecentesca," in *Nel regno dei poveri: arte e storia dei grandi ospedali veneziani in età moderna 1474–1797*, Aikema, B. and Mejers, D. (eds.), Venezia, 1989, pp. 19–34.

———, "Poveri, mendicanti e vagabondi (secoli XIV–XVII)," in *Storia d'Italia, Annali*, Romano, R. and Vivanti, C. (eds.), Turin, 1978, I, pp. 981–1047.

———, "Support and Redeem: Charity and Poor Relief in Italian Cities from the Fourteenth to the Seventeenth Century," in *Poverty and Charity: Europe, Italy, Venice, 1400–1700*, Aldershot, 1994, pp. 177–208.

Re, L., *Enrico Toti: profilo*, Piacenza, 1923.

Reeve, M.D., "The Rediscovery of Classical Text in the Renaissance," in *Itinerari dei testi antichi*, Pecere, O. (ed.), Rome, 1991, pp. 115–157.

Ribton-Turner, C.J., *A History of Vagrants and Vagrancy and Beggars and Begging*, London, 1887.

Ricci, A., "'Nel catalogo dei santi': riflessioni sulla santità di Omobono," in *Strenna dell'ADAFA*, new series, I, Cremona, 2001, pp. 77–93.

Riis, T., "I poveri nell'arte italiana (secoli XV–XVIII)," in *Timore e carità: i poveri nell'Italia moderna*, Politi, G., Rosa, M. and della Peruta, F. (eds.), Cremona, 1982, pp. 45–58.

Riosa, M., "Comitati locali e potere politico: i caratteri della committenza," in *La memoria perduta: i monumenti ai caduti della Grande Guerra a Roma e nel Lazio*, Vidotto, V., Tobia, B. and Brice, C. (eds.), Rome, 1998, pp. 11–27.

Ripa, C., *Iconologia*, Siena, 1613.

———, *Iconologia*, Buscaroli, P. (ed.), Milan, 1992.

Robertson, C., *The Invention of Annibale Carracci*, Cinisello Balsamo, 2008.

Rodley, L., *Byzantine Art and Architecture: An Introduction*, Cambridge, 1994.

Rodocanachi, E.P., *Les corporations ouvrières à Rome depuis la chute de l'empire romain*, 2 vols., Paris, 1894.

Roettgen, S., *Italian Frescoes: The Early Renaissance 1400–1470*, New York, 1996.

Rosa, M., "Chiesa, idee sui poteri e assistenza in Italia dal Cinque al Settecento," *Società e storia*, 10 (1980): 775–806.

———, "Pauperismo e riforme nel Settecento italiano: linee di ricerca," in *Povertà e carità dalla Roma tardo-antica al '700 italiano*, Brown, P., Capitani, O., Cardini, F. and Rosa, M. (eds.), Padua, 1983, pp. 93–125.

———, "Poveri ed emarginati: un problema religioso," *Ricerche per la storia religiosa di Roma*, 3 (1979): 11–41.

Rosa, S., *Satire e vita di Salvator Rosa*, Florence, 1833.

Rose, M.L., *The Staff of Oedipus: Transforming Disability in Ancient Greece*, Ann Arbor, 2003.

Rosenberg, P., "Da Ribera a Ribot, dal naturalismo all'accademismo: la fortuna di un pittore alla ricerca della sua nazionalità e della sua definizione stilistica," in *Jusepe de Ribera, 1591–1652*, Pérez Sánchez, A.E. and Spinosa, N. (eds.), Naples, 1992, pp. 81–104.

Russell, H.D., *Jacques Callot: Prints and Related Drawings*, Washington, 1975.

Salvante, M., "Italian Disabled Veterans between Experience and Representation," in *Men After War*, McVeigh, S. and Cooper, N. (eds.), New York, 2013, pp. 111–129.

———, "The Italian Associazione Nazionale Mutilati e Invalidi di Guerra and Its International Liaisons in the Post Great War Era," in *The Great War and Veterans' Internationalism*, Eichenberg, J. and Newman, J.P. (eds.), London and New York, 2013, pp. 162–183.

San Juan, R.M., *Rome: A City Out of Print*, Minneapolis and London, 2001.

Saxer, V., under "Martirio," in *Dizionario patristico e di antichità cristiane*, Di Berardino, A. (ed.), 2 vols., Casale Monferrato, 1984, II, pp. 2135–2149.

Scanarolo, G.B., *De visitatione carceratorum*, Rome, 1655.

Scharf, F., "La retorica figurativa e il significato politico-sociale degli affreschi del Pellegrinaio in S. Maria della Scala a Siena," in *Armut und Armenfürsorge in der italinischen Stadtkultur zwischen 13. und 16. Jahrhundert: Bilder, Texte und Soziale Praktiken*, Helas, P. and Wolf, G. (eds.), Frankfurt am Main, 2006, pp. 141–160.

Sebregondi, L., "Carità palese e carità occulta: le vesti confraternali nell'esercizio delle opere di misericordia," in *Armut und Armenfürsorge in der italinischen Stadtkultur zwischen 13. und 16. Jahrhundert: Bilder, Texte und Soziale Praktiken*, Helas, P. and Wolf, G. (eds.), Frankfurt am Main, 2006, pp. 97–112.

Selmi, E., "Cultura e committenza artistica: il 'caso' di Giacomo Ceruti," in *La società bresciana e l'opera di Giacomo Ceruti*, Brescia, 1988, pp. 227–248.

Semi, F., *El parlar s'ceto e neto de Capodistria: testi antichi e moderni, glossario*, Venice, 1983.

Seneca the Elder, *Ad Lucilium Epistulae Morales*, 3 vols., Gummere, R.M., Cambridge and London, 1989.

———, *Controversiae*, Winterbottom, M. (tr.), Cambridge and London, 1974.

———, *De Beneficiis*, in *Moral Essays*, John W. Basore (tr.), Cambridge and London, 1989.

Shearman, J., *Raphael's Cartoons in the Collection of Her Majesty the Queen and the Tapestries for the Sistine Chapel*, London, 1972.

Shirley, O., *A Cry for Health: Poverty and Disability in the Third World*, Third World Group and ARHTAG, Rome, 1983.

Silvan, P.L., *Roma 1300–1875: l'arte degli anni santi*, Fagiolo, M. and Madonna, M.L. (eds.), Milan, 1984, pp. 357–363.

Simoncelli, P., "Origini e primi anni di vita dell'ospedale romano dei poveri mendicanti," *Annuario dell'Istituto Storico Italiano per l'età moderna e contemporanea*, XXV–XXVI, 1973–1974 (1976), pp. 121–172.

Smith, M., *Jesus the Magician*, New York, 1978.

Sonnino, E. (ed.), *Popolazione e società a Roma dal medioevo all'età contemporanea*, Rome, 1998.

Soranus' Gynecology, Temkin, O. (tr.), Baltimore and London, 1991,

St. Bonaventure, *The Life of St. Francis*, Gurney Salter, E. (tr.), New York, 1904.

St. John Chrysostom, *On Repentance and Almsgiving*, Christo, G.G. (tr.), Washington, 1998.

St. Maximus the Confessor, *The Ascetic Life, The Four Centuries on Charity*, Sherwood, P. (tr. and ed.), Westminster, MD, and London, 1955.

Stahl, J., "Physically Deformed and Disabled People," in *Social Relations in the Roman World*, Peachin, M. (ed.), Oxford, 2011, pp. 715–733.

Stiker, H.-J., *A History of Disability*, Ann Arbor, 1999.

Strong., J. (ed.), *The New Strong's Exhaustive Concordance of the Bible*, Nashville, 1990.

Suetonius, *Lives of the Caesars*, Rolfe, J.C. (tr.), 2 vols., Cambridge and London, 1979.

Sullivan, E.J., "Ribera's *Clubfooted Boy*: Image and Symbol," *Marsyas*, 19 (1977–1978), 17–21.

Sutherland Harris, A., "Ludovico, Agostino, Annibale: . . . l'abbiam fatto tutti noi," *Accademia Clementina: atti e memorie*, 33–34 (1994): 69–84.

Swediaur, F., *Complete Treatise on the Symptoms, Effects, Nature and Treatment of Syphilis*, Hewson, T.T. (tr.), Philadelphia, 1815.

Sydenham, E.A., *The Coinage of the Roman Republic*, London, 1952.

Terence, *The Eunuch*, Sargeaunt, J. (tr.), Cambridge and London, 1994.

Thacker, A., "*Loca Sanctorum*: The Significance of Place in the Study of the Saints," in *Local Saints and Local Churches in the Early Medieval West*, Thacker, A. and Sharpe, R. (eds.), Oxford, 2002, pp. 2–43.

———, "Rome of the Martyrs: Saints, Cults and Relics, Fourth to Seventh Centuries," in *Roma Felix: Formation and Reflections of Medieval Rome*, Carragáin, É.Ó. and Neuman de Vegvar, C. (eds.), Aldershot and Burlington, 2007, pp. 13–49.

The Book of Pontiffs (Liber Pontificalis), Davis, R. (tr.), Liverpool, 1989.

The Code of Justinian, in *The Civil Law*, Scott, S.P. (tr.), Cincinnati, 1932.

The Defensor Pacis of Marsilius of Padua, Previté-Orton, C.W. (ed.), Cambridge, 1928.

The Illustrated Bartsch, 108 vols., Strauss, W.L., Spike, J.T. and de Ramaix, I. (eds.), New York, 1978–.

The Institutio Oratoria of Quintilian, 4 vols., Butler, H.E. (tr.), Cambridge, MA, and London, 1989.

The Jerusalem Bible, Jones, A. (ed.), Garden City, 1966.

The Old Testament Pseudepigrapha, Charlesworth, J.H. (ed.), New York, 1983.

The Oxford Classical Dictionary, Hammond, N.G.B. and Scullard, H.H. (eds.), Oxford, 1984.

The Treatises of Cyprian, in *The Ante-Nicene Fathers*, 10 vols., Cleveland Coxe, A. (comp.), Roberts, A., Donaldson, J., Schaff, P. and Wace, H. (eds.), Grand Rapids, 1990.

Thunø, E., "The Golden Altar of Satn'Ambrogio in Milan," in *Decorating the Lord's Table*, Kaspersen, S. and Thunø, E. (eds.), Copenhagen, 2006, pp. 63–78.

Tierney, B., *Foundations of the Conciliar Theory*, Leiden, 1998.

———, "The Decretists and the 'Deserving Poor,'" *Comparative Studies in Society and History*, 1 (1959): 360–373.

Tobia, B., "Dal Milite ingonto al nazionalismo monumentale fascista (1921–1940)," in *Guerra e pace*, Barberis, W. (ed.), Turin, 2002, pp. 593–642.

Tommaseo, N., *Dizionario della lingua italiana*, Turin, 1916.

Tours, Bibliothèque Municipale, MS 1018, fol. 18r.

Tranfaglia, N., *La prima Guerra Mondiale e il fascismo*, Turin, 1995.

Trentin, L., "Deformity in the Roman Imperial Court," *Greece and Rome*, 58 (2011): 195–208.

———, "What's in a Hump? Re-examining the Hunchback in the Villa Albani-Torlonia," *Cambridge Classical Journal, Proceedings of the Cambridge Philological Society*, 55 (2009): 130–156.

Trexler, R.C., "The Bishop's Portion: Generic Pious Legacies in the Late Middle Ages in Italy," *Traditio*, 28 (1972): 433–436.

Valdecio, D., *Lo scoglio dell'umanità [. . .] per cautelarsi contro le male qualità delle donne cattive*, Venice, 1774.

Valenti, C., "I poveri in Sicilia nella seconda metà del Settecento," in *Timore e carità: i poveri nell'Italia moderna*, Politi, G., Rosa, M. and della Peruta, F. (eds.), Cremona, 1982, pp. 283–296.

Valerius Maximus, *Facta et Dicta Memorabilia*, 2 vols., Shackleton Bailey, D.R. (tr.), Cambridge, MA, and London, 2000.

Valla, L., *On the donation of Constantine*, Bowersock, G.W. (tr.), Cambridge, 2007.

Van Dam, R., *Saints and their Miracles in Late Antique Gaul*, Princeton, 1993.

van Os, H.W., "St. Francis of Assisi as a Second Christ in Early Italian Painting," *Simiolus*, 7 (1974): 115–132.

Varchi, B., "Della maggioranza delle arti," in *Scritti d'arte del Cinquecento*, 3 vols., Barocchi, P. (ed.), Milan and Naples, 1971, I, p. 14.

Vaticanus graecus 1613, Biblioteca Apostolica Vaticana.

Vauchez, A., *Omobono di Cremona (1197): laico e santo, profilo storico*, Cremona, 2001.

———, *Sainthood in the Later Middle Ages*, Cambridge, 1997.

———, *Saints, prophètes et visionnaires: le pouvoir surnaturel au Moyen Âge*, Paris, 1999.

———, *The Spirituality of the Medieval West: The Eighth to the Twelfth Century*, Friedlander, C. (tr.), Kalamazoo, MI, 1993.

Velmans, T., *Le Tétraévangile de la Laurentienne*, Paris, 1971.

Venchi, A.I., "Il messaggio teologico della cappella Niccolina," in Buranelli, F. (ed.), *Il Beato Angelico e la cappella Niccolina: storia e restauro*, Novara, 2001, pp. 45–62 and 63–76.

Venturi, F., *Settecento riformatore: da Muratori a Beccaria*, Turin, 1969.

Vernant, J.P., "From Oedipus to Periander: Lameness, Tyranny, Incest in Legend and History," *Arethusa*, 15:I (1982): 19–38.

Vidotto, V., "La Vittoria e i monumenti ai caduti," in *Mélanges de l'École Française de Rome: Italie et Méditerranée*, 112:2 (2000): 505–513.

Vignini Paloschi, M., *Enrico Toti. La centuria di ferro: la pattuglia dei combattenti*, Milan, 1940.

Villani, G., *Cronica*, 3 vols., Florence, 1847.

Vives, J.L., *On Assistance to the Poor*, Tobriner, A. (tr.), Toronto, Buffalo and London, 1999.

Vivès, L., *Il modo di sovvenire a' poveri*, Venice, 1545.

von Kraemer, E., "Le type du faux mendiant dans les littératures romanes depuis le moyen âge jusqu'au XVIIe siècle," *Societas Scientiarum Fennica Commentationes Humanarum Litterarum*, 13:6 (1944): 1–338.

von Pastor, L., *Geschicte der Päpste*, Freiburg, 1886.

———, *The History of the Popes from the Close of the Middle Ages*, 40 vols., Kerr, R.F. (tr.), London, 1891–1941.

von Wilpert, J., *Die römischen Mosaiken und Malereien der kirchlichen Bauten vom 4. bis 13. Jahrhundert*, 4 vols, Freiburg, 1924.

Vuolanto, V., "Infant Abandonment and the Christianization of Medieval Europe," in *The Dark Side of Childhood in Late Antiquity and the Middle Ages*, Mustakallio, K. and Laes, C. (eds.), Oxford, 2011, pp. 3–19.

Waterhouse, E., "Introduction," in *Jusepe de Ribera: lo Spagnoletto, 1591–1652*, exhibition catalogue, Felton, C. (ed.), Fort Worth, 1982.

Weinstein, D. and Bell, R.M., *Saints and Society: The Two Worlds of Western Christendom, 1000–1700*, Chicago and London, 1982.

Weitzmann, K. (ed.), *Age of Spirituality: Late Antique and Early Christian Art, Third to Seventh Century*, Princeton, 1979.

———, *The Miniatures of the Sacra Parallela Parisinus Graecus 923*, Princeton, 1979.

Weitzmann, K. and Galavaris, G., *The Monastery of Saint Catherine of Mount Sinai: The Illuminated Greek Manuscripts*, Princeton, 1990.

Whitman, N., *Roma Resurgens: Papal Medals from the Age of the Baroque*, Ann Arbor, 1981.

Winckelmann, J.J., *Briefe*, 4 vols., Berlin, 1952.

———, *Reflections on the Painting and Sculpture of the Greeks*, Füssli, J.H. (tr.), London, 1765.

Wind, B., *"A Foul and Pestilent Congregation": Images of "Freaks" in Baroque Art*, Cambridge, 1998.

Wolff, R., *Der Heilige Franziskus in Schriften und Bildern des 13. Jahrhunderts*, Berlin 1996.

Woolf, S.J., "Problems in the History of Pauperism in Italy, 1800–1815," in *Timore e carità: i poveri nell'Italia moderna*, Politi, G., Rosa, M. and della Peruta, F. (eds.), Cremona, 1982, pp. 317–329.

Wormald, F., "Some Illustrated Manuscripts of the Lives of the Saints," *Bulletin of the John Rylands Library*, 35 (1952–1953): 248–266.

Zander, P., *Il ciborio degli apostoli*, Città del Vaticano, 2010.

Zanker, P., *The Power of Images in the Age of Augustus*, Shapiro, A. (tr.), Ann Arbor, 1988.

Zorzi, M., "Anni Santi, 'mendicità provveduta' e l'Ospizio Apostolico dei Poveri Invalidi," in *L'arte per i giubilei e tra i giubilei del Settecento*, Debenedetti, E. (ed.), Rome, 1999, pp. 23–39.

Index

For the artists, works of art and pagination of the black and white images in this volume, see the list of *Figures*.

For Product Safety Concerns and Information please contact our EU
representative GPSR@taylorandfrancis.com
Taylor & Francis Verlag GmbH, Kaufingerstraße 24, 80331 München, Germany

www.ingramcontent.com/pod-product-compliance
Ingram Content Group UK Ltd
Pitfield, Milton Keynes, MK11 3LW, UK
UKHW050754180926
475701UK00007B/1041
9780367200268